Neurology and Neurobiology

EDITORS

Victoria Chan-Palay
University Hospital, Zurich

Sanford L. Palay
The Harvard Medical School

ADVISORY BOARD

Albert J. Aguayo
McGill University

Günter Baumgartner
University Hospital, Zurich

Masao Ito
Tokyo University

Tong H. Joh
Cornell University Medical
College, New York

Bruce McEwen
Rockefeller University

William D. Willis, Jr.
The University of Texas,
Galveston

Please contact publisher for information about previous titles in this series.

(MAL)NUTRITION AND
THE INFANT BRAIN

(MAL)NUTRITION AND THE INFANT BRAIN

Proceedings of an International Symposium
Held in Montréal, Québec, Canada,
May 11-12, 1989

Editors

Nico M. van Gelder

Centre de Recherche
en Sciences Neurologiques
Dép. Physiologie
Université de Montréal
Montréal, Québec, Canada

Roger F. Butterworth

Laboratory of Neurochemistry
André-Viallet Clinical Research Centre
Department of Medicine
Université de Montréal
Montréal, Québec, Canada

Boris D. Drujan

Instituto Venezolano de Investigaciones Cientificas
Laboratorio de Neuroquimica
Caracas, Venezuela

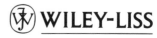

A JOHN WILEY & SONS, INC., PUBLICATION
NEW YORK • CHICHESTER • BRISBANE • TORONTO • SINGAPORE

While the authors, editors, and publisher believe that drug selection and dosage and the specifications and usage of equipment and devices, as set forth in this book, are in accord with current recommendations and practice at the time of publication, they accept no legal responsibility for any errors or omissions, and make no warranty, express or implied, with respect to material contained herein. In view of ongoing research, equipment modifications, changes in governmental regulations and the constant flow of information relating to drug therapy, drug reactions and the use of equipment and devices, the reader is urged to review and evaluate the information provided in the package insert or instructions for each drug, piece of equipment or device for, among other things, any changes in the instructions or indications of dosage or usage and for added warnings and precautions.

The publication of this volume was facilitated by the authors and editors who submitted the text in a form suitable for direct reproduction without subsequent editing or proofreading by the publisher.

Library of Congress Cataloging-in-Publication Data

(Mal)nutrition and the infant brain : proceedings of an international
  symposium held in Montréal, Québec, Canada, May 11-12, 1989 /
  editors, Nico M. van Gelder, Roger F. Butterworth, Boris D. Drujan.
      p.   cm. -- (Neurology and neurobiology ; v. 58)
   Includes index.
   ISBN 0-471-56823-6
   1. Infants--Nutrition. 2. Brain--Growth. 3. Intellect-
  -Nutritional aspects. 4. Malnutrition in infants. 5. Developmental
  neurology.   I. Van Gelder, Nico M.   II. Butterworth, Roger F.
  III. Drujan, Boris D.   IV. Series.
      [DNLM: 1. Brain--growth & development--congresses. 2. Infant
  Nutrition Disorders--complications--congresses. 3. Placenta
  Diseases--complications--congresses.   W1 NE337B v. 58 / WL 300
  M2564 1989]
  RJ216.M285   1990
  618.92'8--dc20
  DNLM/DLC
  for Library of Congress   90-12720
                                                                   CIP

Contents

Contributors and Participants

Kurt D. Ackerman, Department of Neurobiology and Anatomy, University of Rochester Medical Center, Rochester, NY 14642 **[313]**

Yudieth Alizo, Special Research Division of Pediatric Neurology, Family Nutrition Research Division, FUNDACREDESA, Chacao-Caracas 1060-A, Venezuela **[285]**

G. Harvey Anderson, Department of Nutritional Sciences, Faculty of Medicine, University of Toronto, Toronto, Ontario M5S 1A8, Canada **[41]**

Nancy Angulo-Rodriguez, Special Research Division of Pediatric Neurology, Family Nutrition Research Division, FUNDACREDESA, Chacao-Caracas 1060-A, Venezuela; present address: Apartado 80474, Codigo 1080-A Caracas, Venezuela **[285]**

Miriam Banay-Schwartz, Center for Neurochemistry, The Nathan S. Kline Institute for Psychiatric Research, Orangeburg, NY 10962 **[191]**

Wail A. Bengelloun, Unité de Neuroscience, Département de Biologie, Faculté des Sciences, Université Mohamed V., BP 1014 Rabat, Morocco **[65]**

Virgilio Bosch, FUNDACREDESA: Center for Studies on Growth and Development of the Venezuelan Population, Chacao-Caracas 1060-A, Venezuela **[269]**

Roger F. Butterworth, Laboratory for Neurochemistry, André-Viallet Clinical Research Centre, Hôpital St-Luc, Montréal; Department of Medicine, Université de Montréal, Montréal, Québec H2X 3J4, Canada **[xv, 207]**

Marilyn Cabedo, Special Research Division of Pediatric Neurology, Family Nutrition Research Division, FUNDACREDESA, Chacao-Caracas 1060-A, Venezuela **[285]**

Kenneth J. Carpenter, Department of Nutrition, University of California, Berkeley, CA 94720 **[127]**

The numbers in brackets are the opening page numbers of the contributors' articles.

Arianna Carughi, Department of
Nutrition, University of California,
Berkeley, CA 94720 **[127]**

John B. Clark, Biochemistry Department, St. Bartholomew's Hospital
Medical College, University of London, London EC1M 6BQ, United
Kingdom **[237]**

Marian C. Diamond, Department of
Physiology-Anatomy, University of
California, Berkeley, CA 94720 **[127]**

Boris D. Drujan, Instituto Venezolano de Investigaciones Cientificas,
Laboratorio de Neuroquimica, Caracas
1010-A, Venezuela **[xv, 267]**

David Dunlop, Center for Neurochemistry, The Nathan S. Kline Institute for Psychiatric Research,
Orangeburg, NY 10962 **[191]**

Michael A. Edwards, Department of
Developmental Neurobiology, E.K.
Shriver Center, Waltham, MA 02154
[111]

Reha S. Erzurumlu, Department of
Developmental Neurobiology, E.K.
Shriver Center, Waltham, MA 02154
[111]

David L. Felten, Department of
Neurobiology and Anatomy, University of Rochester Medical Center,
Rochester, NY 14642 **[313]**

Suzanne Y. Felten, Department of
Neurobiology and Anatomy, University of Rochester Medical Center,
Rochester, NY 14642 **[313]**

Marlene Fossi, FUNDACREDESA:
Center for Studies on Growth and
Development of the Venezuelan Population, Chacao-Caracas 1060-A, Venezuela **[269]**

Bernard Haber, Neurochemistry
Section, Marine Biomedical Institute,
University of Texas Medical Branch,
Galveston, TX 77550

Anders Hamberger, Institute of
Neurobiology, University of Göteborg,
POB 33 031, S-400 33 Göteborg,
Sweden

Alfred E. Harper, Departments of
Nutritional Sciences and Biochemistry,
University of Wisconsin, Madison,
WI 53706 **[301]**

George A. Hashim, Department of
Immunology, St. Luke's Hospital
Center, New York, NY 10025

Sami A. Hashim, Department of Metabolism and Nutrition, St. Luke's
Hospital Center, New York, NY 10025

Gerald Huether, Max-Planck-Institut
für experimentelle Medizin, Forschungsstelle Neurochemie, 3400
Göttingen, Federal Republic of Germany **[141]**

Sonal Jhaveri, Department of Brain
& Cognitive Sciences, Massachusetts
Institute of Technology, Cambridge,
MA 02139 **[111]**

Carl L. Keen, Department of Nutrition, University of California, Davis, CA 95616 **[225]**

Abel Lajtha, Center for Neurochemistry, The Nathan S. Kline Institute for Psychiatric Research, Orangeburg, NY 10962 **[191]**

Maritza Landaeta-Jimenez, FUNDACREDESA: Center for Studies on Growth and Development of the Venezuelan Population, Chacao-Caracas 1060-A, Venezuela **[269]**

Paul D. Lewis, Department of Histopathology, Charing Cross & Westminster Medical School, University of London, London W6 8RF, United Kingdom **[89]**

Mercedes López-Blanco, FUNDACREDESA: Center for Studies on Growth and Development of the Venezuelan Population, Chacao-Caracas 1060-A, Venezuela **[269]**

Kelley S. Madden, Department of Neurobiology and Anatomy, University of Rochester Medical Center, Rochester, NY 14642 **[313]**

Maria Mendéz, FUNDACREDESA: Center for Studies on Growth and Development of the Venezuelan Population, Chacao-Caracas 1060-A, Venezuela **[269]**

Hernan Méndez-Castellano, FUNDACREDESA: Center for Studies on Growth and Development of the Venezuelan Population, Chacao-Caracas 1060-A, Venezuela **[269]**

Sheldon L. Miller, The Wistar Institute, Philadelphia, PA 19104 **[175]**

Patricia Oteiza, Department of Nutrition, University of California, Davis, CA 95616 **[225]**

David K. Rassin, Department of Pediatrics, The University of Texas, Medical Branch at Galveston, Galveston, TX 77550 **[57]**

Lois M. Roeder, Department of Pediatrics, University of Maryland School of Medicine, Baltimore, MD 21201 **[253]**

John M. Rogers, Developmental Toxicology Division, MD-67, HERL, US Environmental Protection Agency, Research Triangle Park, NC 27711 **[225]**

Pedro R. Rosso, Departments of Pediatrics and Endocrinology, Nutrition and Metabolic Diseases, School of Medicine, Catholic University, Santiago, Chile **[25]**

Armando Sanchez, Special Research Division of Pediatric Neurology, Family Nutrition Research Division, FUNDACREDESA, Chacao-Caracas 1060-A, Venezuela **[285]**

Arnold B. Scheibel, Department of Anatomy and Cell Biology and Psychiatry and Biobehavioral Sciences and the Brain Research Institute, University of California, Los Angeles, Center for the Health Sciences, Los Angeles, CA 90024 **[83]**

Gerald E. Schneider, Department of Brain & Cognitive Sciences, Massachusetts Institute of Technology, Cambridge, MA 02139 **[111]**

Mervyn Susser, Gertrude H. Sergievsky Center, Columbia University, New York, NY 10032 **[1]**

Nico M. van Gelder, Centre de Recherche en Sciences Neurologiques, Dép. Physiologie, Université de Montréal, Montréal, Québec H3C 3J7, Canada **[xv, xvii, 21, 157, 161, 249, 327]**

Foreword

On May 11, 12, 1989, the Centre de recherche en sciences neurologiques, Université de Montréal, held its 11th International Symposium on "(MAL)NUTRITION AND THE INFANT BRAIN". The two-day conference was organized by RF Butterworth (Montréal), BD Drujan (I.V.I.C., Venezuela); NM van Gelder (Montréal). The participants came from 8 different countries and four continents: Morocco, F.R. Germany, Sweden, the U.K., Canada, U.S.A., Venezuela, Chile. The symposium (18 speakers, 4 chair persons) was divided into four sections: Dietary Requirement; Neuroanatomical Factors; Neurochemical Integration; the Nurture Factor: Environment, and had the following theme.

The proper maturation of the brain and the development of optimum intelligence in a child depend on three essential factors: the inborn genetic directives, the complexity of the environment, and an adequate nutrition. Humans all belong to the same species and it must be assumed therefore that only subtle variations in the genome distinguishes one individual from another. On the other hand, the quality of nutrition and the nature of its social and intellectual environment may be unique for each infant. To a large extent both the anatomical as well as the functional maturation of the brain occurs after birth, and is almost completed by age three. This relatively short period of neonatal brain development is therefore of critical importance for the success of an individual to adapt to the social environment, his/her ease of learning and the ability to assimilate new knowledge, and to properly care for the next generation.

Genetic directives are not likely to become altered after birth, barring special circumstances. On the other hand, the nature of social and intellectual stimuli to which the growing infant is exposed, in combination with the quality of nutrition, is infinitely variable and, indeed, not entirely controllable. Nutritional and environmental conditions thus are crucial, in that they superimpose upon the framework of genetic directives the final anatomic and functional integration of neurons with various types of glial cells, and their metabolic interconnectivity. This conference examined the impact of nutritional and social parameters on the anatomic and neurochemical maturation of the infant brain.

The organizers gratefully acknowledge the generous financial contributions by the following organizations: Fondation Savoy pour l'Epilepsie, International Society for Neurochemistry, Ministère de la Santé et des Services sociaux (Québec), Fonds de la Recherche en Santé du Québec, Health and Welfare/Santé et Bien-être social (Canada), and the Faculté de Médecine, Université de Montréal. Some financial aid from H.J. Heinz Co, Canada and Squibb Canada was also greatly appreciated.

Finally, we wish to especially acknowledge the collaboration of two persons who were indispensable for the success of the symposium and the publication of the proceedings. To Mdme Helene Auzat our deep appreciation for her unstinting and skillful help in organizing the meeting. Mlle Michelle Piché has been largely responsible for uniforming these proceedings into a cohesive publication. Her assistance and support has been invaluable.

Nico M. van Gelder
Roger F. Butterworth
Boris D. Drujan

Introduction

A growing child needs food, shelter and care. It seems so simple. From the reports that follow it is evident however that the simplicity is more apparent than real. How much food is needed, what type, what is implied by care, is there a danger in providing too much (emotional) shelter? The uncertainties and insufficient knowledge in these areas of child development are profound.

The theme of these proceedings is best summarized by Susser, in discussing the influence of diet and the social impact on the mental performance of the child. After extensively reviewing 5 large studies dealing with the rehabilitation of intellectual performance among children in nutritionally and socioeconomic disadvantaged communities, he sums up the data in three conclusions:

1. Undernutrition in pregnant women will preferentially spare foetal brain development . Provided post-partum nutrition is restored soon after birth (6 mo.), few lasting functional deficits are observed.

2. Nutritional rehabilitation alone in malnourished children becomes ineffective after approximately 40 months following birth, but prior to that period is effective.

3. Psychosocial intervention past this 40 months growth phase is, on the other hand, still markedly effective.

These conclusions provide hope for millions of infants who, through no fault of their own, are born and grow up in societies where the psychosocial environment is less than ideal due to grinding poverty, violence, and family or community dislocation. It is no accident that these same communities often also experience undernutrition and/or malnutrition, with the latter posing the greater threat to foetal as well as infant brain development and for resulting mental performance deficits. However, successful intervention in this viscious cycle formed by nutritional and social impoverishment, and the formulation of effective strategies for rehabilitation, requires insight into the biological and mental processes which are at risk of underdevelopment. In the following reports an attempt has been made to address some of the problems associated with nutritional and social insufficiencies in the child and, based on present knowledge, what type of rehabilitation method(s) might be most effective.

Nico M. van Gelder

(Mal)Nutrition and the Infant Brain, pages 1–19

NUTRITION, BRAIN DEVELOPMENT AND MENTAL PERFORMANCE: THE CHALLENGE OF CAUSALITY*

Mervyn Susser

Gertrude H. Sergievsky Center, Columbia University, New York, NY 10032, USA

The causal relations of nutrition and mental development have been a matter of concern and dispute for the past two decades. The five major studies analyzed here permit conclusions specific to the exposures and the stage of life observed in each. When taken together a limited role for nutrition in mental performance emerges. Although less striking than education, it is a role that cannot be ignored in prudent public policies.

Disputation stems more from interpretations of what constitutes valid evidence than from the actual results in the literature. This paper begins, therefore, with a framework for considering the properties of causes before proceeding to consider data selected from a few crucial tests of the hypothesis that nutrition affects the development of mental competence.

Causes and their Attributes

In a common place perspective that suits epidemiology, a cause is something that makes a difference. Thus causes include all determinants of an outcome, and they may be either *active agents* or *static conditions*. Implicit in this concept of determinants is a model of multiple causes. If the determinant is an active agent, it produces change; the determinant is an intended or unintended intervention, or a natural force or an accident, or the removal or absence of something that is needed, like vitamins. If the determinant is a static condition, it is an unchanging antecedent in a given set of circumstances; outcomes differ as the nature or quality of the condition differs. Usually, conditions are fixed attributes or circumstances, like sex, heritage or geography. Sometimes they may be attributes, like poverty or rural isolation, that are potentially changeable but unchanging in all the given circumstances open to study.

---

* This paper was published in The Bulletin of the New York Academy of Medicine (in press) and is reprinted here with permission.

One must still ask how to know a cause on seeing one, and how not to confuse the real thing with an impostor. Three attributes of any cause - association, time order, and direction - are sine qua none.

Association: A causal factor (X) must occur together with the putative effect (Y). Association is judged by the criterion of probability in relation to preset expectations of chance occurrences e.g., the conventions of statistical testing. If no grounds for an association can be shown to exist, causality has been rejected and we proceed no further. The presence of association, whether certain or uncertain, allows testing to continue.

Time order: If association is present, then a suspect causal factor (X) must precede the effect (Y). If the reverse can be shown to hold, again causality has been refuted and we proceed no further. Failure to refute, i.e. (X) does precede (Y) or it may possibly do so, allows testing to continue.

Direction: Direction is the crux of causal inference. We often reach firm decisions about both association and time order, but decisiveness about direction is another matter. Even though in a given instance both association and time order are appropriate for causality, the relation between two variables may yet be without direction (as with the sun daily preceding the moon, or with two persons responding in mutual communication, or with any association produced by a common cause or third variable).

With either active or static determinants, direction requires the presence of *consequential change*. An active agent (X) brings about the effect (Y). With a static determinant (X_1), the effect (Y) changes in consequence of a change in a prior condition, say male or female sex. Given association and time order, direction can be judged by such logical criteria for causal associations as magnitude, specificity, consistency, survivability, predictive performance, and coherence.

How Study a Cause?

To establish the attributes of a putative cause, the scientific strategy is to simplify the conditions of observation by design. In epidemiological and clinical science, this is done by two familiar general approaches: the scientist observes the relations between the cause (X) and the effect (Y) under circumstances chosen to be revealing; or the scientist experiments, which is to produce change in the effect (Y) by introducing or removing (X) from the field of observation.

Research designs implement these approaches. Every study challenges the survival of a hypothesis more or less severely. Design governs the severity of the challenge. The more rigorous the tests withstood by a hypothesis, the greater its survivability and the more likely it is to be causal.

Survivability and Research Design

In the light of the criterion of survivability, forms of design can be roughly ranked by the confidence they generate about the presence of the definitive attributes of causes. Given competent execution and *a priori* hypotheses, this confidence is a function of two elements of design, both bearing on the determinant under study. One element is the amount of *activity* in the determinant mobilized by the design. A second element is the degree of *isolation* of the determinant achieved by the design. Briefly, I list only the three strongest available designs, ranked by strength, since I shall not draw on weaker designs to test the causal interpretations at issue.

Controlled experiment yields the strongest assurances about association, time order and direction. Experiments allow the maximum activity in the determinant to be mobilized, since exposure to the hypothesized cause is a creation of the design. Experiments also allow the maximum isolation of the determinant, since direct control over the conditions simplifies observation. A critical factor for control is that experimental and comparison groups are selected before the intervention in order to neutralize the heavy bias that selection after the event can produce.

Quasi-experiment describes studies of intervention effects when comparison groups unexposed to the intervention have not been preselected by the systematic design of the researcher. Often quasi-experiments can give knowledge of the time of the intervention as secure as in the classic experiment. What is less secure is the knowledge of direction. Because initial entry to observation is not according to the neutral plan of the experimenter, it is open to the choices of the subjects and the vagaries of the social situation.

Natural experiment is a term I reserve for the observation of the effects of non-routine, well-defined changes in environment. Such changes will best be events that are major, sharp, and out of the ordinary. Natural experiments yield strong inference about time order but, also, introduce potential problems of bias and confounding in comparisons with unexposed groups.

EARLY NUTRITION AND MENTAL PERFORMANCE

By 1967, animal studies had found exquisitely timed effects of nutritional deprivation on brain development during the phase of maximum brain growth (Winick and Noble, 1967). In particular, in the early phase of rapid brain growth produced by cellular hyperplasia, acute protein deprivation resulted in irreversible brain cell depletion; in the later phase produced by cellular hypertrophy, it resulted in cellular growth retardation that was reversible. The effects of such deprivation on behavior in animals and on mental performance in human beings were much less clearcut.

Both poor nutrition and poor mental performance typically go together with poverty and poor education. In this common complex, it is a difficult task to isolate the factor of interest from the others. Yet, after a seminal conference that ranged from cellular to epidemiological studies (Scrimshaw and Gordon, 1967) the world at large was quick to make the leap of extrapolation from neuropathological and biochemical studies of the brain to the human situation. Hundreds of millions of malnourished children in the less developed world (220 to 250 million under 6 years by some estimates at the time) were widely believed to be the victims of irreversibly depressed mental performance.

The Dutch Famine Study

Several investigators, including Zena Stein and myself, felt it necessary to face up to this situation. We hoped to carry out the epidemiological analogue of the "crucial experiment" in order to discover the ultimate effects of severe prenatal undernutrition. The hypothesis to be tested was that severe deprivation in the second half of pregnancy would lead to irreversible brain cell depletion and hence to intellectual dysfunction. The first of two designs we chose for this purpose was based on the natural experiment of the Dutch Famine of 1944/45 (Stein et al 1972, 1975). The second was a randomized controlled trial of diet supplements during pregnancy in a New York City population of poor, black women; the data are presented elsewhere (Rush et al 1980 a,b).

We knew already that exposure to the Dutch famine in the third trimester had produced low birth weight; (Smith, 1947). The famine was sharply defined in both time and place: it was initiated by an embargo on transport in West Holland imposed in reprisal by the German occupying forces, and it was ended with the liberation of Holland by the Allied Forces six months later, on May 7 1945. Food rations declined to as little as 500 calories per person daily, but remained balanced in proteins, carbohydrates and fats. The affected population lived in the cities of West Holland; unaffected cities served as controls. Well-nourished before the war, the Dutch had been sparely nourished but not malnourished for the three years of the German occupation previous to the famine.

The study used an historical cohort design, that is, a longitudinal study reconstructed from available data. For this purpose, records or other data must be sufficient l) to assign exposures and 2) to determine outcome. Because this famine was so well demarcated in time and place, any record set could serve that gave date and place of birth on the one hand and the outcome of interest on the other.

Exposure could be specified from date and place of birth; it could also be quantified from the daily food ration published weekly for each region throughout the war. Outcomes came from several sources: births and deaths both from local population registers and the Central Bureau of Statistics, maternities from teaching hospitals and, crucially, mental test scores (and many other data) from military induction examinations of all 19-year old men.

Birth cohorts over four years for the entire study population were reconstructed in relation to exposure to the famine at different stages of gestation, with unexposed comparison groups from before and after the famine and also from the unaffected regions of the country (Fig. 1). The birth cohorts B1 and B2 were exposed to the famine in the second half of gestation, C in mid-gestation and D1 and D2 in the first half of gestation. A1 and A2 and E1 and E2 escaped the famine.

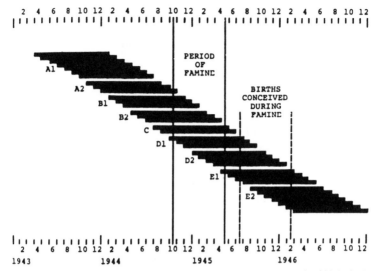

Figure 1. Design of study. Cohorts by month of conception and month of birth, in the Netherlands, 1943 through 1946, related to famine exposure. Solid vertical lines bracket the period of famine, and broken vertical lines bracket the period of births conceived during famine

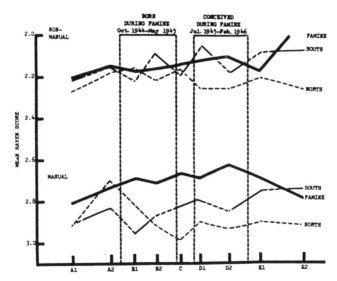

Figure 2. Raven scores by area and class (mean Raven scores by cohort in famine, Northern control, and Southern control areas, comparing manual and non-manual occupational classes)

Since we were looking for the effects of neurone depletion and slowed cell growth during rapid brain growth in the second half of pregnancy, the appropriate outcome is intellectual dysfunction, manifest either in depressed IQ or in raised frequency of mild mental retardation. No effect on any of the several measures available to us was detected (see Fig. 2). (Frank brain disorders did occur in excess with first trimester exposure to famine, but are not germane to the hypothesis under test.)

Can this study then be taken as a definitive refutation of the hypothesis posed? Problems that need to be considered are 1) Measures of exposure, 2) Measures of outcome, 3) Control of confounding 4) Interpretation.

First, the **exposure variables**, although detailed in terms of nutritional quantities available daily, are based on the fluctuations in food rations by region and therefore apply to groups and not to individuals. It is always possible with such variables that some individuals and not others are affected, so that an association present in individuals but misclassified could be suppressed in groups.

This possibility falls away in the face of strong effects of prenatal nutritional deprivation in the third trimester on fertility, on fetal growth including head circumference as measured at birth, and on mortality in the first three months of life. The likelihood of detecting change is considerably less with infant mortality, which is relatively rare, than with IQ, which can be measured in everybody. Thus it is not obvious why effects on IQ should be suppressed when effects harder to detect are not.

As to **measures of outcome**, one might ask if the group tests of mental performance used are sufficiently sensitive to detect the effects of prenatal nutrition on deprivation in 19-year old men. The riposte to this is that the measures were sufficiently sensitive to detect subtle variations of IQ with such factors as birth order, height, and family size.

Confounding of the results by other factors is a third major question that must be weighed, in this as in any study. Control of confounding rests in the first place on apt comparison. In this design, in the absence of preselected comparison groups, the double-edged control by both time and place protects against the potential confounding by historical change in comparisons over time on the one hand, and by local differences in populations in comparisons by place on the other.

Among possible confounding factors, the stressful effects of a war waged more savagely at some times and places than others immediately come to mind, only to be as quickly dismissed. Confounding which would spuriously attribute a war effect to the famine hardly pertains to the absence of an effect.

More important confounders are social factors that affect both development and mental performance. Social class, for example, modifies reproductive behavior and also relates strongly to both mortality and mental performance. A startling example of confounding by social class indeed appeared. Conception at the height of the famine seemed to be beneficial; IQ was higher in the relevant birth cohorts (D1, D2). Analysis of fertility explained this result. A sharp decline in conceptions at the height of the famine, greatest in the lowest social classes, had changed the balance of conceptions in favor of the higher classes, who invariably score better than the lower classes on IQ tests. The change in class composition had given the appearance of an improved average IQ level for the entirety of the affected cohorts.

Finally, in the matter of **interpretation**, at least three explanations are possible alternatives to the absence of a causal relation between nutritional deprivation and later mental performance:

(1) Effects of famine manifested early in life might have disappeared as social and nutritional conditions improved. The results rule out dysfunction from irreversible damage during a critical period if, as postulated in the initial hypothesis, gestation is such a period. They do not rule out the possibility of damage with subsequent recovery.

(2) Prenatal nutritional deprivation limited at most to a six-month period of gestation might have been insufficient to produce detectable effects on mental performance. Subsequent to the launching of the Dutch Famine study, indeed, the maximum brain growth spurt was found to extend beyond the first six months of life and well into the third year (Dobbing and Sands, 1974). To eliminate this alternative, the nutritional deprivation also needs to extend well into postnatal life.

(3) The type of exposure in this study may not have been salient for exploring the vulnerability of human beings to malnutrition. The Dutch Famine exposure fits closely the model of severe and acute short-term exposure to early nutritional deprivation, namely, the experiment of Winick and Noble (1967) on which we based our hypothesis. Neither the natural nor the animal experiments, however, test the effects of the pervasive form of malnutrition in the less-developed world and in most deprived social situations, which is chronic. To eliminate any of these alternative hypotheses, further studies are required.

The INCAP study in Guatemala

Concurrently with the initiation of the Dutch Famine Study in the mid 1960s, an intervention experiment was planned in Guatemala. The study was able in principle to address the hypotheses left open by the Dutch study.

Four villages were chosen to represent a rural area in which diets were mildly to moderately deficient in protein and calories and where stunting and underweight were common. In all four villages, women and children were encouraged to visit a depot twice daily to partake of a beverage ad libitum. In two of the villages, the beverage was a protein/calorie mixture; in the other two, the supplement contained no protein and rather few calories. At each visit, the amount consumed by each individual was recorded. The children were evaluated at each birthday from three to seven years of age.

Associations between level of supplementation and outcome were found (Freeman et al, 1980). Supplementation of both mother and child correlated with psychometric test scores and with growth; consumption by the children themselves correlated most strongly. Time order is left in doubt, however. In the postnatal period, the intake of the supplement continued concurrently with the tests of cognitive performance; from the major analysis of cognitive development, with positive associations throughout, one cannot be sure whether the postulated effects should be ascribed solely to supplementation early in life, or to continuing or concurrent supplementation.

Direction is even more in doubt; the results immediately raise a question of confounding by self-selection and social selection. The initial design aimed at controlled comparisons of villages preselected for different levels of supplementation. The data were neither analyzed nor presented in terms of that design. The analytic procedure converted the Guatemala Study into a quasi-experiment. The measure of exposure is the total nutritional supplementation of each mother and child (regardless of treatment or village) and, from birth on, children are compared with each other in terms of supplement intake. Since villages and not children were preselected and assigned to a given level of treatment, *within* the villages each pregnant woman and each child was a volunteer for supplemented diet according to their own choices. Moreover, the main strategy for analyzing cognitive development converts the design into a cross-sectional study, based as it is on correlations between concurrent measures of height and head circumference as nutritional indices, three social status indices, and mental performance.

Therefore, one must ask, was the child who took more supplement livelier because of the food, or was the livelier child the one who took the most supplement? Language was the test measure associated most consistently with supplement. This test also related positively to behavior and social interaction outside the testing situation. The finding points to initiative in the bright child, which enhances the threat of bias from self-selection and could be the underlying cause of the association (Fig. 3).

The Guatemala study established associations between nutrition and cognition , but neither the time order nor the direction of the causal sequences. Hence this study did not give answers to the three alternative explanations for the absence of effects left open by the Dutch study, namely, early effects with recovery, a too short exposure, and the absence of chronic malnutrition.

The Cali Intervention Trial

Some of the questions left open by the Dutch study were addressed by a Colombian study in Cali (McKay et al 1978). The ingenious design of the study is illustrated in Figure 4.

Three hundred (300) representative lowest income families--each with a 3-year old child who belonged in the category of the smallest and most malnourished children--were assigned, from randomized residential blocks, to different treatment groups. The better-off remainder were left untreated. The

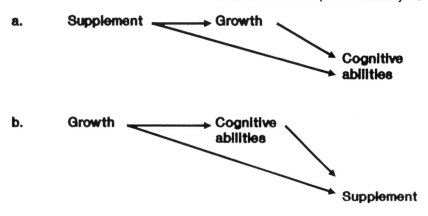

Fig. 3. Alternative causal pathways for associations between nutrition and outcome demonstrated in the Guatemala INCAP study.

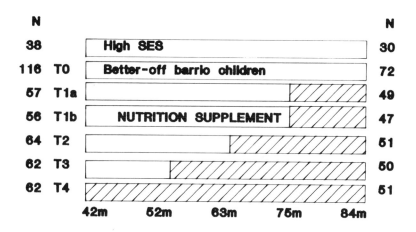

Fig. 4. Treatment groups (T0, T1a, T1b, T2, T3, T4) in the Cali experiment indicating ages at entry to program, numbers at entry and numbers at completion (constructed from McKay et al., 1978).

treatment was a daily six-hour, five-day week integrated curriculum focussed on education, health and nutrition.

The randomization was literally a lottery. The draw assigned successive groups to treatment one after the other at roughly equal intervals over the 42 months of the program. Thus each successive group entered at an older age and experienced a shorter program. The fourth and last age-group to enter, at 75 months of age, was assigned to two treatment groups: one was given nutritional supplementation at home (of a form and content not specified in the description) from the start at 42 months of age; the other, like all the rest awaiting entry to the program, was not. To these five treatment groups, a sixth group recruited from well-off homes was added; although outside the treatment program, the children were tested at the same intervals as the groups from the barrio. The results are shown in Figure 5. The main points are the following:

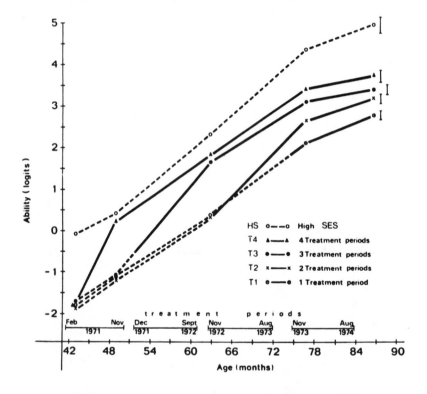

Fig. 5. Cognitive ability in four groups of children (T1, T2, T3, T4) in the Cali experiment who entered the treatment program successively at 42 to 75 months, with a high socioeconomic group for comparison. Drawn from McKay et al., 1978.

1. All the treated groups were superior to the initially better off and untreated barrio group (not shown in the figure).

2. In relation to the well-off children, the gap in performance of the treated children was narrowed, although never closed.

3. Each successive treatment group had a sharp upward spurt in cognitive ability in the first period on entering the program, and then sustained a position in advance of, but parallel with, those entering later.

4. After the treatment ended (when the children entered primary school), each group retained its advantage relative to the others, but performance fell off relative to the high socioeconomic group.

5. Previous nutritional supplementation from ages 42 to 75 months made no perceptible difference to the performance of the children who were the last to enter treatment (in presenting results, the analysts therefore combined the two groups who entered last).

The Bogotá Intervention Trial

The studies discussed so far leave a hiatus, in direct observations of consequential change, between birth and 3 years of age. The hiatus is filled by two randomized trials of diet that meet most requirements for tests of survivability. One, to be described, is the Bogotá trial (Waber et al 1981); it begins prenatally and ends at 36 months. The second, the New York City trial (Rush et al 1980 a,b), is of prenatal supplements only; it provides additional observations up to 12 months of age.

The Bogotá study, like the Cali study, aimed to test the effects of early nutrition and social stimulation, and families were identified by door-to-door survey in the barrios. In eligible familes, the mother was up to 6 months pregnant, and a majority of one or more children under 5 years of age were undernourished (weight for age <85 percentile for Colombia). A total of 456 families were randomly assigned to six treatment groups (not equal in size, for reasons unstated) with permutations on the period of nutritional supplementation and indirect social stimulation through education of the mother. The substantial nutritional supplements were provided for the whole family; the maternal education component, however, was not reported in terms of intensity and exact content.

The main results relating to cognition presented by the investigators are shown in Table 1. They concluded that nutritional supplements had a beneficial effect on mental performance (from a repeated measures analysis of variance of four groups--A, D, E, F--which had the same treatment throughout). They also concluded that the effect was "contemporaneous," in that group C, in which diet supplements ceased at six months of age, performed less well thereafter than group D, in which supplements continued throughout.

It is not clear that these "repeated measures" analyses of variance provide a straightforward address that plays to the strengths of the initial design. For this reason, the data in Table 1 were reanalyzed. The data from Table 1 were recompiled and reanalyzed by multiple regression analysis to test *a priori* hypotheses derived from the study design; standard errors were obtained for the scores in each relevant cell. From the initial structure of the design, four separate hypotheses relating to the timing and content of the intervention can each be tested by two comparisons. The results of the reanalysis for each hypothesis follow:

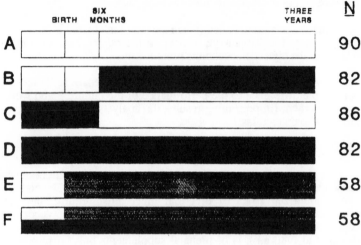

Fig. 6. Bogotá Intervention Study Design: Six randomized blocks assigned to A. Health care only. B. Diet supplements from six to 36 months of age. C. Diet supplements from the third trimester to six months of age. D. Diet supplements from the third trimester to 36 months of age. E. Maternal education from birth to 36 months of age. F. Maternal education from birth to 36 months of age and diet supplementation from the third trimester to 36 months of age. After Waber et al., (1981)

Prenatal diet supplementation, continued to *six months of age,* had no detectable effect. (This result, shown in Fig. 7, was consistent with both the Dutch and the New York City studies).

Prenatal diet supplementation, continued to *36 months of age*, had an effect (of about 6 points on the Griffiths overall scale) first detectable at 12 months and persisting till supplementation stopped (Fig. 8).

The whole effect of diet, continued to 36 months of age, resides in the supplementation given from 6 months on (Fig. 9).

Maternal education had no detectable persisting effects up to 36 months of age, although some effect seems to be present at the 12 month mark (Fig. 10).

TABLE 1. GRIFFITHS GENERAL QUOTIENT SCORES BY TREATMENT GROUP* (AFTER WABER ET AL.)

Treatment group	Sex(N)	4 m.	6 m.	12 m.	18 m.	24 m.	36 m.	Mean
A (no S)	M (29)*	98.2	105.8	95.2	94.5	95.0	82.9	95.3
	F (25)	105.0	105.3	88.3	79.5	103.2	94.0	95.9
B (S 6-36m)	M (24)	107.7	109.0	101.9	87.3	104.7	90.2	100.1
	F (36)	103.2	104.7	105.4	89.6	96.0	92.7	98.6
C (S prenatal-6m)	M (25)	108.0	106.3	103.0	82.5	93.3	94.9	98.0
	F (32)	110.2	103.9	97.4	86.3	85.2	91.1	95.7
D (S prenatal-36m)	M (29)	94.0	103.1	101.4	96.2	98.9	99.6	98.9
	F (28)	105.1	105.7	105.1	98.0	102.0	94.7	101.8
E (E 0-36m)	M (15)	96.4	102.8	105.8	79.8	95.5	92.5	95.5
	F (19)	101.6	105.5	100.8	75.3	99.0	85.6	96.4
F (0-36m;S prenatal-36m)	M (20)	112.3	100.1	104.3	81.1	94.1	95.4	97.9
	F (22)	114.8	106.8	111.4	90.5	109.4	95.6	104.7

*S = supplements. E = Maternal education
(N) = number of subjects

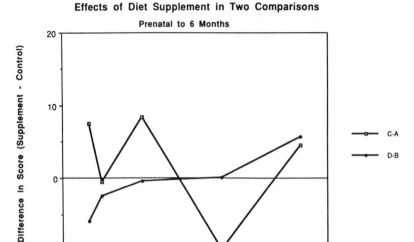

Fig. 7. Bogotá Intervention Study: Effects of *diet supplements* from **third trimester to 6 months of age** (Z scores for overall Griffiths scores from 6 to 36 months of age in two comparisons, C versus A and D versus B).

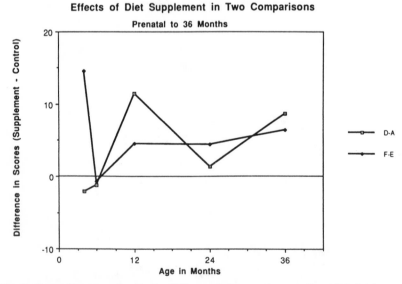

Fig. 8. Bogotá Intervention Study: Effects of *diet supplements* from **third trimester to 36 months of age** (Z scores for overall Griffiths scores from 6 to 36 months of age in two comparisons, D versus A and F versus E).

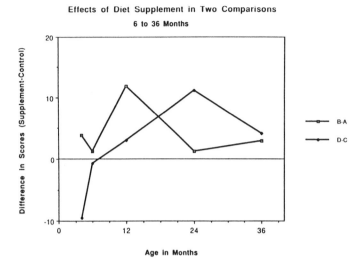

Fig. 9. Bogotá Intervention Study: Effects of *diet supplements* from **6 to 36 months of age.** (Z scores for overall Griffiths scores from 6 to 36 months of age in two comparisons, B versus A and D versus C.)

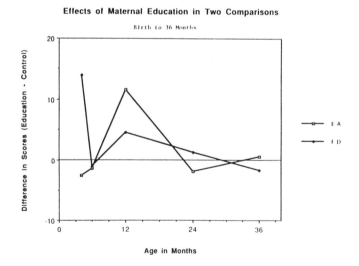

Fig. 10. Bogotá Intervention Study: Effect of *maternal education* from **birth to 36 months of age.** (Z scores for overall Griffiths scores from 6 to 36 months of age in two comparisons (E versus A and F versus D.)

Taken successively through the life course from conception to adulthood, the Dutch Famine study, the New York City study, the Bogotá study and the Cali study afford severe tests of several hypotheses relating successive phases of early nutrition to cognitive performance over the life course. We can interpret their combined results as follows:

1. *Effects of Nutrition on Mental Performance.*

1.1 Nutritional changes during gestation (as in the Dutch, New York City and Bogotá studies) and up to 6 months of age postnatally (as in the Bogotá study) produced no effects detectable between birth and three years of age or in young male adults.

1.2 Diet supplements from 6 months of age produced an effect by 12 months of age which persisted, contemporaneously with the supplements, up to 36 months of age (as in the Bogotá study). About possible persisting effects beyond 36 months, no data are available.

1.3 Diet supplements from 42 months to 75 months (as in Cali) produced no detectable effects.

2. *Effects of Psychosocial Intervention on Mental Performance:*

2.1 Educational intervention from birth to 36 months of age indirectly through the mother (as in Bogotá) produced no detectable effect up to 36 months.

Note that direct intervention at these ages has produced marked effects (Garber 1975; Campbell & Ramey, 1984), and indirect effects have also been reported (Grantham-McGregor, 1987).

2.2 Direct intervention from 42 to 84 months (as in Cali) produced marked effects.

3. *Nutritional and Psychosocial Factors in Combination or Interaction*

The evidence so far, in the main, is negative.

3.1 In good social conditions, no effects of poor nutrition have been demonstrated (Lloyd-Still 1976).

3.2 In poor social conditions, effects demonstrated have been either nutritional (as in Bogotá) or psychosocial (as in Cali), but not both.

The challenge remaining might best be addressed to two main questions:

1. Does the effect of nutritional supplements on mental performance at 6 to 36 months persist beyond the period of supplementation?

1.1 If the effect does persist, this would argue for a vulnerable and possibly critical period of brain development between six and 36 months.

1.2 If the effect does not persist, this would argue that food is needed to keep a child happy and performing well, but that lack of food sufficient to limit physical growth does not produce cumulative intellectual dysfunction nor irreversible dysfunction.

2. Do dietary and psychosocial effects interact either during or after the period of nutritional exposure?

2.1   If there is no interaction, the effects of diet on mental performance may not be a major issue.

2.2   If there is interaction, then these effects continue to present a major research and policy challenge.

In the world at large, however, nutritional and social deprivation go hand in hand. Regardless of our ultimate understanding of these research questions, in the matter of public policy prudence as well as humanity enjoin that we rear children under the most favorable conditions, both social and nutritional.

ACKNOWLEDGEMENTS

I am indebted to Patrick Shrout whose collaboration was critical to the reanalysis of the Bogotá data, and to Zena Stein whose reading was critical to my writing. The Bulletin of the New York Academy of Medicine kindly allowed me to reprint this paper which was printed as part of the proceedings on Nutrition, Children and Health sponsored by the Academy and the New York State Department of Health on March 9, 1989.

REFERENCES

Birch HG, Gussow, JD (1970). "Disadvantaged Children: Health, Nutrition and School Failure." New York: Harcourt Brace & World, and Grune & Stratton.

Cravioto J, DeLicardie ER (1975). Environmental and nutritional deprivation in children with learning disabilities. In Cruickshank WM, Hallahan DR (eds.): Syracuse: University Press, pp 3-102.

Dobbing J (1974). The later growth of the brain and its vulnerability. Pediatrics 53:2-6.

Dobbing J and Sands J (1973). Quantitative growth and development of the human brain. Arch Dis Childh 48:757-767.

Freeman HE, Klein RE., Townsend JW, Lechtig A (1980). Nutrition and cognitive development among rural Guatemalan children. Am J Public Health 70:1277-1285.

Garber HL (1975). Intervention in infancy: a developmental approach. In Begab MJ, Richardson SA (eds.): "The Mentally Retarded and Society: A Social Science Perspective." Baltimore: University Park Press, pp 287-304.

Grantham-McGregor S, Schofield W, Powell C.(1987). Development of severely malnourished children who received psychosocial stimulation: Six-year follow-up. Pediatrics 79:247-254.

Hertzig ME, Birch HG, Richardson SA and Tizard J (1972). Intellectual levels of school children severely malnourished during the first two years of life. 49:814-823.

Lloyd-Still J (1976). Clinical studies on the effects of malnutrition during childhood. In Lloyd-Still J. (ed): "Nutrition and Mental Development". Lancaster, England: Medical and Technical Publishers, 103-159.

McKay H, Sinisterra L, McKay A, Gomez H, Lloreda P. (1978). Improving cognitive ability in chronically deprived children. Science 200:270-278.

Ramey CT, Campbell FA (1984). Preventive education for high-risk children: Cognitive consequences of the Carolina Abecedarian project. Am J Ment Defic 88:515-23.

Richardson SA (1976). The relation of severe malnutrition in infancy to the intelligence of school children with differing life histories. Pediat Res 10:57-61.

Rush D, Stein Z, Susser M. (1980a). A randomized controlled trial of prenatal nutritional supplementation. Pediatrics 65:683-97.

Rush D, Stein Z, Susser M. (1980b). "Diet in Pregnancy: A Randomized Controlled Trial of Prenatal Nutritional Supplementation." National Foundation-March of Dimes Birth Defects Original Article Series, Vol. XVI, No. 3. New York: Alan Liss.

Scrimshaw N and Gordon JE (1968). "Malnutrition, Learning, and Behavior." Proceedings from the International Conference on Malnutrition, Learning and Behavior, co-sponsored by the Nutrition Foundation, Inc. and Massachusetts Institute of Technology, March 1-3, 1967. Boston: MIT Press.

Smith CA (1947). Effects of wartime starvation in Holland on pregnancy and its products. Amer J Obstet Gynec 53:599-608.

Stein ZA and Kassab H (1970). Nutrition. In Wortis J (ed): "Mental Retardation. II". New York: Grune & Stratton pp 92-116.

Stein Z, Susser M, Saenger G, Marolla F (1972). Nutrition and mental performance. Science 178:708-713.

Stein Z, Susser M, Saenger G, Marolla F (1975). "Famine and Human Development: The Dutch Hunger Winter of 1944/45." New York: Oxford University Press.

Susser M, Stein Z (1977). Prenatal nutrition and subsequent development. In Reed DM, Stanley FJ (eds): "The Epidemiology of Prematurity." Baltimore: Urban and Schwarzenberg, pp 311-3S26.

Waber DP, Vuori-Christiansen L, Ortiz N, Clement JR, Christiansen N, Mora JO, Reed RB, Herrera MG (1981). Nutritional supplementation, maternal education, and cognitive development of infants at risk of malnutrition. Amer J Clin Nutr 34:807-813.

Winick M and Noble A (1966). Cellular response in rats during malnutrition at various ages. J Nutr 89:300-306.

Discussion

Q (van Gelder): In the study of the social interaction or the education of the mother, what type of intervention was this actually?

A: In Bogota you mean. Nico, we have a problem in that the Bogota Study which did both kinds of intervention, the social intervention is very poorly documented. I don't know the answer to that. How often the mothers were visited, I don't know what was done when they were visited, I don't know how long it went on. It is not a study - as published, it may be that actually the data is much stronger - but as published we don't know the answer to that.

Similarly, with the Cali Study, they document exceptionally well the psychosocial intervention - it is fully documented - but they tell us very little about the nutritional intervention. Again, it may be a perfectly solid, sound intervention but they don't tell us enough. So, those questions are a bit gray.

Q (Audience): Inaudible (study by Craviotto?)

A: Yes, that was a pioneering study. I read it again some while ago because I always had shunted it aside. It was carefully done and very carefully thought out for its time. This was published in the early sixties. The problem is the comparison groups chosen for this study. They had a group of malnourished children with Kwashiorkor and severe nutritional deficiencies in the first couple of years of life and followed them up. They showed marked differences between those children and a comparison group. So it was one of the few studies which had a comparison group. Unfortunately, the comparison group was distinctly better off than the malnourished group, clearly from the social indicators that were presented in the paper. And because we know that socioeconomic status, family size, a dozen different family factors are so powerful in determining cognitive performance, that was fundamentally confounding. So it is a study which is difficult to interpret.

Section I: THE DIETARY REQUIREMENTS OF DEVELOPING BRAIN

In this first section the nutritional needs of the growing child have been divided into three stages: foetal development, preparation for birth, neonatal maturation. Rosso reports on data dealing with the perinatal nutritional requirements of the foetus. His discussion is concentrated on the effects of the most common biochemical deficits which affect brain development. These are the deficiencies of specific trace minerals or vitamins. Among a number of issues raised, several are of particular importance.

Chronic nutritional insufficiency in the mother, before pregnancy, puts the infant at greater risk than when malnutrition is confined to the gestational period only. In concordance with experimental results and by extrapolation, underweight women exhibit a decreased plasma volume, and uterine as well as placental perfusion may become inadequate. This implies that umbilical provisions essential for foetal growth are decreased. Further, an imbalance between maternal energy intake and needs alters glucose homeostasis, with the final consequence that glucose-energy transfer to the foetus is reduced. Finally, when head circumference is smaller than the norm before the 26th week of gestation, the infant subsequently demonstrates a diminished mental performance whereas if head size reduction occurs in the later stages of pregnancy, intelligence appears less affected. The decreased or reduced growth of an undernourished foetus to some extent causes the neonate to exhibit many of the developmental characteristics associated with prematurely born infants. Such infants, in order to survive, require special nutritional care. These special dietary needs are discussed in the next report.

Anderson highlights some of the biological challenges which confront the premature infant. Oxidative mitochondrial metabolism, probably (see Clark), and lung structure, certainly, are still underdeveloped. Hence, a number of oxidative transformations of nutrients normally occurring in full-term neonates are not possible in premature infants, or are far less efficient. The nutritional requirements of these infants may differ importantly from the normal diet (milk) a newborn needs. Midway between foetal and neonatal life, many anatomical phases of brain development are as yet incomplete. These phases, which usually occur during *in utero* development, quite likely are in part influenced or triggered by alterations in the nutrient composition of the umbilical circulation (or *vice versa*). Part of the nutritional control of brain development is thus exercised by the mother, and is lacking in the premature.

As Anderson points out, the diet(s) formulated to meet the special nutritional demands of the premature infant, at the present time are still quite imprecise. He expresses reservations and warns of the dangers which may be associated with setting too broad minimum and maximum nutrient requirements or advice, in the face of an obvious incomplete knowledge. In areas where solid scientific data is lacking, it may be prudent not to set fixed standards but, rather, to make every effort to set a safe range of intake for a nutrient. This avoids giving a sense of false security that the present nutrient formulations for the premature are entirely scientifically based and need no further modification. Not that all is negative, however. His report also indicates how far the medical care

21

of the premature infant has progressed to allow not merely survival, but also subsequent normal intellectual development of the prematurily born infant.

That not only the precocious neonate is at risk from malnutrition due to incomplete knowledge, is brought out in the discussion presented by Rassin. It is evident that the nutrient composition of human milk is very complex; the milk formulas serving to substitute for the natural product are under continuous revision to improve their nutritional value. Because the neonate in this case is biologically ready to assume a terrestrial life, the problem of defining the nutrient requirements of a new-born baby is far easier. If it were possible to quantitatively analyze all nutrients present in human milk, reconstitution of this diet in a bottle would assure that the infant receives a formula which in all respects fully meets the biological needs of the neonate. Unlike the uncertainties associated with defining the nutritional requiremens for the premature infant, in the case of the normal new-born the ideal nutritional goal to reach is at least well defined, although not attainable for the time being.

Rassin indicates that one of the greatest obstacles to the artificial reconstitution of breast milk is the fact that there is no substitute for human milk protein. Different species supply milk of a unique protein composition, with distinct qualitative properties and in characteristic relative amounts. The difference resides, among others, in (genetic) variations of amino acid structure of the proteins, which implies that after intestinal absorption the relative proportions of free amino acids available to the infant will vary according to the species source of the milk consumed. To add to the complexities, other food factors are present in milk, many as yet unidentified, which give natural milk nutritional advantages beyond those easily recognized: changing composition according to growth stage, the conferring of passive immunities, varying hormonal balances, essential fatty acids composition, ketone and sugar content are only some of the factors which add weight to the notion that no substitute for human milk exists.

It is therefore not surprising, as Rassin reports, that breastfed infants demonstrate greater health and less morbidity than bottle fed infants. There are particular concerns for the nervous system since inappropriate quantities of protein, either too much or too little, or qualitative differences from the natural proteins, have been demonstrated to alter the outcome of neurological development. This is due not only to the effects of protein malnutrition *per se* but the adverse effects are also associated with an imbalance of the free amino acid supply after the ingested proteins have been hydrolyzed. Rassin mentions as examples the specific changes in infant behaviour associated with an increased tryptophan supply (sleep) or valine (reduced sleep). In the light of all these cited disadvantages of bottle feeding, it is striking that most infants on today's baby formulas are doing very well and are thriving. It is both a testimony to the resilience of nature, and to the efforts aimed at improving the formulation of artificial human milk.

The ability of the infant to withstand nutritional imperfections is never more tested than in the case of one of the most commonly occurring and most dangerous forms of malnutrition: Kwashiorkor. The particular health problems associated with a deficiency of protein in the infant diet are severe, rapidly damaging to mental performance and, worse, are usually though not invariably associated with a general food scarcity. The social environment, so important for the developing intellectual competence of the child, is also poor since in societies in which kwashiorkor occurs the adult population is equally affected. This is reflected in the diminished energy of the community, which is needed to extract itself from this situation. Poor health standards, reduced immune resistance, mental and physical lethargy, increased incidence of disease, are all too common phenomena which accompany chronic protein insufficiencies. Bengelloun discusses some of these problems and presents an animal model, the growing rat, which may be useful to study the biological impact of kwashiorkor on behaviour. Although the model is by no means perfect, the data presented nevertheless indicates that such studies will be helpful to plan strategies for rehabilitation.

The differential impact of kwashiorkor on particular stages of neural development may require different approaches for rehabilitation, depending on the length of exposure to this form of malnutrition. Because of the severe debilitating effects of kwashiorkor, external intervention is usually required. The more rapid and efficient the methods of rehabilitation, the more of the infant population may be spared the permanent intellectual sequelae which are still far too prevalent in many parts of the world.

Nico M. van Gelder

(Mal)Nutrition and the Infant Brain, pages 25–40
© 1990 Wiley-Liss, Inc.

PRENATAL NUTRITION AND BRAIN GROWTH

Pedro R. Rosso

Departments of Pediatrics and Endocrinology, Nutrition and
Metabolics Diseases, School of Medicine, Catholic University,
Santiago, Chile.

Over the last two decades a wealth of information has been made
available on the effects of prenatal and postnatal nutrient deficiences on brain
growth and development. This data has greatly expanded our knowledge of
brain nutrient metabolism during early development and, in the process, revealed
various previously unsuspected facts, such as the influence of diet on brain
neurotransmitters. Most importantly, however, it has provided an answer to the
question: "Does undernutrition during infancy inhibit brain growth and
subsequent mental development?" posed nearly three decades ago by two South
African pediatricians: Stoch and Smythe (1963). We have learned since that early
postnatal malnutrition can affect brain growth and mental capacity, but that long-
term consequences can be minimized if proper rehabilitation begins during the
first two years of life (Winick et al., 1975; Lien et al., 1977; Galler et al., 1984).

By contrast, when we ask the same question for the prenatal period our
answer is still tentative, reflecting the fact that important aspects remain
unresolved.

The problem has been approached using different animal models. In
these studies the effect on physical growth, learning capacity and behaviour of
the offspring of mothers submitted to either energy-protein undernutrition or to a
specific nutrient deficiency before and during pregnancy have been examined
(Dobbing, 1971). In most cases the studies have focused on the effects of the
first generation; (Resnick, 1988). Other authors have extended their studies to
the consequences of malnutrition imposed on succesive generations, thus
combining the effects of pre and postnatal undernutrition (Zamenhoff and van
Marthens, 1978; Galler, 1979; Resnick and Morgane, 1984). Overall, the data
coincides in showing that prenatal exposure to either energy-protein malnutrition
or certain specific nutrient deficiencies, such as zinc (Halas et al., 1986), leads to
postnatal growth stunting, and both, depressed performance and behavioural
abnormalities. The behavioural effects and concomitant biochemical changes are
greater when the animals have suffered combined pre- and postnatal malnutrition
(Resnick, 1988). Following nutritional rehabilitation some recovery is attained
in both physical growth and function, but lasting deficits are the norm.

Marked interspecies differences in central nervous system structure and function, as well as rates of prenatal growth and perinatal maturation preclude the possibility of extrapolating animal data to the human situation. In addition, differences in reproductive function between humans and other mammals, including number of fetuses or fetal mass/maternal mass ratios and the severity of experimental malnutrition, limit the possibility of meaningful comparisons with the human situation. On the other hand, for ethical reasons the study of the consequences of prenatal nutritional deficiencies on human brain growth and function cannot be experimentally approached. Thus, most of the available data have been generated by observational studies, quasi-experimental studies, and case studies of "nature's experiments" in which associations between pregnancy conditions and outcomes have been explored. These studies have faced the rather difficult task of isolating the effect of malnutrition on the fetus from other maternal and environmental factors. An additional methodological problem is the lack of well-defined criteria of "maternal malnutrition", including degrees of severity. This lack of definition prevents comparisons between different studies.

Despite the problems mentioned above, some progress has been made on the effects of prenatal exposure to malnutrition and brain growth and subsequent development. By contrast, except for iodine, relatively little is known about prenatal specific deficiencies and brain growth. This area has been rather neglected in the past because it was generally assumed that maternal specific deficiencies did not alter prenatal growth. However, new information suggesting a link between clinically undetected maternal deficiencies and congenital malformations of the central nervous system has created a renewed interest in this area.

The purpose of this review is to critically analyze current information on prenatal nutritional deficiencies and human brain growth and subsequent mental performance. Although in humans nutritional problems are usually of a mixed nature with specific deficiencies coexisting with different degrees of energy-protein malnutrition, they will be separately analyzed for the sake of organizing the available information.

Specific Deficiencies

Despite the lack of epidemiological data on the prevalence of specific nutrient deficiencies in various areas of the world, the overall impression is that they are becoming increasingly rare, except for iron deficiency -which remains the most common specific deficiency world-wide- and zinc deficiency, a previously unsuspected problem whose real magnitude has not been determined yet. The most common specific deficiencies known to affect the human fetus are listed in Table 1, where they have been ordered according to an estimate of their world-wide incidence. Obviously, this order may change drastically for any one region depending on the characteristics of the local diets.

Animal studies, mostly in the rat, have shown that the embryo of the mammalian species is highly sensitive to several vitamin and mineral deficiencies (Giroud, 1968). Most likely, the human embryo is equally sensitive to these

TABLE 1. Maternal Specific Deficiencies Known to Affect   Prenatal
Growth and/or Early Postnatal Development

VITAMINS	MINERALS
1. Folates	1. Iron
2. Vitamin D	2. Zinc
3. Thiamin	3. Iodine
4. Vitamin B_{12}	

deficiencies. The fact that certain specific deficiencies which can alter prenatal growth when induced in animals, such as pantothenic acid, riboflavin, nicotinic acid, pyridoxine, vitamin A, and copper (Giroud, 1968) have not been described in humans may be due to several reasons. Deficiencies severe enough to cause abnormal embryonic growth may not occur in pregnant women or, less likely, that if they do occur they cause infertility.

Vitamin Deficiencies

Folate: The essential role of tetrahydrofolate in one carbon transfer metabolism, thus, indirectly in purine and pyrimidine synthesis, is well known. In addition, thymidylate synthetase requires the presence of 5.10-methylene tetrahydrofolate; therefore, folate deficiency causes arrest or retardation of cell division in a variety of tissues, in particular those with the highest rates of cell multiplication. Prepregnancy maternal folate deficiency, either alone or associated with other specific deficiencies, would affect embryonic growth causing various types of congenital malformations, especially neural tube defects (Fraser and Watt, 1964; Hibbard and Smithells, 1965). The data is far from being conclusive and presently research is being conducted to validate the claims that prenatal supplementation with a multivitamin preparation can prevent the occurrence of neural tube defects in at risk groups (Smithells et al., 1980; Laurence et al., 1981).

The presence of gross congenital malformations reflects cell death, changes in mitotic rate, altered biosynthetic rates or other interference with critical stages of differentiation. These in turn would result in abnormal tissue or organ growth. However, at later stages of development folate deficiency, or other specific deficiencies may cause more circumscribed structural defects and functional abnormalities in specific areas of cognitive development. This possibility has not been explored.

When the mother becomes folate deficient during the course of pregnancy, the infant may be born with reduced liver stores, thus, be at a greater risk of becoming folate deficient him/herself during the first year of life.Breast-feeding by a folate deficient mother may contribute to the severity of the problem (Oski, 1982). Infants with megaloblastic anemia also suffer some degree of growth retardation and delayed pshychomotor development (Cecalupo and

Cohen, 1987). The mechanisms underlying the delayed functional maturation associated with folic acid deficiency are unkown.

Folate supplementation is known to have a positive influence on gestational length (Tchernia et al., 1982) and to reduce the frequency of premature birth in populations with endemic deficiency of this vitamin (Baumslag et al., 1970). Since folate reserves are accumulated during the last few weeks of pregnancy, there is an increased incidence of premature infants and an earlier onset of megaloblastic anemia compared with term infants (Cecalupo and Cohen, 1987).

Vitamin D: The effects of maternal vitamin D deficiency on the fetus reflect a reduced calcium availability. The resulting changes in calcium metabolism lead to an altered composition of the dental enamel in the deciduous teeth (Purvis et al., 1973), neonatal hypocalcemia (Roberts et al., 1973) and, in more severe cases, to congenital rickets (Russell and Hill, 1974). Infants with neonatal hypocalcemia exhibit neurological symptoms ranging from minor tremors to generalized convulsions. However, there is no evidence of lasting developmental changes.

Vitamin B_{12}: Cases of vitamin B_{12} deficiency have been described in breast-fed infants of strictly vegetarian mothers (Lampkin and Saunders, 1969; Higginbotton et al., 1978). These infants would be born with very low vitamin B_{12} stores and the low concentration of this vitamin in maternal milk would precipitate vitamin B_{12} deficiency much earlier than the pernicious anemia syndrome associated with postnatal deficiency of this vitamin.

The cases described so far involve 4-6 months old infants and central nervous system symptoms, including a comatose state, are the most salient features. Recovery of both brain and peripheral nerve function is apparently total after vitamin B_{12} is administered.

Thiamin: Diet-induced thiamin deficiency has practically disappeared in Western countries, but it continues to be a potentially important health problem in various areas of the world. Maternal thiamin deficiency during the course of gestation is often asymptomatic. However, the reduced plasma levels of this vitamin determine reduced thiamin stores in the neonate. This may lead to one of the various forms of infantile beri-beri, including the nearly always fatal cardiac form, with rapid progressive congestive heart failure (King, 1967). Thiamin deficiency affects both the mature and developing brain. Lesions associated with infantile beri-beri are focal and mostly located in the thalamus, hypothalamus, pons and mammilary bodies (Davis and Wolf, 1958).

Studies in thiamin-deficient rats suggest that these lesions may be secondary to a decreased synthesis of neuro-transmitters such as GABA and acetylcholine (Hamel et al., 1979). In addition, offspring of thiamin-deficient rats also have a reduced accumulation of galactolipids, phospholipids and phasmalogens, but myelination appears unaffected (Reddy and Ramakrishnan, 1982).

Mineral Deficiencies

Iron: Increasing evidence indicates that iron deficiency during pregnancy leads to reduced iron stores in the neonate. The data contradicts the assumption that the fetus is not affected by iron deficiency, which was based on the observation that cord blood hemoglobin concentration was normal in infants of anemic mothers. A reduced iron availability in the mother would result in a reduced placental transfer of iron and, thus, reduced iron stores in the neonate. Inadequate iron content of weaning food would be a contributing factor (Rosso and Lederman, 1985).

Postnatal iron deficiency leads to delayed motor development and it may determine a variety of symptoms such as generalized weakness, irritability, easy fatigue, anorexia and pica even prior to the appearance of classical hematological abnormalities (Cecalupo and Cohen, 1987). The concomitant behavioral and intellectual changes, including decreased perceptive skills, decreased attention span and decreased intellectual performance described by some authors in iron deficient infants has generated great interest in this field (Oski and Honig, 1978; Walter et al., 1983; Lozoff et al., 1987). The functional abnormalities are partially corrected by iron therapy, but data support the possibility that severe and prolonged deficiency of this mineral may have lasting effects. In one of the studies, children who had been anemic between 6 and 18 month of age had significant deficits when assessed in terms of motor coordination at 7-9 years of age (Cantwell, 1974).

A series of studies in rats, iron deficient during early growth, have shown that this deficiency induced a deficit in brain iron content and behavioural changes that persisted into adulthood despite iron therapy (Weinberg et al., 1979; Williamson and Ng, 1980; Dallman and Spirito, 1977). The functional and/or structural abnormalities caused by iron deficiency in the developing brain remain poorly understood.

Zinc: During the last decade an increasing number of studies have linked zinc deficiency during pregnancy to congenital malformations of the central nervous system and to fetal growth retardation (Solomons, et al., 1986; Keen and Hurley, 1987; Swanson and King, 1987). In addition, studies in rats and subhuman primates have shown that marginal zinc deficiency may depress learning capacity and cause behavioural abnormalities (Golub et al., 1985; Halas et al., 1986).

The biochemical lesions underlying these effects are for the most part unknown. Within the cells there are a wide variety of metabolic defects which may occurr as a result of zinc deficiency, including abnormal nucleic acid metabolism. Zinc deficient rat embryos have lower activities of both DNA polymerase and thymidine kinase (Swenerton et al., 1969; Eckhert and Hurley, 1977). In the fetal brain abnormal DNA synthesis could alter critical periods of cellular growth resulting in abnormal histogenesis of focal areas.

Besides abnormalities in nucleic acid metabolism, marginal zinc deficiency has been shown to decrease the rate of tubulin polymerization in the rat brain of mothers and their offspring at 21 days of age (Oteiza et al., 1987). Reduction in tubulin assembly in brain supernatants has also been reported in adult rats and pigs fed severely zinc deficient diets (Hesketh, 1981).

Iodine: Prenatal exposure to iodine deficiency may cause cretinism with or without hypothyroidism. The main characteristics of this syndrome are physical growth retardation and severe mental retardation. Some patients, usually those without congenital hypothyroidism, may also present deaf-mutism and diplegia (Pharoah et al., 1980).

The effects of iodine deficiency on the developing brain have been explored in several experimental models. The postnatally thyroidectomized rat has been the subject of a considerable number of studies. In this animal, iodine deficiency causes brain growth retardation and marked histologic abnormalities, including decreased size of cortical neurons, decreased number of cortical axons, reduced dentritic arborization, and delayed myelination (Hamburgh et al., 1971).

These profound morphologic changes reflect altered protein synthesis. Thyroid hormones are known to influence RNA polymerase II activity (Krawiec et al., 1977), to influence t-RNA sulfur transferase which confers codon specificity to transfer RNA (Wong et al., 1977), and to affect the release of polypeptide chains from ribosomes (Sokoloff, 1977). A reduced rate of protein synthesis also affect the rate of cell proliferation, which explains the reduced brain DNA content of hypothyroid animals (Hetzel and Querido, 1980).

Extensive studies of electric and behavioural activity of hypothyroid rats have shown electroencephalograms of low amplitude and delayed appearance of evoked response (Meisami et al., 1970).

Protein-Energy Malnutrition

The fetal consequences of an inadequate maternal intake of energy and protein during gestation are strongly influenced by the nutritional status of the mother before pregnancy (Rosso and Lederman, 1985). In a non-pregnant woman a deficient energy intake determines a decreased body weight for height (Grande and Keys, 1980). This reflects a reduced quantity of body fat, which can be quantitated by skinfold measurements, and a reduced lean body mass, whose main component is muscle. Mid-arm circumference is one of the anthropometric variables most commonly used to assess muscle mass. In undernourished subjects both skinfold thickness and midarm circumference are reduced proportionate to the severity of the condition (Grande and Keys, 1980).

During the course of pregnancy, an inadequate energy intake determines a smaller weight gain. Well-nourished women of average size gain 11-13 Kg during gestation (Hytten and Leitch, 1971). Smaller weight gains indicate that the energy needs of pregnancy are not being met. Absolute weight gains of pregnant women are proportional to their height, therefore, assessment of adequacy of maternal weight gain must consider height (Rosso, 1985). For example, a 9 Kg weight gain is normal for a woman whose height is 149 cm, but certainly insufficient for a 175 cm woman.

At present well-defined criteria to diagnose maternal undernutrition are lacking. This fact has been the source of considerable confusion since many of the available studies concerning the effects of maternal malnutrition on fetal growth are hardly comparable. Based on maternal weight for height before pregnancy and weight gain during pregnancy, the following types of maternal malnutrition can be recognized (Rosso, 1990): 1) prepregnancy malnutrition; 2) gestational malnutrition and 3) combined prepregnancy and gestational malnutrition.

Women with prepregnancy malnutrition have a weight for height below 90 percent of standard weight. Since during the first 12 weeks of gestation most women gain little weight , and some may even lose weight, anthropometric measurements performed during this period reflect rather closely prepregnancy nutritional status. Prepregnancy malnutrition will affect fetal growth unless the initial weight deficit is corrected during the course of gestation (Rosso, 1985).

In developing countries a significant number of mothers are very short due to malnutrition during childhood and, probably, the effects of undernutrition in previous generations. Maternal height also influences fetal growth, and for this reason, these mothers should be considered in a special category of "chronic undernutrition".

Gestational malnutrition can be recognized by an inadequate weight gain during the course of pregnancy. Well-nourished women with a normal weight/height at conception should experience a 20 percent increase in body weight during the course of pregnancy (Rosso, 1985). Failure to reach this goal is indicative of energy deficiency.

Consistent with the previous definitions, women suffering combined prepregnancy and pregnancy malnutrition exhibit a weight for height at conception below 90 percent of standard weight ("prepregnancy malnutrition") and a weight gain less than 20 percent of standard weight during the course of gestation.

These various types of maternal malnutrition interfere with fetal growth. However, the characteristics of the fetal growth retardation depends on the type and severity of maternal malnutrition (Table 2).

Chronic malnutrition leads to an approximately 250 g to 350 g decrease in mean birth weigth in mild and severe forms, respectively, and to a small decrease in body length. By contrast, head circumference is only significantly reduced in the most severe cases (Rosso, 1987). Mild cases are those in which maternal weight for height at conception corresponds to 80-90% of standard. Severe cases are those with body/height below this range.

Prepregnancy malnutrition determines a smaller drop in mean birth weight than chronic malnutrition. Fetal body length is affected only in severe cases (also defined as weight/height at conception less than 80% of standard weight). However, head circumference is not affected by this type of maternal malnutrition (Rosso, unpublished).

TABLE 2. Effects of Type and Severity of Maternal Malnutrition on Birth Weight, Body Length and Head Circumference (HC).

Type	Severity	Birth weight*	Body length**	HC**
1. Chronic	Mild	-250***	R	N
	Severe	-350***	R	R
2. Prepregnancy	Mild	-100***	N	N
	Severe	-200***	R	N
3. Gestational	Mild	-150	N	N
	Severe	-300	R	N
4. Combined	Mild	-350	R	R
(2 & 3)	Severe	-500	R	R

* Compared with well-nourished women
** N = >10th percentile
   R = <10th percentile
*** a "normal" weight gain assumes a 9-13 kg increase, depending on maternal height.

TABLE 3. Effects of Severe Gestational Malnutrition Caused by Famine on the Anthropometric Characteristics of the Newborn (1).

Group	Birth wt (g)	Body length (cm)	Head Circ. (cm)
Pre-famine	3 418 ± 517 (110)	50.3 ± 5.3 (107)	34.9 ± 1.7 (27)
Famine	3008 ± 557 (116)	48.9 ± 4.4 (114)	34.8 ± 1.6 (30)
	p<0.001	p<0.03	N.S.

1. Adapted from Stein et al., (1975)

Gestational undernutrition in a previously well-nourished woman, may lead to a 150-300 g decrease in average birth weight depending on its severity, but it does not affect head circumference. In this respect data in Chilean women (Rosso, unpublished) coincides with the Dutch famine data (Stein et al., 1975)

(Table 3). Mild cases are those gaining between 12 and 15 percent of standard weight and severe cases those gaining less than 12 percent of standard (Rosso, 1985).

Finally, when prepregnancy and pregnancy undernutrition are combined average birth weight may be reduced by as much as 500 g and at birth both body length and head circumference are reduced (Rosso, unpublished).

Thus, the only types of maternal malnutrition which affect brain growth are severe chronic malnutrition and combined prepregnancy (including chronic) and gestational undernutrition. Other types of malnutrition may affect fetal body length, but head circumference remains within normal limits.

Mechanisms of Fetal Growth Retardation

While some specific deficiencies directly affect fetal growth by intefering with cell division and/or protein synthesis, the mechanisms by which maternal energy-protein malnutrition leads to fetal growth retardation are still under investigation.

Studies in rats, food restricted during pregnancy, have shown that uterine and placenta blood perfusion are markedly reduced when compared with well-fed animals (Rosso and Kava, 1980). This change has been linked to a limited plasma volume expansion and decreased cardiac output, both present in the food restricted rat (Rosso, 1981). Underweight women also have a reduced plasma volume near term, thus suggesting that hemodynamic changes similar to those described in the rat may be taking place in humans (Rosso et al., 1983). A reduced placental blood flow is known to retard fetal growth in animals (Wigglesworth, 1964; Creasy et al., 1972) and explains the common occurrence of fetal growth retardation when the mother suffers conditions such as preclampsia and chronic hypertension, which cause vasoconstriction in various tissues and organs, including the gravid uterus.

Depending on the severity and time of gestation when uterine blood flow becomes limiting for the growing fetus, fetal weight, length and head circumference can be differentially affected. Thus, the newborn may be very small and proportionately affected in all his body segments (Type I fetal growth retardation) or he may have a reduction in body weight proportionately greater than the reduction in either length and head circumference, (Type II fetal growth retardation) (Rosso and Winick, 1974; Villar and Belizan, 1982) In some cases, where presumably growth retardation had a late onset and the relative reduction in uterine blood flow was only moderate, head circumference, thus brain size, may be within normal limits.

Besides the hemodynamic changes leading to fetal growth retardation and, eventually, brain growth retardation, several adaptive metabolic changes are taking place in the malnourished mother which may also affect fetal growth. This aspect which is particularly relevant for mothers suffering from gestational undernutrition has not been investigated.

Based on animal studies and on pregnant women submitted to prolonged fasting during the first trimester of pregnancy, it is known that the imbalance between maternal energy intake and needs trigger various metabolic adjustments required to maintain plasma glucose homeostasis (Felig and Lynch, 1970; Felig et al., 1972; Freinkel, 1972). These include increased fat mobilization, decreased maternal glucose consumption and increased gluconeogenesis from amino acids provided mostly by muscle. In this situation, post-prandial and post-absorptive plasma glucose values are lower than normal, thus determining a reduced placental glucose transfer. The fetus would react to this diminished availability of its main energy fuel by reducing insulin secretion and, consequently, the rate of fat deposition and protein synthesis. The net results of these metabolic changes would be a reduced fetal growth rate. Additional growth retarding factors could be a reduced maternal free aminoacids pool or, as suggested by Metcoff (1983), an altered plasma amino acids profile caused by a reduced protein intake.

Maternal Malnutrition and Brain Growth

As previously discussed, human data indicates that maternal malnutrition can cause brain growth retardation, but only when fetal growth is affected. On the other hand, the altered metabolic profile of a malnourished mother could, conceivably, affect the brain by reducing the availability of certain amino acids. The effect of maternal malnutrition on the infant's subsequent mental capacity could be mediated by brain growth retardation, and the resulting irreversible histologic and functional changes or, without brain growth retardation taking place, by the altered milieu caused by the maternal metabolic changes brought about by her reduced energy intake.

The Dutch famine study by Stein et al., (1975) has clearly shown that gestational undernutrition severe enough to cause an approximately 300 g drop in mean birth weight, but not a significant reduction in head circumference, does not have any subsequent functional sequelae, at least when occurring in an affluent Western population. This evidence has resisted the test of time and, unless otherwise proven, should be considered a conclusive result.

Comparable data concerning the possibility that maternal metabolic changes caused by malnutrition may lead to a subsequent decrease in mental capacity is lacking. In this respect, it is worth mentioning the study by Naeye and Chez (1981) on the effects of maternal acetonuria and low prepregnancy weight on children's psychomotor development. These authors, using the database of the U.S. Collaborative Perinatal Project, revised an earlier study by Churchill and Berendes (1969) in which acetonuria during gestation was associated with lower mental and motor scores at 8 months of age and lower IQ values at 4 years of age. The more recent studies found no differences in various performance tests between control children and those prenatally exposed to acetonuria.

Thus, available evidence would indicate that when maternal malnutrition does not affect brain growth, subsequent mental development is not affected.

What is the situation when brain growth has been retarded by maternal malnutrition? Unfortunately, we don't have clear answers to this question since the problem has not been investigated from this perspective. As discussed earlier, maternal malnutrition does not always cause brain growth retardation.

None of the available studies on maternal nutrition and postnatal development have compared infants according to their head circumference at birth and/or the type of malnutrition suffered by the mother.

We can turn, however, as a source of alternative information to the follow-up studies of small-for-gestational age infants. This type of growth retardation and the one caused by malnutrition have in common a reduced placental blood flow as a major determinant; however, they may differ in other respects, i.e. perinatal events, including intra- partum complications.

All studies conducted so far on subsequent mental development of Type I and Type II infants, which include studies by Fancourt et al., (1876); Harvey et al., in England (1982) and Villar et al., in Guatemala (1984), consistently show that Type II infants exhibit a better rate of postnatal growth and perform better than Type I infants when tested with various developmental and intelligence tests.

These results can be exemplified by those reported by Harvey et al., (1982). In this study, small-for-date infants were divided into two groups: one whose head sizes were below the 25th percentile of a cephalometry chart before the 26th week of gestation, which corresponds to Type I prenatal growth retardation, and a second group of infants in which serial ultrasound measurements demonstrated a fall in head size values after the 26th week of pregnancy, in most cases around week 30 of gestation. Thus, they suffered a Type II growth retardation. When these groups were compared at 3.9-7 years of

TABLE 4. McCarthy Scales Scores in 3.9-7 Year Old Infants Who at Birth Had Type I or Type II Intrauterine Growth Retardation, Determined by Ultrasonic Cephalometry[1].

Scale Item	Type I	Type II	P
Verbal	53.4 ± 11.4	56.7 ± 11.6	NS
Perceptual Performance	51.5 ± 7.0	58.0 ± 10.9	<0.05
Quantitative	49.2 ± 6.6	55.7 ± 8.4	<0.02
Motor	45.1 ± 6.8	51.5 ± 11.3	<0.05
Memory	46.8 ± 9.0	52.5 ± 9.7	NS
Gener.Gognitive Index	102.9 ± 11.7	113.2 ± 16.4	<0.05

[1] Adapted from Harvey et al., (1982).

age using a McCarthy scale, Type I infants had significantly lower scores than Type II in the following items: perceptual-performance, quantitave, motor and general cognitive index (Table 4). When each of these groups was separately compared with infants fully grown at term matched by age, sex, social class and birth order, Type I infants had lower scores for perceptual performance, motor and general cognitive index. By contrast, scores in Type II and their matched controls were not significantly different.

These results coincide with those of Fancourt et al., (1976) who also used ultrasonic measurement to establish the type of prenatal growth retardation, and those of Villar et al., (1984) who compared infants according to their ponderal index. Considered together, they strongly support the concept that prenatal brain growth retardation can affect mental performance during childhood, but in order to cause this effect it must be severe and/or last a critical length of time. More moderate cases of brain growth retardation with a shorter duration apparently have no lasting consequences. If these findings hold for the brain growth retardation caused by maternal malnutrition, negative consequences for mental performance should be expected only in the most extreme cases of combined chronic and gestational undernutrition.

REFERENCES

Baumslag N, Edelstein T, Metz J (1970). Reduction of incidence of prematurity by folic supplementation In pregnancy. Br Med J 1:16-17.

Cantwell, RJ (1974). The long term neurological sequelae of anemia in infancy. Pediatr Res 8:342 (Abstract)

Cecalupo AJ, Cohen HJ (1987). Nutritional anemias. In: Grand RJ, Sutphen JL and Dietz WH (eds): Pediatric Nutrition, Therapy and Practice. Boston: Butterworth, pp 493-495.

Churchill JA, Berendes HW (1969). Intelligence of children whose mothers had acetonemia during pregnancy. Pan Am Health Org Sci Publ 185:30-36.

Creasy RK, Barrett CT, de Swiet M, Kahangaa KV, Rudolph AC (1972). Experimental intrauterine growth retardation in the sheep. Am J Obstet Gynecol 112:566-573.

Dallman PR, Spirito RA (1977). Brain iron in the rat: extremely slow turnover in normal rats may explain long-lasting effects of early iron deficiency. J Nutr 107:1075-1081.

Davis RA, Wolf A (1958). Infantile beri-beri associated with Wernicke's encephalopathy. Pediatrics 21:409-420.

Dobbing J (1971). Undernutrition and the developing brain: the use of animal models to elucidate the human problem. Psychiatr Neurol Neurochir 74:433-442.

Eckhert CD, Hurley LS (1977). Reduced DNA synthesis in zinc deficiency: Regional differences in embryonic rats. J Nutr 107:855-861.

Fancourt R, Campbell S, Harvey D, Norman AP (1976). Follow-up study of small-for-dates babies. Br Med J 1:1435-1437.

Felig P, Lynch V (1970). Starvation in human pregnancy: hypoglycemia, hypoinsulinemia, and hyperketonuria. Science 170:990-993.

Felig P, Kim YJ, Lynch V, Hendler R (1972). Amino acid metabolism in starvation in human pregnancy. J Clin Invest 51:1195-1202.

Fraser JL, Watt HJ (1964). Megaloblastic anemia in pregnancy and the puerperium. Am J Obstet Gynecol 89:532-534.

Freinkel N (1972). Accelerated starvation and the mechanisms for conservation of maternal nitrogen during pregnancy. Israel J Med Sci 8:426-439.

Galler JR (1979). Behavioral development following inter- generational and postnatal malnutrition. In Brozek J (ed): Behavioral Effects of Energy and Protein Deficits. NIH Publication NB79-1906, pp 22-38.

Galler JR, Ramsey F, Solimano G (1984). The influence of early malnutrition on subsequent behavioral development. III. Learning disabilities as a sequel to malnutrition. Pediatr Res 18: 309-313.

Giroud A (1968). Nutrition of the embryo. Fed Proc 27:163-184.

Golub MS, Gershwin ME, Hurley LS, Saito WY (1985). Studies of marginal zinc deprivation in rhesus monkeys. VII Infant Behavior. Am J Clin Nutr 42: 1229-1239.

Grande F, Keys A (1980). Body weight, body composition and calorie status. In Goodhart RS and Shils M (eds): Modern Nutrition in Health and Disease, Philadelphia: Lea & Febiger, pp 3-34.

Halas ES, Hunt CD, Eberhardt MJ (1986). Learning and memory disabilities in young adult rats from medly zinc deficient dams. Physiol Behav 37:451-458.

Hamburgh M, Mendoza LA, Burkart JF, Weil F (1971). Thyroid dependent processes in the developing nervous system. In Hamburgh M and Barrington EJW (eds): Hormones in Development. New York: Appleton-Century-Crofts, pp 403-415.

Hamel E, Butterworth RF, Barbeau A (1979). Effect of thiamin deficiency on levels of putative amino acid transmitters in affected regions of the rat brain. J Neurochem 33:575-577.

Harvey D, Prince J, Bunton J, Parkinson C, Campbell S (1982). Abilities of children who were small-for-gestational age babies. Pediatrics 69:296-300.

Hesketh JE (1981). Brain microtubule assembly in zinc deficiency. In Howell JMcC, Gawthorne JW, White CL (eds): Trace Elements Metabolism in Man and Animals. Netley: Griffin Press, pp 613-616.

Hetzel BS, Querido A (1980). Iodine deficiency, thyroid function and brain development. In Stanbury JB, Hetzel BS (eds): Endemic Goiter and Endemic Cretinism. New York: Wiley, pp 461-472.

Hibbard ED, Smithells RW (1965). Folic acid metabolism and human embryopathy. Lancet 1:1254.

Higginbotton MC, Sweetman L, Hyhan WL (1978). A syndrome of methylmalonic aciduria, homocystinuria, megaloblastic anemia and neurologic abnormalities in a vitamin B12-deficient breast-fed infant of a strict vegetarian. N Engl J Med 29:317-323.

Hytten FE, Leitch I (1971). Weight gain in pregnancy. In Hytten FE and Leitch I (eds): The Physiology of Human Pregnancy. Oxford: Blackwell, pp 265-285.

Keen CL, Hurley LS (1987). Effects of zinc deficiency on prenatal and postnatal development. Neurotoxicology 8:379-388.

King EQ (1967). Acute cardiac failure in the newborn due to thiamin deficiency. Exp Med Surg 25:173-177.

Krawiec L, Montalbano CA, Duvilanski BH, de Guglielmone AER,Gomez CJ (1977). Influence of neonatal hypothyroidism on brain RNA synthesis. In Grave GD (ed): Thyroid Hormones and Brain Development. New York: Raven Press, pp 315-324.

Lampkin BC, Saunders EF (1969). Nutritional vitamin B12 deficiency in an infant. J Pediatr 75:1053-1055

Laurence KM, James N, Miller MH, Tennant GB, Cambell H (1981). Double-blind randomized controlled trial of folate treatment before conception to prevent recurrence of neural-tube defects. Br Med J (Clin Res) 282:1509-1511.

Lien NM, Meyer KK, Winick M (1977). Early malnutrition and "late" adoption: A study of their effects on the development of Korean orphans adopted into American families. Am J Clin Nutr 30:1734-1739.

Lozoff B, Brittenham GM, Wolf AW, McClish DK, Kuhnert PM, Jiménez E, Jiménez R, Mora LA, Gomez I, Krauskoph D (1987). Iron deficiency anemia and iron therapy effects on infant developmental test performance. Pediatrics 79:981-995.

Massaro TF, Levitsky DA, Barnes RH (1977). Protein malnutrition induced during gestation: Its effect on pup development and maternal behavior. Dev Psychobiol 10:339-345.

Meisami E, Valcana T, Timiras PS (1970). Effects of neonatal hypothyroidism on the development of brain excitability in the rat. Neuroendocrinology 6:160-166.

Metcoff J, Cole T, Lunn P, Salem S (1983). Fetal growth retardation caused by maternal dietary amino acid imbalance. In Dretchmer N and Minkowski A (eds): Nutritional Adaptation of the Gastrointestinal Tract of the Newborn. New York: Raven Press pp 151-161.

Miller M, Resnick O (1980). Tryptophan availability: The importance of prepartum and postpartum dietary protein on brain indolamine metabolism in rats. Expt Neurol 67:298-314.

Naeye RL, Chez RA (1981). Effects of maternal acetonuria and low pregnancy weight gain on children's psychomotor development. Am J Obstet Gynecol 139:189-193.

Oski FA, Honig AS (1978). The effects of therapy on the developmental scores of iron-deficient infants. J Pediatr 92:21-25.

Oski FA (1982). Nutritional anemias of infancy. In Lifshitz F (ed): Pediatric Nutrition. New York: M Dekker, pp 123-138.

Oteiza PI, Keen CL, Lonnerdal B, Hurley LS (1987). Marginal Zn deficiency affects maternal brain microtubule assembly in rats. Fed Proc 46:596.

Pharoah P, Delange F, Fierro-Benitez R, Stanbury JB (1980). Endemic cretinism. In Stanbury JB and Hetzel BS (eds): Endemic Goiter and Endemic Cretinism. New York: Wiley, pp 395-421.

Purvis RJ, Barrie WJ, McKay GS, Cocklourn F, Barrie WJMcK, Wilkinson EM, Berton NR (1973). Enamel hypoplasia of the teeth associated with neonatal tetany: a manifestation of maternal vitamin D deficiency. Lancet 3:811-814.

Reddy TS, Ramakrishnan CV (1982). Effects of maternal thiamin deficiency on the lipid composition of rat whole brain, gray matter and white matter. Neurochem Int 4:495-499.

Resnik O, Morgane PJ (1984). Generational effects of protein malnutrition in rat. Dev Brain Res 15:219-227.

Resnik O (1988). Nutrition, neurotransmitter regulation, and developmental pharmacology. In Menolascino FJ and Stark JA (eds) Baltimore: PH Brookes, pp 161-175.

Roberts SA, Cohen MD, Forfar JD (1973). Antenatal factors associated with neonatal hypocalcaemic convulsions. Lancet 2:809-811.

Rosso P, Winick M (1974). Intrauterine growth retardation. A new systematic approach based on the clinical and biochemical characteristics of this condition. J Perinat Med 2:147-159.

Rosso P, Kava R (1980). Effects of food restriction on cardiac output and blood flow to the uterus and placenta in the pregnant rat. J Nutr 110:2350-2354.

Rosso P (1981) Nutrition and maternal-fetal exchange. Am J Clin Nutr 34:744-755.

Rosso P, Arteaga A, Foradori A, Grebe G, Lira P, Torres J, Vela P. (1983). Physiological adjustments and pregnancy outcome in low-income chilean women. Fed Proc 17:138A (Abstract).

Rosso P, Lederman SA (1985). Nutrition and fetal growth. Adv Perinat Med 4:1-61.

Rosso P (1985). A new chart to monitor weight gain during pregnancy. Am J Clin Nutr 41:644-652.

Rosso P (1987). Maternal nutrition and fetal growth: implications for subsequent mental competence. In Rassin DK, Haber BH, Drujan B (eds): Basic and Clinical Aspects of Nutrition and Brain Development. New York: AR Liss, Inc, pp 339-357.

Rosso P (1990). Maternal calorie intake and fetal growth. In Rosso P (ed): Nutrition and Fetal Growth. New York: Oxford U Press (in press).

Russell JGB, Hill LF (1974). True fetal rickets. Br J Radiol 47: 732-734.

Smithells RW, Sheppard S, Schorah CJ, Fielding DW, Seller MJ, Nevin NC, Harris R, Head AD (1980). Possible prevention of neural tube defects by periconceptional vitamin supplementation. Lancet 1:339-340.

Sokoloff L (1977). Biochemical mechanisms of the action of thyroid hormones: Relationship to their role in brain. In Grave GD (ed): Thyroid Hormones and Brain Development. New York: Raven Press, pp 73-88.

Solomons NW, Helitzer-Allen DL, Villar J (1989). Zinc needs during pregnancy. Clin Nutr 5:63-71.

Stein Z, Susser M, Saenger G, Marolla F (1975). Famine and Human Development. New York: Oxford Univ Press.

Stoch MB, Smythe PM (1963). Does undernutrition during infancy inhibit brain growth and subsequent mental development? Arch Dis Child 38:546-552.

Swanson CA, King JC (1987). Zinc and pregnancy outcome. Am J Clin Nutr 46:763-771.

Swenerton H, Shrader R, Hurley LS (1969). Zinc-deficient embryos: Reduced thymidine incorporation. Science 166:1014-1015.

Tchernia G, Blot I, Rey A, Kaltwasser JP, Zittoun J, Papiernik E (1982). Maternal folate status, birthweight and gestational age. Dev Pharmacol Ther 4 (Suppl 1):58-65.

Villar J, Belizan JM (1982). The timing factor in the pathophysiology of the intrauterine growth retardation syndrome. Obstetrical and Gynecol Surv 37:499-505.

Villar J, Smeriglio V, Martorell R, Browne CH, Klein R (1984). Heterogeneous growth and mental development of intrauterine growth retarded infants during the first three years of life. Pediatrics 74:783-791.

Walter T, Kovalskys J, Stekel A (1983). Effect of mild iron deficiency on infant mental development scores. J Pediatr 102:519-522.

Weinberg J, Levine S, Dallman PR (1979). Long-term consequences of early iron deficiency in the rat. Pharmacol Biochem Behav 11:631-638.

Wigglesworth JS (1964). Experimental growth retardation in the foetal rat. J Path Bact 88:1-13.

Williamson AM, Ng KT (1980). Behavioural effects of iron deficiency in the adult rat. Physiol Behav 24:561-567.

Winick M, Meyer KK, Harris RC (1975). Malnutrition and environmental enrichment by early adoption. Science 190:1173-1175.

Wong T, Harris SL, Harris MA (1977). Some factor controlling the activity of t-RNA sulfurtransferase. In Grave GD (ed): Thyroid Hormones and Brain Development. New York: Raven Press, pp 345-366.

Zamenhoff S, van Marthens E, Granel L (1973). Prenatal nutritional factors affecting brain development. Nutr Rep Int 7:371-382.

DISCUSSION

Q (van Gelder): I am not quite sure what the difference is between gestational and chronic malnutrition.

A: In chronic malnutrition the woman is undernourished before pregnancy and then does not gain weight (during pregnancy). In contrast, in gestational undernutrition she may have had a normal W/H ratio during the pre-pregnancy period but then fails to gain weight when pregnant. This means she did not have an adequate energy-protein intake (during gestation).

(Mal)Nutrition and the Infant Brain, pages 41–55
© 1990 Wiley-Liss, Inc.

NUTRIENT REQUIREMENTS OF THE PREMATURE INFANT

G. Harvey Anderson

Department of Nutritional Sciences, Faculty of Medicine, University of Toronto, Toronto, Ontario,Canada. M5S 1A8

In North America the largest group of newborn infants at risk of impaired neurological development is the premature. Of these, infants born at 1500 g body weight or less are of particular interest. During the 1920's to 1950's most low-birth-weight infants died, but in the 1960's and 1970's survival rates increased greatly so that now more than 85% of infants born within the weight range of 1000 to 1500 g survive.

Quality, in addition to quantity, of survival must also be considered. The majority of follow-up studies have shown that low-birth-weight infants are more likely than healthy, term infants to sustain sensorimotor and intellectually handicapping conditions. Some follow-up studies suggest morbidity rates have risen rather than fallen in recent years (Ross, 1983). However the role of diet in influencing clinical outcome remains uncertain (Lucas, 1987).

Much of the improved survival rate for low-birth-weight infants can be attributed to more aggressive and appropriate approaches to nutritional support. The support includes total parenteral nutrition, and use of milk feeds, preferably the infant's own mothers milk or of formula designed for the premature infant.

With the recognition that nutritional support was a strong determinant of survival came attempts to define the nutrient requirements of the premature infant, and to develop recommendations for the composition of parenteral and enteral feeds. Several recent reviews are available (American Academy of Pediatrics, Committee on Nutrition, (AAP-CON) 1985; Brooke, 1987; European Society of Paediatric Gastroenterology and Nutrition, Committee on Nutrition, (ESPGAN-CON) 1987; Galeano and Roy, 1985; Tsang, 1985; Whitelaw, 1986). An analysis of these reviews and the inconsistencies among them in their recommendations suggests that knowledge of the nutrient requirements of premature infants is much less complete then that required to ensure that the premature infant receives optimal nutrition.

The purpose of this review is to suggest that statements of the recommended nutrient intakes of the premature infant should be formulated through a systematic approach based on an understanding of the goals of recommended intakes. To do so I will discuss the general principles assumed in setting recommended nutrient intakes for healthy populations, the approaches taken in determining nutrient requirements of the premature infant, the current recommendations for advisable intakes, and the current enteral feeds recommended for the premature infant.

Recommended Nutrient Intakes: General Principles

The goal of defining nutrient requirements for all age and sex groups in the population is to derive a recommended intake of nutrients that is adequate to meet the requirements of the majority of individuals within a specific classification (Anderson et al., 1982; Beaton, 1988). The nutrient requirements for each individual are those which maintain optimal growth rates and tissue levels and physiological functions of each nutrient.

The recommended intake for a nutrient takes into account that there is a variability in nutrient requirements among individuals and is set at two standard deviations above the average need (Fig. 1). This, for most nutrients, is 120-130% of the estimated average requirement. Or, put another way, it is an overestimate of the nutrient requirements of the majority of individuals in the population. For energy, the estimated average requirement is described, because this is one component of food intake which is regulated by physiological control systems of the individual (Anderson, 1988). Clearly most individuals will eat to meet their energy requirements, but have no physiological mechanisms that helps them identify nutrient needs. The absence of such mechanisms is the reason that recommended intakes for nutrients must be set at a level that assures an adequate intake for those individuals with the highest requirements.

Based on the recommended intakes, diets can be constructed that meet the requirement, or the adequacy of dietary intakes can be assessed (Anderson et al., 1982; Beaton, 1988).

Nutrient requirements for humans beyond infancy are derived from a combination of experimental and epidemiological studies (Beaton, 1988). Experimental approaches to define nutrient requirements are generally short-term and include feeding the nutrient under question in amounts from deficient to excess with dependent measures including growth, nutrient balance, body stores, enzyme function, plasma and tissue concentrations and any other measure that is specifically reflective of the nutrient under study.

Epidemiologic data are useful in describing intakes of nutrients which are consistent with the maintenance of health in a population. Epidemiological data are used to check recommendations derived from experimental studies or in the absence of these data, may be used to provide an estimate of a safe level of intake at which nutrient deficiencies are unlikely to occur.

The most reliable estimates of nutrient requirements are probably for the young adult, for the simple reason that this age group is most likely to be available for experimental studies in university settings and presents the least difficulties in terms of ethics of experimentation. Requirement estimates for many other age groups are based on extrapolation from this age group.

For the healthy newborn infant the estimates of nutrient requirements have little support from experimental data because of the obvious inappropriateness of experimental studies on this age group. On the other hand estimates of requirements can be derived from the composition and volume of intake of human milk (Beaton, 1985). These estimates have been derived by adding a variability estimate of 30%, equivalent to two standard deviations of the mean, to the average nutrient intake, calculated from the average nutrient concentrations in milk and average volume of milk consumed. The composition of milk formula is based on the recommended intakes for the newborn infant. However, it should be noted that this approach leads to much higher nutrient intakes by infants fed milk formula instead of their own mother's milk.

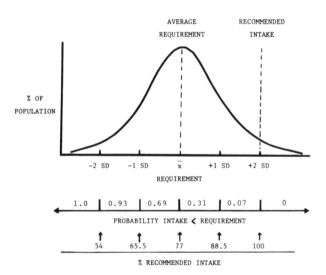

Fig. 1. Description of distribution of nutrient requirements and the probability of intakes being less than the individual's requirement within given intervals below the Recommended Daily Nutrient Intake (RDNI). It is assumed that the distribution of requirements is Gaussian in nature, and that the coefficient of variation is about 15%, Anderson et al., (1982). The RDNI, at plus two standard deviations of the mean, is above the actual requirement of 97.5% of the individuals in a population. For the individual, the risk of inadequate intake increases as intake falls below the RDNI, as shown by the probability of intake requirement. In developing recommended intakes it is very important to identify the mean requirement, and the variability in requirement among individuals. As well, it is important to specify the measure of requirement.

The implication of setting the recommended intakes for newborn infants at an intake level of the mean plus two standard deviations of the nutrient intake from human milk in turn leads to the illogical conclusion that most human milk won't meet the needs of newborn infants (Anderson, 1985). Considering that there is no evidence that human milk is nutrient inadequate, it seems likely that currently stated, recommended intakes for term infants are overestimates.

Estimated nutrient requirements of the low-birth-weight infant have not been based on the composition and intake of human milk primarily because many early studies in which pooled banked human milk was fed found it to be inadequate in energy and many nutrients. On the other hand, because they require extensive hospital care, they have been a captive audience for experimental studies.

Nutrient Requirements of the Premature Infant

The major determinants of requirements for energy and nutrients of infants are 1) maintenance of existing body tissues, a function of body size 2) the rate of deposition of new tissue, a function of growth rate and composition of tissue and 3) individual variability in requirement (Beaton, 1985).

An infant of 28 weeks gestation weighs approximately 1000 g. Of this 860 g is water, 10 g is fat and 88 g is protein and other nitrogen containing compounds. By contrast a term infant of 3500 g contains 2400 g water, 560 g fat and 387 g of protein and other nitrogen containing compounds. Clearly, without a source of energy and nutrients, the premature infant will survive for only a few days. Maintenance energy requirements, that needed for resting metabolism in a thermoneutral environment are met with 45-60 kcal/kg (Brooke, 1986). Protein requirements of the non-growing infant have been estimated to be 1.0 g/kg/day. Water and electrolyte requirements for maintenance are also known, because these are the first to be provided during any medical crisis. Premature infants are initially given a 10 per cent dextrose solution with electrolytes until the respiratory status of the infant is clear. Gastric feeds, preferably the baby's own mother's milk, are then started. If gastric feeds are not tolerated, total parenteral nutrition is initiated.

For nutrients other than water and electrolytes there is little basis for estimating a maintenance requirement. Furthermore it is unlikely that such data will be derived from experimental data because maintenance of the premature infant should not be the goal of nutritional support.

The greatest determinant of nutrient requirements of the premature infants is the requirement for growth. Growth of the fetus proceeds rapidly, with a linear velocity (gain in weight per unit of time) to approximately 34 weeks and then slows. This slowing of growth rate is primarily due to the decreased rate of deposition of water in lean body tissue, whereas deposition of fat and nitrogen proceeds on a linear velocity (Widdowson et al., 1988). From 28 weeks to 40 weeks of gestation the fetus increases it weight 3.5 fold, body fat 56 fold and body nitrogen by 4.5 fold, with an overall average tissue increment of 25-30 g/d. Based on analyses of the composition of fetuses estimates have been made for the total amount of water, fat, nitrogen, and minerals in the body of the developing fetus from 13 to 40 weeks of fetal age (Zeigler et al., 1981).

The goal of nutritional support for the premature infant has been the subject of some debate. However, the AAP-CON, 1985 has defined the optimal diet for the LBW infant as one that supports a rate of growth close to that of the third trimester of intrauterine life without imposing stress on the developing metabolic or excretory systems.

Estimates of the advisable or recommended energy and nutrient intakes of premature infants made by the AAP-CON (1985) have been strongly guided by the factorial approach to deriving requirements, an approach described by Zeigler et al (1976). This approach requires an identification of each of the components of the requirement. Information on these individual factors may be derived from several sets of experimental data and are seldom completely described within any one experiment. Estimates based on this approach are acknowledged to be imprecise, and not suitable for all nutrients. However, the approach has been useful for describing requirements for energy, protein, and many major minerals, including calcium, phosphorus, magnesium, sodium, potassium and chloride especially when these estimates can in turn be compared with experimental balance and growth data.

In the factorial approach the advisable intake is based on the sum of the maintenance requirement which is estimated from urine and dermal losses, the growth requirement which is estimated from tissue accretion rates based on analysis of autopsy materials, the intestinal absorption of food and nutrients based on experimental data and a 10% addition to allow for individual variability of requirements among infants. The addition of only 10% to the average requirement estimate is a conservative estimate of variability in requirements among infants. The coefficient of variation in requirements is more likely 15% but the rationale for the low estimate is based on concern for overloading the metabolic capacities of some infants if the full variability in requirement among infants was recognized (Zeigler et al, 1981).

Recommended or Advisable Nutrient Intakes

In this present examination of recommended intakes for premature infants several assumptions have been made. It assumed that the infant was born at 28-29 weeks of gestational age, is now 3-4 weeks of age and in a stable condition in a thermoneutral environment and presently weighs approximately 1200 to 1300 g and has a potential growth rate of 20-30 g/day. The reason for making these assumptions is to bring a focus to the presentation.

There is no doubt that recommended nutrient intakes need to be defined for the management of the newly born low-birth-weight infant. However a definition of the nutrient intakes required to support the initial and stable phases of development should logically be approached as separate issues. The focus of this discussion is on the stable (at least relatively so) phase of development.

In the tables that follow the recommended intakes of three groups are shown for each of the nutrients, and are contrasted with the average composition of milk derived from mothers giving birth prematurely and after four weeks of lactation (Anderson, 1985), and with the range in composition of three formulas (Enfamil Premature, SMA Preemie, Similac Special Care) designed for feeding low-birth-weight infants (Galeano and Roy, 1985; AAP-CON, 1985). Ranges in the summaries of recommendation for nutrient intakes are illustrated by taking data from a report arising from a workshop on the vitamins and mineral requirements in preterm infants edited by Tsang (1985), and from the AAP-CON, (1985), and from the ESPGAN-CON, 1987. The latter report has been published in full (Wharton, 1987) and in summary (ESPGAN-CON, 1987). Other reviews on the subject (e.g. Brooke, 1987, Galeano and Roy, 1985, Whitelaw, 1986) are not utilized because these reviews usually reflect the authors' summary of previous committee recommendations or a focus on a few selected nutrients or aspects of feeding the premature infant.

For comparative purposes the data are uniformly expressed in units per 100 kcal because the nutrient content of human milk and formula is usually expressed on a volume or energy basis. A conversion of all numbers as intake or requirement per kilogram of body weight can be easily made. Based on the recommended energy intake of 120 or 130 kcal/kg body weight all numbers in the table, if multiplied by 1.2 or 1.3, would reflect requirement or intake on a body weight basis.

Numbers for presentation in the tables were obtained by utilizing the lowest nutrient intake advised within each report. Often a range was presented, but in principle this is an inappropriate approach to stating a recommended intake. If the lowest intake specified is accurate and has any merit in being stated it must be assumed that the intent of the recommended intake is that it will provide for the requirement of the majority of premature infants. The higher level in the recommendation of a safe range of intake would logically be that level which does not present a danger of excess. However the purpose of stating a range is not explicitly clear with respect to its intended interpretation (e.g. Tsang, 1985).

Energy Requirements

Energy requirements have been derived from the sum of expenditures for maintenance of basal metabolic rate, activity, response to cold stress, specific dynamic action of food, fecal loss and for growth (AAP-CON, 1985; Brooke, 1986). A average of 120 (AAP-CON, 1985) or 130 (ESPGAN-CON, 1987) kcal/kg/d is recommended as this amount allows most infants in a carefully maintained thermoneutral environment to achieve satisfactory rates of growth of between 15-20 g per day. Greater energy input does not appear to lead to increments in lean body mass but rather, to large increments in fat deposition, well above the 14% of total weight gain which occurs *in utero* (Putet et al., 1987).

Macronutrients: Recommended Intakes vs Human Milk and Formula

The recommended intake for protein based on the factorial approach as calculated by Zeigler et al (1981) is 3.1 and 2.7 g/100 kcal for the 800-1200 g and 1200-800 g infant, respectively (AAP-CON, 1985) (Table 1). There is also good experimental evidence that protein intakes in this range provide in utero growth rates with energy intakes of 120-130 kcal/kg (e.g. 3.5 g protein/kg) (Zeigler, 1986). The ESPGAN-CON, (1987) makes a lower recommendation of 2.2 g/100 kcal for protein. Preterm human milk would provide less protein then the recommended intake of the AAP-CON (1985) whereas formulas designed for premature infants approximate the recommended intake.

There is no known requirement *per se* for either fat or carbohydrate, other than the amount required to provide essential fatty acids and prevent hypoglycemia, respectively. The balance of these energy sources in human milk

TABLE 1. Macronutrients: Recommended Intakes vs Human Milk and Formula

	Recommended Intake[1]			
	AAP	ESPGAN	Preterm Milk[2]	Formula[3]
(g/100 kcal)				
Protein	3.1	2.2	2.2	2.6- 3.0
Fat	6.0	3.6- 7.0	6.3	5.0- 5.4
Carbohydrate	8.0	7 -14	8.7	10.6-10.9

[1] AAP-CON, (1985) recommended energy intake is 120-130 kcal/kg; ESPGAN (1987) recommended energy intake is 130 kcal/kg; data expressed per 100 kcal.

[2] Average composition, Anderson (1985).

[3] Enfamil Premature, SMA "Preemie", Similac Special Care, AAP-CON (1985).

guides the recommendation for the total amount of fat and carbohydrate recommended and in infant formulas (Table 1). Human milk is high in fat, over 50% of the energy, and contains 35% of the energy as carbohydrate. Recently developed special formulas contain fat in the form of medium chain triglycerides and predominantly polyunsaturated fatty acids to enhance lipid digestion. The carbohydrate source is provided by both lactose and glucose polymers, again as a result of consideration of immaturity of the prematures gastrointestinal tract for lactose digestion to reduce osmotic load.

Macrominerals: Recommended Intakes vs Human Milk and Formula

Guided by the factorial approach to estimates made by Zeigler et al., (1981) and combined with some experimental data the various committees have made recommendations for sodium, chloride, potassium, calcium, phosphorus and magnesium (Table 2). In general there are considerable differences in recommendations among the committees.

Human milk and formula would meet the recommended intakes for sodium as proposed by Tsang (1985) but not by the AAP-CON (1985), or the ESPGAN-CON (1987).

Calcium and phosphorus accretion is very rapid in utero and human milk is very inadequate in these nutrients (Atkinson et al., 1983). Their concentrations in formula for prematures has been increased to amounts which are sufficient to achieve normal bone mineralization (Anonymous, 1989). Again there is considerable variation in the recommended intakes stated by the three committees.

Iron stores are very low in premature infants and supplements are recommended for the low-birth-weight infant who has achieved two months of age. Whether or not the range of 1.5 to 1.8 mg per 100 kcal meets or exceeds the requirement for iron is not well defined by the experimental data despite the fact that there is reasonable agreement among the committees on the recommendation (Table 2). Formula and human milk contain much less iron than the recommended intake.

TABLE 2. Minerals: Recommended Intakes vs Human Milk and Formula

Mineral (per 100kcal)	Tsang	AAP	ESPGAN	Preterm[2] Milk	Formula[3]
Sodium, mmol	0.8	2.7	1.0	1.7	1.7- 1.8
Chloride, mmol	1.0	2.4	1.3	1.9	1.8 - 2.3
Potassium, mmol	0.8	1.7	1.8	2.1	2.3 - 3.2
Calcium, mg	150	160	70	40	92 - 177
Phosphorus, mg	87	108	50	21	49 - 89
Magnesium, mg	4.2	7.5	6.0	4.9	8.6 - 12
Iron, mg	1.3	1.7	1.5	0.12	0.16 - 0.37
Zinc, μg	615	500	550	560	615 - 1480
Manganese, μg	8.0	5.0	2.1	(0.5)	4.0 - 30
Copper, μg	77	90	90	90	86 - 246
Iodine, μg	3.0	5.0	10	(25)	7.0 - 18
Molybdenum, μg	1.5	?	?	(0.3)	?
Selenium, μg	1.2	?	?	(2.4)	?
Chromium, μg	1.5	?	?	(0.04)	?

Recommended Intake[1]

[1] Tsang (1985), p VII, assuming energy intake of 130 kcal/kg AAP-CON (1985), as stated for 800-1200 g infant ESPGAN-CON (1987), Wharton (1987) as stated guidelines for formula composition.
[2] Anderson (1985). Those numbers in ( ) are from Beaton (1985) and are values for term milk.
[3] Enfamil Premature, SMA "Preemie", Similac Special Care, taken from AAP-CON (1985).

Recommended intakes made by Tsang (1985) for zinc and manganese are uniformly higher than those recommended by the AAP-CON (1985) and the ESPGAN-CON (1987). Preterm milk would not meet the recommended intake, but formulas would. Recommended copper intakes would be met by both formula and preterm milk.

Estimates of the premature's need for iodine, molybdenum, selenium and chromium cannot be made with confidence at the present time, although estimates were reported by Tsang (1985). There is also uncertainty with respect to the amount of most of these nutrients in formula, or human milk.

Vitamins: Recommended Intakes vs Human Milk and Formula

There is little agreement among the committees in the recommended intakes for the fat soluble vitamins (Table 3). In general the recommended intakes are not provided by human milk, nor are they provided uniformly by specially designed formulas.

Recommended intakes for the water soluble vitamins vary greatly among the three committees. Preterm human milk would be inadequate to provide the recommended intakes. Special formulas are more likely to provide the recommended intakes, although not consistently.

Feeding of the Premature Infant.

Based on the foregoing, it is clear that human milk does not provide most nutrients in amounts to meet the recommended intakes and that formulas would fail to do so in some instances. The lack of confidence that the recommended intakes reflect requirements of the premature infant is evident from the fact that these same committees recommend human milk or formula as preferred feeds for the premature infant and this seems to be the practise (Churella et al., 1985). It is generally recommended that preterm milk is the preferred enteral feed if supplements are provided to correct for hyponatremia, if it occurs, and to provide calcium and phosphorus. This recommendation is rationalized by the evidence that human milk has a number of positive factors including anti-infective properties and easy digestibility. Furthermore there is a general lack of evidence that it is grossly deficient in the majority of nutrients as would be implied from the recommended intakes.

In the late 1970's considerable interest in feeding the premature infants own mother's milk was stimulated by a report that preterm milk might have some unique nutritional advantages over term milk (Atkinson et al., 1978). Early preterm milk from mothers giving birth at 26-31 weeks is higher in protein and fat and lower in lactose then term milk (Anderson et al., 1981) although these advantages have not been demonstrated for milk from mothers giving birth after 32 weeks (Lepage et al, 1984). However preterm milk has been found inadequate in calcium and phosphorus (Atkinson et al., 1983) and the trace elements zinc and iron (Mendelson et al., 1983). As well, it can be of highly variable composition, perhaps because it must be expressed under unusual and stressful circumstances. Thus it is clear that preterm milk cannot be safely relied

TABLE 3. Vitamin: Recommended Intakes vs Human Milk and Formula

Vitamin (per 100kcal)	Recommended Intake[1]			Preterm[2] Milk	Formula[3]
	Tsang	AAP	ESPGAN		
A, (RE) μg	320	420	90	200	94 - 203
D, IU	310	400	160	?	62 - 120
E, mg	4.0	0.5	0.6	1.1	2.0 - 4.0
K, μg	4.0	?	4.0	?	9.0 - 12
Ascorbic Acid, (mg)	30	27	7.5	6.0	9.0 - 37
Thiamine, μg	250	230	20	13	77 - 247
Riboflavin, μg	335	307	60	38	91 - 617
Niacin, mg	4.0	4.6	0.8	0.3	0.8 - 4.9
Pyridoxine, μg	250	230	35	9.0	62 - 247
B_{12}, μg	0.15	0.4	0.15	0.03	0.25 - 0.56
Folic Acid, μg	15	40	60	4.0	12- 36
Pantothenic Acid, μg	800	1540	300	32	?
Biotin, μg	0.5	27	1.5	0.8	?

[1]Tsang (1985), p VII, assuming energy intake of 130 kcal/kg AAP-CON (1985), as stated for 800-1200 g infant ESPGAN-CON (1987), Wharton (1987) as stated guidelines for formula composition.
[2]Anderson (1985). Those numbers in ( ) are from Beaton (1985) and are values for term milk.
[3]Enfamil Premature, SMA "Preemie", Similac Special Care, taken from AAP-CON (1985).

upon to meet the nutrient needs of the majority of preterm infants. The development of fortification mixtures to add to preterm human milk allows the safe use of preterm milk to achieve nutrient balance goals and at the same time provide the non-nutrient benefits of human milk (Ehrenkranz et al., 1989).

Formulas for premature infants have an advantage in that they can be designed in accordance with the specific physiological needs of the preterm infant. However their composition is heavily dependent on the interpretation of experimental data relating to nutrient requirements of preterm infants. The weakness of experimental data and the lack of consistency among reports in which statement of recommended intakes are made, make it unlikely that formulas provide very closely the premature infant's requirements for several nutrients.

DISCUSSION

Based on this review it can be suggested that the recommended nutrient intakes for the infant who is 1200 g, 3-4 weeks old, in a stable medical condition and born at 28-29 weeks gestation do not reflect very closely the true requirements of the infant.

The recommended intakes for the macronutrients and the macrominerals may be within ±30% of the true requirement of the premature infant. In contrast, one can have very little confidence in the recommended intakes for trace elements and water soluble vitamins. It is possible that they are several factors, up to 10X too low or too high, more likely the latter, in relation to true requirements. This leads to uncertainty as to whether or not intakes, as derived from formula, are within a safe range. The recommended intake of fat soluble vitamins may be somewhat closer to that required, but again may not be within several factors of the true requirement.

The large variations in recommended intakes set by the committees cited herein are difficult to explain except on the basis of inconsistency in understanding the goal of setting the recommended intakes and their relationship to requirements. For example the goal of the ESPGAN-CON (1987) appears to have been to provide estimates that would serve as a basis for the composition of formula. However it is very uncertain as to whether the goal was to provide excesses for most nutrients in relation to the requirements of most premature infants, or if they were to reflect or approximate requirements. The AAP-CON (1985) clearly set a goal of defining requirements based on the systematic approach advocated by Zeigler et al (1981) and of extending these estimates to recommended intakes. However the approach was used for some nutrients and not for others, and there is no explanation for this. Finally, the group assembled by Tsang (1985) arrived at a consensus for the recommended intakes but the purpose of the numbers which appear in the summary table is not described.

It is clear then that there is a need for careful committee review of the recommended nutrient intakes of premature infants. In undertaking such a review it would be helpful if the committee defined a clear goal for the outcome of its deliberations and developed a systematic approach to evaluating the existing literature. The committee should be instructed to define nutrient requirements and should have a clear understanding of the need to determine from the literature average requirements and the variations of requirements among prematures in order to set a recommended intake adequate for the majority of prematures. Attempts should be made to define safe ranges of intake, and if the requirement can not be stated with confidence than at least a safe range of intake should be stated. If the data are inadequate to define a recommended intake, this should be clearly stated. Of course there must be a definition of the age, size and state of development of the infant for which the requirements are being derived.

One aspect of the developing infant that requires considerable thought by committees setting recommended nutrient intakes is the relationship between the nutrient composition of enteral and parenteral feeds and the requirements of the central nervous system. The brain, which is 12-14% of body weight, is growing very rapidly in the premature infant, and *in utero* would average a weight gain of 2.5 g/day. It is well accepted that the brain has a high energy requirement, approximating 50% of the resting energy expenditure, and that these energy needs must be met. Less attention, however, has been given to the nutrient needs of the brain for the development of *in utero* composition. This may be an important consideration in the prevention of neurological deficits.

While it can be easily recognized that premature infants are much better fed now then twenty years ago it remains possible that nutrient imbalances, especially excesses of trace elements and the water soluble vitamins could affect neuronal development. In addition, the brain may have a unique requirement for nutrients that are not needed for the normal growth and development of peripheral tissues. For example in the last trimester the fetal brain rapidly accumulates long chain polyenoic fatty acids (Clandinin and Chappell, 1985; Heim, 1985). These fatty acids are provided in human milk, but not in formula. Whether or not the presence of polyenoic fatty acids in the central nervous system of term infants at birth and in human milk indicates a requirement, or is simply the result of maternal diet and metabolism remains to be established. Nevertheless data relating to nutrient requirements of the central nervous system require careful review and incorporation into statements of the recommended nutrient intakes for the premature infant.

Finally, it would be most helpful if committees would identify research needed to allow a systematic development of safe and complete recommended nutrient intakes for the premature.

REFERENCES

American Academy of Pediatrics, Committee on Nutrition (1985). Nutritional needs for low-birth-weight infants. Pediatrics 75:976-986.

Anderson GH (1988). Metabolic regulation of food intake. In Shils ME, Young VR (eds): "Modern Nutrition in Health and Disease", Philadelphia: Lea and Febiger pp 557-569.

Anderson GH (1985). Human milk feeding. In Pencharz PB (ed): "The Pediatric Clinics of North America, Vol 32, No. 2," Philadelphia: Saunders, pp 335-353.

Anderson GH, Peterson RD, Beaton GH (1982). Estimating nutrient deficiencies in a population from dietary records: the use of probability analyses. Nutr Res 2:409- 415.

Anderson GH, Atkinson SA, Bryan MH (1981). Energy and macro-nutrient content of human milk during early lactation from mothers giving birth prematurely and at term. Am J Clin Nutr 34:258-265.

Anonymous (1989). Optimal mineral intakes by very-low-birth-weight infants. Nutr Rev 47:73-75.

Atkinson SA, Radde IC, Anderson GH (1983). Macromineral balances in premature infants fed their own mother's milk or formula. J Pediatr 102:99-106.

Atkinson SA, Bryan MH, Anderson GH (1978). Human milk: Differences in nitrogen concentration in milk from mothers of term and preterm infants. J Pediatr 93:67-69.

Beaton GH (1988). Criteria of an adequate diet. In Shils ME, Young VR (eds): "Modern Nutrition in Health and Disease" Philadelphia: Lea and Febiger, pp 649-665.

Beaton GH (1985). Nutritional needs during the first year of life. Some concepts and perspectives. In Pencharz PB (ed): "The Pediatric Clinics of North America, Vol 32, No. 2," Philadelphia: Saunders, pp 275-288.

Brooke OG (1987). Nutritional requirements of low and very low birthweight infants. In Olson RE, Beutler E, Broquist HP (eds): "Annual Reviews of Nutrition, Volume 7," Palo Alto, California: Annual Reviews Inc., pp 91-116.

Brooke OG (1986). Energy needs in infancy. In Fomon SJ, Heird WE (eds): "Energy and Protein Needs during Infancy," Orlando, Florida: Academic Press, Inc, pp 3-17.

Churella HR, Bachhuber WL, MacLean WC Jr (1985). Survey: Methods of feeding low-birth-weight infants. Pediatrics 76:243-249.

Clandinin MT, Chappell JE (1985). Long chain polyenoic essential fatty acids in human milk: are they of benefit to the newborn? In Schaub J (ed): "Composition and Physological Properties of Human Milk," New York: Elsevier Science Publishers, pp 213-222.

Ehrenkranz RA, Gettner PA, Nelli CM (1989). Nutrient balance studies in premature infants fed premature formula or fortified preterm human milk. J Pediatr Gastroenterol Nutr 8:58-67.

European Society of Pediatric Gastroenterology and Nutrition, Committee on Nutrition (1987). Nutrition and Feeding of preterm infants. ACTA Paediatr Scand, Suppl 336:3-14.

Galeano NF, Roy CC (1985). Feeding of the premature infant. In Lifshitz F (ed): "Nutrition for Special Needs in Infancy." New York: Marcel Dekker Inc, pp 213-228.

Heim T (1985). How to meet the lipid requirements of the premature infant. In Pencharz PB (ed): "The Pediatric Clinics of North America, Vol. 32, No. 2," Philadelphia: Saunders, pp 289-317.

Lepage G, Collet S, Bougle D, Kein LC, Lepage D, Dallaire L, Darling P, Roy CC (1984). The composition of preterm milk in relation to the degree of prematurity. Am J Clin Nutr 40:1042-1049.

Lucas A (1987). Does diet in preterm infants influence clinical outcome? Biol Neonate 52: Suppl 1, 141-146.

Mendelson RA, Bryan MH, Anderson GH (1983). Trace mineral balances in preterm infants fed their own mother's milk. 3 J Pediatr Gastroenterol Nutr 2:256-261.

Putet G, Senterre J, Ringo J, Salle B (1987). Energy balance and composition of body weight. Biol Neonate 52: Suppl 1, 17-24.

Ross G (1983). Mortality and morbidity in very low birthweight infants. Pediatric Annals 12:32-44.

Tsang RC (1985). "Vitamin and Mineral Requirements in Preterm Infants." New York: Marcel Dekker, Inc, pp v-vii.

Wharton, BA (1987). Nutrition and feeding of preterm infants: Blackwell Scientific Publications

Whitelaw A (1986). Feeding the very-low-birthweight infant.. Hum Nutr: Appl Nutr 40A: Suppl 1, 19-26.

Widdowson EM, Southgate DAT, Hey E (1988). Fetal growth and body composition. In Lindblad BS (Ed): "Perinatal Nutrition," San Diego: Academic Press, pp 3-14.

Zeigler EE (1986). Protein requirements of preterm infants. In Fomon SJ, Heird WE (eds): "Energy and Protein Needs During Infancy," Orlando, Florida: Academic Press, Inc., pp 69-85.

Ziegler EE, Biga RL, Fomon SJ (1981). Nutritional requirements of the premature infant. In Suskind RM (ed): "Textbook of Pediatric Nutrition," New York: Raven Press, pp 29-39.

Ziegler EE, O'Donnell AM, Nelson SE, Fomon SJ (1976). Body composition of the Reference Fetus. Growth 40:329-341.

DISCUSSION

Q (Harper): What are the principles for estimating the requirements of the premature infant. What, for example, is the estimation of the efficiency of fetal utilization of the ingested material. Is there any information about survival.

A: There is a little bit, for example, in terms of energy. If you raise energy intake much above 120-130 cal/Kg, the efficiency of utilization, certainly of the protein, tends to decrease. The problem is that you no longer get the normal distribution that you would get in fetal growth: 15% gain of protein mass and 15% of adipose tissue gain. The adipose gain under these circumstances increases tremendously. So there is that factor.

  Also, there are lots of metabolic problems in terms of efficiency of utilization: For example, lactose is not a preferred carbohydrate, and is utilized in relatively only small amounts by premature infants from the milk formulas, because they have problems absorbing and utilizing that form of energy. Same thing with fat. There are a number of such considerations which makes estimating individual requirements a problem. When, (even though premature) an infant is born at 2000 g or more, you will not be dealing with so many of these immaturity factors. Also, infants vary tremendously in their ability to catabolize and convert, for example, methionine to cystein in terms of liver enzyme activity. How do you account for all these (individual) variables?

  I don't think that the committees, in making recommendations, have tried to wrestle in any detail or systematic manner with these issues.

Q (S. Hashim): Could one say that nutrient requirements of the premature infant represent in effect the sum total of (all the nutrients) it would have had if he had not been born premature? With other words, the mother supplies these nutrients on a 24 hr basis, whereas feeding of the infant after it has come into a terrestrial life, is interrupted. Do you think this has to be looked at.

A: That is an interesting concept. Of course, they are virtually fed continuously, every two hours or it is a continuous intravenous feed. I think the issue is - you are probably right - that we are still in a non-qualitative or quantitative stage (of knowledge) and so are not able to answer your question.

  My objection at this time is that the assumptions underlying some of the statements or recommendations are presented as being right in the absolute sense, and that is incorrect.

Q (van Gelder): Why, in estimating nutrient requirements, are you not going closer to the blood composition of the mother: This is where the food is coming from. To follow up on this, I don't understand why you look at amino acids in milk when the premature infant should get its nutrition at this time by trans-placental transfer from maternal blood.

A: I just answered that, although in an indirect way. If you look at milk or at fetal transfer of, e.g. vitamin E, you must consider flow problems or uptake problems. There are a lot of questions in terms of what is meant by "adequate". Vitamin E is just an example.

I had some very high recommendations for vitamin E intake, 25 mg/day; we only recommend 12-44 mg/day for an adult, for heaven's sake. The reason for that was because of the low plasma vitamin E levels in the premature. It turns out, after having fed these infants such very high doses of vitamin E for many years now, that the reason for the low plasma levels is because vitamin E is not transported in blood. The whole lipoprotein system is different in premature infants. So what you get actually is that vitamin E is deposited in red blood cells and other tissues. Is that good or bad? But that's where it has all been going. So I think that it is a complex issue.

Comment (Rassin): I think that we may be looking at the problem somewhat simplistically. Plasma amino acid patterns of the foetus are very different from anything you can achieve *ex-utero*. In fact, the foetus is functioning in a relatively anaerobic state of metabolism. And to achieve the kind of plasma amino acid patterns *ex-utero*, you would have to feed extremely abnormal proteins, or amino acids, probably also other nutrients.

Take that argument one step further. The foetus is in water and obtains its oxygen supply via the umbilical artery. The opposite is true for the infant *ex-utero*. That is a whole new being, one really has to think about this. You can't just treat the premature as if it is still living in the uterus. It has come out and that resulted in a lot of changes. It is now a terrestrial organism.

Q (S. Hashim): I can speak about fatty acids, which are quite different between the infant and the mother. But the question is - while the mother is supplying, the infant is not just storing; it is modifying it. I should hope that the amino acid composition is different, just as the fatty acid composition is.

The newborn premie has a fatty acid complement which is all solid fat. Oxidation of double bonds must occur, i.e. the infant must have modified the fatty acids, of course. It is not simple.

I think you are absolutely right Dr. Anderson. Your final comment?

A: I agree. You can see the point. My objection is that the committees which have made recommendations seem compelled to make these, despite the fact that there are on very soft grounds, experimental or logical. On the one hand they make these recommendations for advisable intake, on the other hand they are saying that the baby's own pre-term mother's milk is the preferable feed.

I am a little bit extreme in these statements, but I think, nevertheless, that there has to be a little more thought being given (to this issue). There should not be this compulsion to recommend intakes, for the sake of recommending. They should point out where there is an absence of data to make recommendations. That would be a more useful approach.

(Mal)Nutrition and the Infant Brain, pages 57–64

QUALITY OF HUMAN MILK VERSUS MILK FORMULAS: PROTEIN COMPOSITION

David K. Rassin

Department of Pediatrics, The University of Texas, Medical Branch at Galveston, Galveston, Texas 77550, USA

The amino acid requirements of most neonates are satisfied by proteins supplied either from the milk of the breastfeeding mother or formulas prepared from cow milk. Considerable effort has gone into the development of formulas for human infants that simulate human milk but a basic problem that remains to be solved is that the quality, or amino acid composition, of cow milk proteins is different from that of human milk. Both milks are composed of two classes of proteins, casein or acid precipitable proteins and whey or acid-soluble proteins. These classes of proteins consist of a number of different individual proteins, the pattern of which differs from species to species (Blanc, 1981).

The implication of the fact that milks from different species supply different proteins is that the infant does not receive the same relative amount of each amino acid when the source of milk protein is varied. This difference is of particular importance with respect to the functions of amino acids other than as protein precursors. In particular, the amino acids play an important role in central nervous system function as both neurotransmitters and as precursors of neurotransmitters. The influence of dietary variation on these important amino acid functions is one that is only beginning to be appreciated.

The present discussion will briefly review the protein and amino acid composition of human milk and formulas, the potential mechanisms by which variability in protein composition may influence the neonate, and some long-term outcome data to support the view that formula feeding and breastfeeding do indeed influence neurological outcome.

Milk Protein Composition

The major proteins found in human and cow's milk are similar in classification, whey or casein, but differ in individual composition. Cow milk casein proteins are primarily a_{s1}- with lesser contributions from ß- and Kcaseins, while human casein proteins are primarily ß- with some K- and no α_{s1}-caseins (Jenness, 1974). In like manner the major cow whey proteins are ß-lactoglobulin with a contribution from α-lactalbumin, while the major human whey proteins are α-lactalbumin with contributions from lactoferrin and IgA (Hambraeus, 1977). Other whey proteins, such as other immunoglobulins, contribute to this category in lesser amounts.

The variability in quality of protein (different types of protein with varying amino acid compositions) is accompanied by a variability in the quantity of protein. Cows milk contains about 3.3 g of protein per dl while human milk contains about 1.0 g of protein per dl (Hambraeus, 1977). Compounding this difference is the much larger pool of nonprotein nitrogen found in human milk (23% of the pool of nitrogen) compared to that found in cow's milk (5%) (Lonnerdal et al., 1975). Formulas prepared from cow's milk normally contain 1.5g of protein per dl, an amount less than that found in whole milk but more than that found in human milk. When protein intakes have been calculated in healthy term infants of about three months of age it has been found that formula fed infants consume about 2.25g per kg body weight per day of protein while human milk fed infants consume about 1.65g per kg per day (Rassin et al., 1989).

Typical formula preparations available for human infants consist of cow's milk proteins present in either the usual whey to casein ratio found in cow's milk (18:82%) or reformulated to a ratio more similar (but not the same as) human milk (60:40%). Human milk has a whey to casein ratio of approximately 70:30 (Hambraeus, 1977). Even the reformulated cow milk preparation (60:40) is still made up of cow milk whey and casein proteins, and so is different from human milk. These differences are expressed in the amino acid composition of these various preparations.

For the purposes of the following discussion only data for the large neutral class of amino acids will be presented. This group of amino acids is particularly important to the central nervous system because these amino acids compete with one another for a common active transport carrier at the blood brain barrier (Christensen, 1979), and because several of them serve in the central nervous system as precursors to neuroactive compounds (such as tyrosine for the catecholamines and tryptophan for serotonin).

Many of the remaining amino acids also have a variety of other functions in the body. For example the paucity of cysteine in cow's milk proteins (63% in whey protein predominant and 35% in casein protein predominant formula compared to equal amounts of human milk protein) may explain why so much formula protein is necessary to sustain adequate growth in neonates. Cysteine may be rate limiting for protein synthesis during early development (Snyderman et al., 1971). As can be seen (Table 1), formula proteins are relatively low in their content of tryptophan and higher for many other large neutral amino acids when compared to human milk (Rassin et al., 1977a). These differences are exacerbated when the amino acid composition is corrected for the actual intakes of the infants.

Table 1: Large Neutral Amino Acid Composition of Typical Term Infant
Formulas and Human Milk

Amino Acid	Human Milk	Formulas Whey	Casein	Formulas Whey	Casein
		(μmoles)		(%)	
Valine	932	1161	1093	219	205
Isoleucine	836	955	772	200	161
Leucine	1594	1779	1605	196	177
Threonine	796	1097	805	242	177
Methionine	214	304	241	248	198
Tryptophan	186	111	124	103	117
Phenylalanine	614	605	669	173	191
Tyrosine	652	559	677	150	182
Histidine	314	317	344	177	192
Cysteine	402	253	143	110	61

Amino acid composition for typical term infant formulas composed of either predominantly whey proteins at a 60:40 ratio (Whey) or casein proteins at an 18:82 ratio (Casein). The first three columns are presented as μmoles per 2 g of milk protein (μmoles) while the last two columns are presented as actual intake as a percent of intake from infants fed human milk (%).

Infant Responses

These human milk and formula amino acid patterns influence the plasma free amino acid pools of the infant in a manner generally reflective of the amino acid constituents of the proteins (Table 2). Most amino acids are increased in concentration in the plasma of such infants. Noticeable differences between the formulas are seen in the higher threonine observed in the whey- versus the casein-protein predominant formula, while the converse is true for tyrosine. Plasma threonine increases have been related to only marginal toxicity (decreased growth) in animals (Benevenga, 1974), however, increased plasma methionine and aromatic amino acids (Jarvenpaa et al., 1982) may be of more concern (Benevenga, 1974). Plasma threonine concentrations may be used as a biochemical marker for infants fed whey-protein predominant formulas while plasma tyrosine concentrations may serve the same purpose for infants fed casein-protein predominant formulas (Rassin, 1987).

Thus, the plasma amino acid pools that supply the precursors for transport across the blood brain barrier vary as a function of the type of feeding in the infant. The large neutral amino acids compete for a single carrier (Pardridge, 1977) which has been characterized by use of the "brain uptake index" technique of Oldendorf (1971). Using this technique the K_m and V_{max} for each amino acid has been determined in the rat (Pardridge, 1977, 1986) and a mathematical approach used to calculate a K_m apparent for each amino acid that reflects varying amounts of precursor amino acids for the carrier. The individual

Table 2: Large Neutral Amino Acid Concentrations in the Plasma of Term Infants

Amino Acid	Human Milk	Whey Formula	Casein Formula
Valine	202	255 (126)	321 (159)
Isoleucine	79	102 (129)	95 (120)
Leucine	156	172 (110)	175 (112)
Threonine	168	275 (164)	217 (129)
Methionine	42	51 (121)	49 (117)
Tryptophan	38	47 (124)	36 (95)
Phenylalanine	59	67 (114)	80 (136)
Tyrosine	109	98 (90)	142 (130)
Histidine	88	109 (124)	116 (132)
Cysteine	112	107 (96)	118 (105)

Data presented in μmoles per liter (% of human milk fed infants).

influx of each amino acid into the central nervous system reflecting current plasma amino acid concentrations of each amino acid in the group may then be calculated. The calculated rate of influx into the central nervous system is generally higher for the infants fed formulas with differences between the formulas reflecting the plasma concentrations of these amino acids.

Table 3: Calculated Influx of Large Neutral Amino Acids into the Central Nervous System in Infants Fed Human Milk and Formulas

Amino Acid	Human Milk	Whey Formula	Casein Formula
Valine	3.05	3.47 (114)	4.01 (131)
Isoleucine	2.69	3.14 (117)	2.73 (101)
Leucine	5.85	5.86 (100)	5.51 (94)
Threonine	1.68	2.45 (146)	1.83 (109)
Methionine	1.44	1.59 (110)	1.43 (99)
Tryptophan	1.87	1.71 (91)	1.59 (85)
Phenylalanine	2.77	2.86 (103)	3.13 (113)
Tyrosine	5.68	4.76 (84)	6.18 (109)
Histidine	2.35	2.28 (97)	2.32 (99)

Calculated influx into the central nervous system expressed as $\mu mol \cdot min^{-1} \cdot g^{-1}$ (percent of the rate for human milk fed infants).

As can be seen (Table 3) the increased plasma threonine in infants fed whey-protein predominant formulas results in a relative increased influx of threonine and a concomitant decrease in tryptophan (a serotonin precursor) and tyrosine (a catecholamine precursor). Conversely in infants fed a casein-protein predominant formula tyrosine and phenylalanine influx is increased and is accompanied by a decreased tryptophan influx. As both the rate limiting enzymes for serotonin synthesis from tryptophan (tryptophan hydroxylase) and catecholanine synthesis from tyrosine (tyrosine hydroxylase) are not saturated with respect to their precursors, changes in the substrate pool may influence the synthesis of these neurotransmitters (Lovenberg, et al., 1968; Gibson and Wurtman, 1978). Thus, changes in amino acid nutrition due to various types of protein intake influence plasma amino acid concentrations and have the potential to alter brain neurotransmitter synthesis.

Implications for the Brain

The overall health of infants fed human milk appears to be better than that compared to infants fed formulas (Report of the Task Force on the Assessment of the Scientific Evidence Relating to Infant Feeding Practices and Infant Health, 1984). Although there has been a great improvement in the health of bottle fed infants due to improvements in the composition of formulas (mortality is no longer obviously greater in this group, Grulee et al., 1934, 1935), there still appears to be significant morbidity associated with formula feeding (Cunningham 1977, 1979, 1981).

The consequences to the central nervous system of formula feeding versus breastfeeding are of particular concern. There is evidence that inappropriately high amounts of protein in infant formulas have adverse neurological consequences (Goldman et al., 1969). Behavioral differences have been noted in preterm infants receiving low amounts of protein (Tyson et al., 1983) or graded amounts of protein (Bhatia et al., 1986) as measured by the Neonatal Brazelton Assessment Scale. Infants that have high plasma tyrosine (especially preterm infants) which is often a consequence of being fed casein-protein predominant formulas (Rassin, et al., 1977b), have been noted to have some neurological dysfunction (Menkes et al., 1972; Mamunes et al., 1976).

The potential association of neurological outcome with changes in the diet and plasma of specific amino acids that compete at the blood brain barrier are strengthened by studies of tryptophan and valine supplementation. Supplementation of infant formulas with tryptophan (a precursor of serotonin which may be the neurotransmitter responsible for sleep regulation) enhanced sleep behavior in infants (Yogman and Feisel, 1983). In contrast, addition of valine (a competitor for transport at the blood-brain barrier with tryptophan) reduced sleep behavior (Yogman and Feisel, 1983). These latter studies provide direct evidence for the role of amino acid nutrients in behavior changes in the infant.

There is little direct evidence for analogous long-term effects of amino acids on behavior outside the devastating changes observed in patients with inherited metabolic diseases of amino acid metabolism. However, there is data that supports a beneficial role for breastfeeding on long-term intellectual outcome. Slightly better verbal and mathematical scores have been observed in intelligence tests done in eight and fifteen year old children who were breastfed compared to those who were formula fed (Rodgers, 1978). Intelligence and language development were rated to be slightly better in seven year olds who were breastfed compared to those who were formula fed (Fergusson, 1982).

In conclusion, there are observable biochemical differences observed in infants who are breastfed versus those who are formula fed. The mechanisms for translating these biochemical differences into differences in neurological outcome are in place. Evidence exists that supports the contention that neurologic development is better in breastfed than formula fed infants. Thus, there is a strong need to develop programs that support improved breastfeeding behavior in the interests of ensuring optimal neurologic outcome in children.

REFERENCES

Benevenga NJ (1974). Toxicities of methionine and other amino acids. Agricultural and Food Chem 22:2-9.

Bhatia J, Cerreto MC, Rassin, DK, et al (1986). Behavioral differences in ow-birth-weight infants fed formulas with differing protein concentrations. Pediatric Research 20:159A.

Blanc B (1981). Biochemical aspects of human milk - Comparison with bovine milk. Wld Rev Nutr Diet 36:1-89.

Christensen HN (1979). Exploiting amino acid structure to learn about membrane transport. Adv Enzymol 49:41-101.

Cunningham AS (1977). Morbidity in breast-fed and artificially-fed infants. J Pediatr 90:726-729.

Cunningham AS (1979). Morbidity in breast-fed and artificially-fed infants. II J Pediatr 95:685-689.

Cunningham AS (1981). Breast-feeding and morbidity in industrialized countries: An update. Adv Int Mat Child Health 1:128-168.

Fergusson DM, Beautrais AL, Silva PA (1982). Breast-feeding and cognitive development in the first seven years of life. Soc Sci Med 16:1705-1708.

Gibson CJ, Wurtman RJ (1987). Psysiological control of brain norepinephrine synthesis by brain tyrosine concentration. Life Sci 22:1399-1406.

Goldman HI, Freudenthal R, Holland B, et al. (1969). Clinical effects of two different levels of protein intake on low birth weight infants. J of Pediatrics 74:881-889.

Grulee CG, Sandford HN, Herron PH (1934). Breast and artificial feeding. Influence on morbidity and mortality of twenty thousand infants. J Am Med Assoc 103:735-739.

Grulee CG, Sandford HN, Schwartz H (1935). Breast and artificially-fed infants. A study of the age incidence in the morbidity and mortality in twenty thousand cases. J Am Med Assoc 10:1986-1988.

Hambraeus L (1977). Proprietary milk versus human breast milk in infant feeding: A critical appraisal from the nutritional point of view. Pediatric Clin/ N A 24:17-36.

Jarvenpaa AL, Rassin DK, Raiha NCR, et al. (1982). Milk protein quantity and quality in the term infant. II. Effects on acidic and neutral amino acids. Pediatrics 70:214-220.

Jenness R (1974). Biosynthesis and composition of milk. J Invest Dermatol 63:109-118.

Lonnerdal B, Forsum E, Hambraeus L (1976). A longitudinal study of the protein, nitrogen, and lactose contents of human milk from Swedish well-nourished mothers. Amer J Clin Nutr 29:1127-1133.

Lovenberg W, Jequier E, Sjoedsma A (1968). A trytophan hydroxylation in mammalian systems. Adv Pharmacol 6A:21-36.

Mamunes P, Prince PE, Thornton NH, et al. (1976). Intellectual deficits after transient tyrosinemia in the term neonate. Pediatrics 57:675-680.

Menkes JH, Welcher DW, Levi HS, et al. (1972). Relationship of elevated blood tyrosine to the ultimate intellectual performance of premature infants. Pediatrics 49:218-224.

Oldendorf WH (1971). Brain uptake of radiolabelled amino acids, amines, and hexoses after arterial injection. Am J Physiol 221:1629-1639.

Pardridge WM (1977). Regulation of amino acid availability to the brain, in Wurtman RJ, Wurtman JJ (eds): Nutrition and the Brain, Vol. 1. New York, Raven Press, pp 141-204.

Pardridge WM (1986). Effects of the dipeptide sweetener aspartame on the brain. In Wurtman RJ, Wurtman JJ (eds): Nutrition and the Brain, vol. 7. New York, Raven Press, pp 199-241.

Rassin DK (1987). Protein nutrition in the neonate: Assessment and implications for brain development, in Rassin DK, Haber B, Drujan B (eds): Basic and Clinical Aspects of Nutrition and Brain Development. New York, Liss, AR, pp 19-39.

Rassin DK, Gaull, GE, Heinonen K, et al. (1977a). Milk protein quantity and quality in low-birth-weight infants. II. Effects on selected essential and non-essential amino acids in plasma and urine. Pediatrics 59:41-50.

Rassin DK, Gaull GE, Raiha NCR, et al.(1977b). Milk protein quantity and quality in low-birth-weight infants. 4. Effects on tyrosine and phenylalanine in plasma and urine. J of Pediatrics 90:356-360.

Rassin DK, Raiha NCR, Minoli I, Mono G (1990). Taurine and cholesterol supplementation in the term infant: Responses of growth and metabolism. JPEN (in press).

Report of the Task Force on the Assessment of the Scientific Evidence Relating to Infant-Feeding Practices and Infant Health (1984). Pediatrics 74:576-762.

Snyderman SE (1971). The protein and amino acid requirements of the premature infant, in Jonxis JHP, Visser HKA, Troelstra JA (eds): Metabolic Processes in the Foetus and Newborn Infant. Stenfert Kroese pp 128-141.

DISCUSSION

Q (Diamond): When you examine neurological differences in the context of formula factors and breast feeding, do you (also) note the care given by the mother when she either gives the formula or the breast. It is easy to just prop the baby up with a bottle and leave him there. These (social) factors play a role in neurological development.

A: That is really a hard confounding variable. It was one reason why we went into the model where we are just looking at different amounts of proteins in formulas. It removes a lot of that variable from the (study) system. Because, if we could demonstrate behavioral differences in a known biochemical situation, without maternal interactions and other factors like that being a factor, we then would have a better foundation to go on to do the same comparisons in breast-fed and bottle-fed infants. There is no way that you can control completely for that (social factors), obviously.

There are investigators who try to do this. You can recruit moms who are feeding via feeding aids, where they give formula through an attachment so that the baby actually suckles at the breast, although the baby gets formula. But it is very difficult to recruit subjects into those kind of studies. Yes, it is a very difficult problem to deal with.

Q (Harper): When do you take the blood sample in relation to the time of feeding?

A: It is our practice to always take our blood sample 2.5 - 3.0 hrs postprandial. It is about as best as I think you can do in terms of a fasting sample in an infant and it gets you about as far away (as is practical) from the effects of the most recent feeding. Patterns of amino acid changes are certainly different depending on when the last feed was. But you seem to reach a fairly good plateau if you choose your sampling after that feeding time.

Q (Harper): That could influence your interpretation because the amino acid ratios can change during that time. At least in the animal studies, if you sample during the absorptive period, all amino acids tend to arrive together. When their levels fall, the branched chain amino acids, for example, fall much more slowly, and that produces a change in the ratio.

A: Well, what you really did not ask me but which is probably the more important question: when did I do my behavioral testing.

All these infants were on these three (different protein) preparations for two weeks, and then for three days they went on a standard formula preparation. So they then were all being fed the same preparation. The behavioural testing was done two hours after that period. Therefore, whatever the effect was, it is something that lasted longer than for just the most recent (the last) feeding period. This effect is something that persisted for several days after we discontinued the process (of protein modified formulas). To me that is the most exciting finding, that the data do not just reflect the most recent feed. The effects persisted and continued into a different feeding regimen which now was the same amongst all groups. The changes persisted longer than one might expect a (specific diet) to have an influence.

Q (Huether): I find this a very nice approach. But you did not show anything about how the (amino acid relative) ratios might change.

A: O.K., but I did show a slide of the influxes, which would be similar to the ratios.

Q (Huether): Can you say anything about the availability of tyrosine or threonine?

A: The tyrosine availability seems to be increasing and that of threonine decreasing. Phenylalanine availability is increased. I don't know about tryptophan.

Tryptophan is causing us problems in terms of analysis. I am very unhappy with the way you measure it by amino acid analysis. At the same time, getting sufficient sample from these infants to analyse tryptophan seperately has posed somewhat of a problem for us.

(Mal)Nutrition and the Infant Brain, pages 65–81
© 1990 Wiley-Liss, Inc.

KWASHIORKOR: BEHAVIORAL INDICES OF NEUROLOGICAL SEQUELAE

Wail A. Bengelloun

Unité de Neuroscience, Departement de Biologie, Faculté des Sciences, Université Mohamed V, BP 1014, Rabat, Morocco

INTRODUCTION AND PERSPECTIVE

Severe malnutrition in infants represents the extreme end of a range of clinical conditions associated with inadaquate nutrition. In the Third World, the extent to which this condition can be detected in a population serves as an indicator of the far more widespread presence of subclinical malnutrition, which often goes undiagnosed and unreported. Based on anthropometric and biochemical data, for example, between 30 and 50% of all Ugandan children suffer from some form of subclinical malnutrition (Winick, 1976). Indeed, chronic subclinical malnutrition of the mother has long been recognized as one of the main causes leading to severe malnutrition in infants (Smith, 1947; Habicht et al., 1974). It is thus evident that any attempt at eradicating severe malnutrition must address the general nutritional state of the community. The magnitude of this challenge is all the more important when placed within the context of a demographic explosion straining the Earth's resources, with a predicted planetary population of six billion in the year 2000. As the population grows, so does the need for a more rational application of technology to food production and a more equitable distribution of resources.

Clinically, severe infant malnutrition is generally classified as marasmus (insufficient caloric intake), kwashiorkor (protein deficiency), or as a combination of the two syndromes (protein-calorie malnutrition: PCM).In marasmus, the insufficient caloric intake is linked to a general decrease in all nutrients (starvation). This condition may lead to a normal (or even slightly elevated) protein/calorie ratio. The complex of clinical symptoms varies as a function of specific severe deficiencies within the syndrome. In general, marasmic children are characterized by low body weight, which may initially be masked by edema when associated also specifically with protein deficiency. In the more severe cases, growth may be completely arrested. At the same time a gradual loss of subcutaneous fat is observed, starting at the upper trunk and eventually affecting all parts of the body, leading to an emaciated and shrivelled aspect.

Kwashiorkor is a state of protein deficiency, with normal (occasionally elevated) overall caloric intake. It is one of the principal causes of infant mortality. Kwashiorkor is generally diagnosed in children after weaning and up to the age of 4 years. It is characterized by a slowing of growth and development, digestive problems, hypotonic muscles and hair changes. The child is subject to recurring infections.Children suffering from kwashiorkor are severely underweight, though edemas may initially mask this. Height is also retarded, but less severely than weight. The early onset of anorexia may lead to a state of combined protein-calorie malnutrition. Chronic diarrhea is often present, with frequent acute bouts linked to digestive tract infections. Hypothermia with shivering may be observed, and bacterial infections are usually unaccompanied by fever. The abdomen is inflated. Among the other classic symptoms of kwashiorkor are skin lesions and changes in hair texture and color. Hair becomes dry, brittle and easily uprooted. Because of the loss of pigmentation, African hair becomes reddish-blond color, or straw-yellow in the South American.A moderate anemia is frequent. Proteins are low, especially serum albumin levels (between 19 and 25 g/l, sometimes less). The ratio of non-essential to essential amino acids is increased, surpassing 2. There is also a hyperaminoaciduria present, characterized by an over abundance of taurine and beta-amino-isobutyric acid in the urine. Serum glucose and cholesterol levels are low, as are various serum enzymes: amylase, lipase, alkaline phosphatases, esterase, creatine phosphokinase. Edemas, the accumulation of extra-cellular water, start at the feet and progress upwards. There is also fat accumulation in the liver. In contrast to marasmus, the sum of these biochemical changes associated with kwashiorkor point to fundamental alterations in metabolism and regulatory functions. Behavioral consequences are also noted: an indifference to the environment (a general state of apathy) and a reduction of physical activity, occasionally interrupted by bouts of irritability and hostility.

The Incidence of Kwashiorkor

A systematic, statistically reliable study of the incidence of kwashiorkor in Morocco has yet to be undertaken. The problem however may be serious in view of the reported admission of 245 cases under the all-inclusive category of "protein-calorie" malnutrition (PCM) from 1980 to 1986 at the Children's Hospital in Rabat (Lahbabi, 1987). Of these, 56.3% were between the ages of 10 and 24 months, and 68% came from urban communities. It is to be noted that PCM cases represent between 2 and 3% of all pediatric admissions in Rabat (El Khaier, 1986), and that 40 to 50% of these cases over the past few years have been diagnosed as kwashiorkor (Khadri, 1987). These percentages probably understate the problem since in most instances diarrhea was the principal motive in seeking hospital care, and not any parental awareness of a nutritional problem. Moreover, the average hospital stay of these children was around 35 days, with no reported systematic follow-up care. There thus exists an urgent need for long-term follow-up projects, to assess the physiological and psychological sequelae of kwashiorkor, especially insofar as they influence learning and intellectual abilities. Developing brain and behavior are particularly vulnerable to modification by a variety of factors. Yet the mechanisms underlying this vulnerability remain to be elucidated. It is known that the reduced growth following protein deficiency is accompanied by lower average brain size (Platt, 1962), and by decreases in total proteins, RNA, cholesterol, phospholipids and DNA (Winick and Rosso, 1969; Rosso et al., 1970). When the protein deficiency is early in life, these effects of malnutrition may be irreversible. The slowed rate of DNA synthesis curtails cell division, reducing the number of cells. If malnutrition extends beyond about 8 months, cell size is also smaller. Thus both proliferative and hypertrophic growth may be hampered.

In rats it has been shown that when dietary protein is limited, there is reduced protein synthesis in brain cells due to the decrease in the availability of amino acids. Moreover, the available amino acids are preferentially converted to nucleotides, which are in turn preferentially incorporated into RNA. The result is an increase in RNA synthesis and a decrease in DNA synthesis after neonatal protein-calorie restriction (Miller, 1969). The rate of RNA degradation must however also increase since there is a net drop in the RNA/DNA ratio.

Social Factors and Kwashiorkor

Several attempts have been made to study the long-term effects of malnutrition on intellectual performance and learning ability in humans. In most cases, however, it has been difficult to separate the effects due to malnutrition per se from those caused by adverse socio-economic factors. Malnourished children generally come from low socio-economic strata with impoverished environments lacking most forms of stimulation, and this in and of itself may severely hamper subsequent learning capacity and behavior.Among the studies specifically concerning kwashiorkor, a classic report by Champakam et al. (1968) may be cited. It was conducted in India on children aged 8 to 11 years who had previously been hospitalized for kwashiorkor at ages ranging from 18 to 36 months. Controls were matched with each case according to a series of parameters: age, sex, religion, socio-educational background. Standardized tests showed that children who had suffered from kwashiorkor were more severely retarded in tasks requiring perceptual and abstracting ability than in those requiring memory or verbal functions, with the problems being most pronounced in children tested at 8 to 9 years of age rather than 10 to 11. Also affected were intersensory tasks. The authors point to an I.Q. difference of about 35 points lasting 6 or more years after recovery from kwashiorkor. Interestingly, although the body weights of previously malnourished children remained inferior to those of controls, their head circumferences were normal.

Another landmark study was reported by Cravioto and Robles (1965). Antecedent kwashiorkor was found to retard sensory integration independently of socio-economic background. In fact a positive correlation was reported between body size (height, weight) and performance.While these studies point to lasting kwashiorkor-induced problems in sensory-perceptual integration, the results should be viewed with some caution since potentially confounding factors such as infections and the degree of apathy during the bout of malnutrition remain difficult to assess and to quantify. Moreover, several studies have shown that environmental enrichment can improve the intellectual capacity of deprived children. In one such report (Skiels, 1966), institutionalized Korean children with an average I.Q. of 70 gained 28 I.Q. points one and a half years after being placed individually in the care of older female inmates, whereas those who remained under traditional institutional care lost 26 points. After two and a half years "adopted" children had an average I.Q. of 101. It is thus highly probable that environmental "enrichment" following exposure to malnutrition may moderate any long-lasting neuro-behavioral effects.

Animal Models

Because of ethical considerations, experimental research into the physiological and behavioral effects of malnutrition has used animal models. Winick and Nobel (1965) undernourished rats for 3 weeks at birth (18 pups suckling each dam), at weaning, or at 65 days of age (by allowing half the required caloric intake for normal growth). These three periods coincided roughly with the three general phases of organ growth: cellular hyperplasia (until weaning), hyperplasia and hypertrophy, and hypertrophy (after about 65 days). Body weight and organ weights were less than normal in all three groups of malnourished animals. Following refeeding, until 133 days, none of the animals undernourished at birth regained normal body or organ weight. In animals of the second group, undernourished for 3 weeks starting at weaning, refeeding to 133 days resulted in only the brain and lung regaining normal weight. In the group malnourished at 65 days, the body and all organs except the thymus regained normal weight. Similarly, whereas the protein content of all organs in the neonatal group failed to regain control levels after refeeding, normal levels were restored in the brain and lung of the weanling group, as well as in all organs (except the thymus) of the 65-day group. When DNA content (an index of cell number) of body organs was examined, the neonate undernourished group exhibited decreased levels both at the end of the dietary treatment and after refeeding. In the weanling undernourished group only the brain and lungs had normal levels of DNA both at the end of dietary restriction and after refeeding; levels were depressed in all other organs at both times of measurement. In animals undernourished at 65 days, only the thymus and spleen exhibited reduced levels of DNA.

The authors interpreted these results as indicating that the effects of malnutrition are irreversible only if they interfere with hyperplasia. Since the brain and lungs are the first organs to shift to hypertrophy, their differential recovery in the weanling group after refeeding is cited in support of this interpretation. With respect to the brain, three sequential developmental phases have been described by Altman et al. (1970): proliferation of the macroneurons (long-axoned nerve cells, differentiating largely prenatally), proliferation of the microneurons (short-axoned interneurons, differentiating largely from birth to weaning), and finally the differentiation of the neuroglia (serving myelination and support functions) during the early post-weaning period. They have suggested that the more severe effects of early malnutrition may be due to the greater disruption of subsequent differentiation of these cell types. Thus malnutrition at the time of weaning would only be expected to retard myelination.

In monkeys malnourished (2-3.5% protein in diet) at 120 days of age (one month after weaning), Geist et al. (1972) reported physiological effects within the first 30 days. These included reductions in serum albumin and total protein as well as suppression of weight gain. Five percent of their animals developed clinical signs characteristic of kwashiorkor: edema of the extremities and face, brittle and depigmented sparse hair, flakiness in skin, genital rashes, hypoalbuminemia and hypoproteinemia.The behavioral data from animals have tended to parallel and amplify those observed clinically in human children. Chamove (1980) reported that monkeys fed a low-protein diet between the ages of 1 and 7 months were less active than controls in tests of social interaction as well as those involving non-social exploratory behavior. When rehabilitated they tended to be more aggressive towards familiar than unfamiliar peers. This is in agreement with the decreased "behavioral curiosity" reported by Aakre et al. (1973) in monkeys fed a 2% protein diet. Additionally, protein-deficient monkeys have been shown capable of discriminating protein content in the diet during a choice situation, preferring the high protein pellets (Peregoy et al., 1972).

Wolf et al. (1986) have reported that rats severely malnourished (6% protein) up to weaning, nutritionally rehabilitated and thereafter, were hyperactive in a stabilimeter and in the early trials of an 8-arm radial maze. Their scores in terms of trials to criterion, however, and in a spatial alternation task were within normal limits. Moderately deprived rats (8% protein) were comparable to controls on all measures. These results are in agreement with the results of Hall (1983) who also failed to obtain a protein-malnutrition effect in the radial arm maze, and support the human data indicating the absence of a long-term effect on memory.Rats fed a tryptophan-poor corn diet exhibited decreased flinch and jump thresholds to electric shock through 14 weeks of testing (Lytle et al., 1975). A return to control thresholds was observed following dietary rehabilitation or systemic injections of tryptophan. Similarly, other reports have shown a sensory hyperreactivity to electric shock following exposure to a protein-deficient diet. Vendite et al. (1985) found that rats that had suckled from dams fed an 8% protein diet were hyperreactive to electric shock when tested at 90 to 120 days of age. The previous protein malnutrition also abolished the neurochemical changes (hypothalamic beta-endorphin release and amino acid incorporation into protein in brain structures) normally observed during footshock avoidance training. Interestingly, under these conditions memory (a retest 24 hours later) was also impaired by protein malnutrition. Within this context, Salbego and Souza (1986) also reported a decreased latency to escape footshock in rats that had been subjected to an 8% protein diet prior to weaning. The diet also resulted in decreased basal levels of phosphoryl-serine in brain nuclear proteins. Although performance in a shuttle avoidance task was normal, no further reduction in phosphoryl-serine was observed following training; controls do exhibit such a decrease during shuttle avoidance sessions. It may be suggested, based on these tentative results, that protein malnutrition in neonatal rats, as in humans, may have long-lasting differential effects on sensory processes.

Some investigators have suggested that the effects of early malnutrition and those of environmental restriction are mediated by common neural mechanisms (Sackett, 1968; Levitsky and Barnes, 1973; Zimmerman et al., 1974). Cordero et al. (1976) have reported data supporting such an hypothesis. Basilar dendrites of pyramidal cells in the occipital cortex of rats fed a low protein diet from weaning show a severe reduction in branching, reminiscent of that observed by Greenough and Volkmar (1973) with environmental restriction. Interestingly, Katz and Davies (1983) failed to find a significant interaction between undernutrition and environmental complexity on macroscopic brain parameters. To expand on these fundings and to further refine on an animal model of kwashiorkor, we established an experimental program, outlined below, with the purpose of determining the lasting behavioral effects of post-weaning protein malnutrition in rats. It was reasoned that behavioral and learning disruptions likely to be observed must ultimately reflect neural dysfunctions. It was also deemed of interest to establish the interactive effects of protein malnutrition and sex, a possibility that has received surprisingly little attention in the literature.

EXPERIMENTAL INVESTIGATION OF THE SEQUELAE OF KWASHIORKOR: AN ANIMAL MODEL

General Method

Animals in the present experiment were the offspring of albino dams of the Sprague-Dawley strain, housed in an air-conditioned animal room (21±1°C) with food (Purina rat chow) and water available ad-lib. Automatically cycling overhead lights were on 0700 to 1900 hours. At 1 day of age pups in each litter were sexed and weighed, and each litter was culled to 7 or 8 pups per dam. At 10 days of age maternal retrieval tests were conducted to determine whether any of the pups were being rejected by the mother, and therefore being malnourished. Weaning took place at 25 days of age.

At this time pups were tested in an open field, then housed 4 animals (of the same sex, from different litters) per standard maternity cage.Half of the animals were assigned to the normal (27%) protein diet, while the other half was maintained on a low (8%) protein diet (Table 1). Both diets were obtained from the Nutritional Biochemicals Corporation (Cleveland, Ohio).These dietary and housing conditions were maintained for 5 weeks (from weaning at 25 days until 60 days of age). The appropriate diet was presented daily in a glass food cup to each cage of 4 animals. Since both diets were of equivalent powdery consistency, wood blocks were available to all animals for gnawing.

At 60 days the rats were separated and housed individually in standard metal cages, the special diets were terminated, and free access to Purina rat chow (protein content: approximately 26%) and water was permitted. At this time open field and passive avoidance tests were conducted. Some of the animals were sacrificed for organ weights.For animals remaining in the experiment, a 7-week period of undisturbed recovery on Purina rat chow was then allowed, following which open field testing took place at 109 days of age in a third, different open field.

TABLE 1. Composition of Diets by Weight

LOW PROTEIN		HIGH PROTEIN
8%	Vitamin supplemented casein	27%
78%	Starch	59%
10%	Vegetable oil	10%
4%	Salt mixture U.S.P. XIV	4%

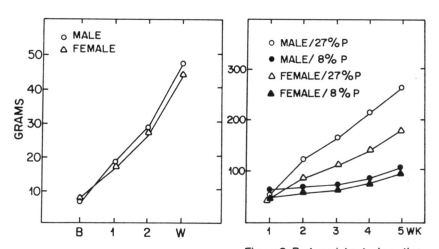

Figure 1. Body weight to weaning

Figure 2. Body weight during diet.

Between 150 and 240 days of age animals were tested on performance under a fixed ratio schedule of reinforcement and, two weeks later, on a second passive avoidance task. The first task required a food deprivation whereas the second a water deprivation. At 283 days of age, all animals remaining in the experiment were sacrificed and, as was the case for the group of animals sacrificed at the end of the dietary treatment (60 days), wet weights were obtained for brain, liver, spleen, adrenal glands, and gonads.

Morphological Results

Body weight:
Newborn pups were assigned to cages so as to equate mean body weights within sex. Up until weaning all animals rapidly gained weight and, by 25 days of age, males as a group tended to be heavier than females (Fig. 1). Figure 2 shows that the high protein (control) male and female groups continued their weight gain during the 5 weeks of post-weaning dietary regimen, with the normally observed difference in growth rate apparent throughout.

The malnourished groups of both sexes, however, exhibited depressed weights (slightly more than 1/3 of controls at 60 days in males, about 1/2 of controls in females), and depressed rates of growth. The low protein diet appears to have supported only a given rate of growth, irrespective of sex.By the fifth week of the diet, approximately 30% of malnourished animals (across sex) had developed kwashiorkor-like symptoms of skin lesions, patches of hair loss covering an area if 1 cm^2 or more and hair discoloration. Typically, the hair loss was first seen around the head and neck, and gradually receded posteriorly. Fig. 3 is a photograph of two female littermates at age 60 days, one maintained on the 27% protein control diet, the other on the 8% low-protein diet and exhibiting hair loss.During the dietary recovery period (60 to 283 days of age), male and female rats previously on the control diet continued to gain weight (Fig. 4) although the rate of weight gain was slowed by the 5th week post-diet. Malnourished animals gained weight at an accelerated rate until about the 5th week post-diet, then also slowed to control levels as they approached normal weight. By the 3rd week post-diet, previously malnourished animals had also started to exhibit a sex difference in body weight. By 32 weeks post-diet the only statistically significant effect is that of Sex ($p < 0.0005$).

Organ weights:
Absolute wet weights of the various organs were measured after sacrifice at the end of the dietary manipulation (60 days), and after recovery (283 days). The brain was separated from the brain stem at the foramen magnum; brain weight included the olfactory bulbs. Care was taken to remove excess fat from the other organs measured. Data was expressed as a ratio of organ weight to body weight.

Except for female gonads, organ weight to body weight ratios at 60 days were statistically greater in malnourished than in well-nourished animals (Table 2). This effect was particularly apparent for brain. After recovery (283 days) these differences tended to disappear (Table 3). Sex differences were obtained at both times of measurement such that adrenal ratios were higher in females whereas liver ratios were higher in males.

Behavioral Protocols and Results

Maternal retrieval test
The mother was removed from the cage when the pups were 10 days of age, and all pups were moved from the nest to the opposite end of the cage using forceps. The mother was then returned to the cage for a 5-minute observation

TABLE 2. Organ weight/Body weight ±SD at 60 days

Sex	Diet	n	$\dfrac{brain}{BW}\!\times\!10^3$	$\dfrac{adrenal}{BW}\!\times\!10^4$	$\dfrac{liver}{BW}\!\times\!10^3$	$\dfrac{spleen}{BW}\!\times\!10^3$	$\dfrac{gonad}{BW}\!\times\!10^3$
Male	27%P	5	7.06±0.17	1.98±0.18	41.00±1.09	2.71±0.71	11.41±1.09
Male	8%P	5	15.55±1.31	2.36±0.16	54.49±3.51	3.42±0.21	13.44±2.23
Female	27%P	3	8.72±0.20	2.50±0.24	34.42±0.90	2.78±0.17	0.43±0.09
Female	8%P	3	15.05±1.26	3.27±0.57	47.60±1.61	3.78±0.12	0.44±0.01

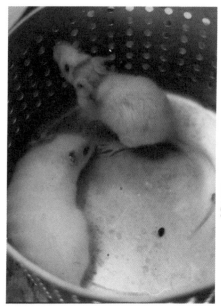

Fig. 3. Diminished body weight accompanied by hair loss in protein deficient female littermate at 60 days.

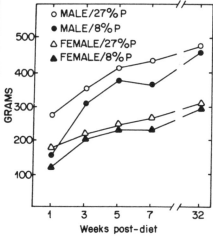

Figure 4. Body weight during recovery

TABLE 3. Organ weight / Body weight ± SD at 283 days

Sex	Diet	n	$\frac{brain}{BW}$x10^3	$\frac{adrenal}{BW}$x10^4	$\frac{liver}{BW}$x10^3	$\frac{spleen}{BW}$x10^3	$\frac{gonad}{BW}$x10^3
Male	27%P	7	4.22±0.14	1.38±0.13	34.49±1.76	2.09±0.38	7.46±0.44
Male	8%P	6	4.18±0.13	1.30±0.13	35.04±1.39	1.86±0.07	8.02±0.20
Female	27%P	5	6.12±0.22	2.25±0.21	29.25±0.88	2.16±0.16	0.47±0.03
Female	8%P	5	6.50±0.16	2.89±0.60	30.02±1.50	2.01±0.03	0.52±0.03

period. In all cases all pups were either retrieved by the mother or returned on their own during the 5 minutes, indicating the absence of rejection.

Open field test at 25 days:

Activity was measured in a 2-level open field. Each level was 30.5 x 30.5 cm, divided into 16 equal squares, with the upper level 30.5 cm above the lower level in step-wise fashion. A wire mesh ladder (5.0 cm wide) at a 45x angle provided access between levels. Measurements during a single 5-minute session consisted of: initial activity (number of crossings) on the lower level (where the session was started by placing the rat in the middle of the area), latency to first reaching the top level, activity on the top level after the first time up, total activity on each of the levels, the number of transitions between the two levels, and the amount of time spent with at least two paws on the ladder.

TABLE 4. Open field activity at weaning

	Lower level		Upper level		Total	Latency to 1st up (sec)	Transitions	Ladder time (sec)
	Initial	Total	Initial	Total				
Male (n=47)	53.23	75.23	6.74	11.38	86.20	183.36	2.09	49.00
Female (n=36)	63.95	74.84	9.26	13.34	88.18	223.50	1.16	47.39

As is traditionally the case in open field tests, females tended to be initially more active on both the lower and upper levels, although this sex difference disappeared in the total measure of activity at the end of the session (Table 4). Males ascended to the upper level earlier, but were comparable to females in terms of number of transitions between levels and in time spent on the ladder.

Open field at 60 days:
At the end of the dietary treatment animals were tested in a second, different open field 56 x 46 cm, divided into 4 quadrants. Attached to this larger compartment was a smaller, covered compartment (12.7 x 2.7 cm) painted flat black. Access to this smaller chamber was blocked during testing by a guillotine door. The animal was placed in the middle of the larger compartment, and activity (number of square crossing) was recorded during a single 5-minute session (illumination in the middle of the field: 1022 meter-candles). The field was placed on a table with the black compartment extending over the edge. Animals not sacrificed for organ weights following open field testing were tested on a passive avoidance task in this apparatus on the next day.

Protein malnutrition significantly increased activity in this test in both males and females ($p < 0.05$; Fig. 5). Additionally, malnutrition did not influence the sex difference in activity: females were generally more active than males ($p < 0.005$).

Passive avoidance at 61 days:
Animals were tested in the same apparatus as the previous day. The rat was placed in the black (dark) compartment with access to the larger open field compartment blocked off. Fifteen seconds later the trap door of the black compartment was opened, dropping the animal a distance of 75 cm to the floor of the testing room. The rat was then picked up and placed in the middle of the large compartment, with free access to the black compartment. Entries (if any) into the black compartment were recorded, and immediately punished by a drop through the trap door. The animal was then returned to the middle of the larger compartment. This test situation therefore served to assess passive avoidance performance in the absence of food or water deprivation, and without the use of electric shock.

Mean number of entries on this test for the different groups ranged from 0.80 ± 0.45 and 1.57 ± 1.62; there were thus no significant differences between groups in terms of passive avoidance performance.

Open field at 109 days:
After a 7-week recovery period on Purina rat chow, tests were conducted to determine the sequelae (if any) of early protein malnutrition. An open field test took place in a 59 x 59 cm apparatus whose floor was divided into nine equidimensional squares, illuminated at 538.2 meter-candles. The bulb was connected to a timer which, when activated, flashed the light at 0.5-second intervals. Each animal was tested in this field for 5 minutes: 2 minutes with the light on, 1 minute with the light flashing, then light on again for 2 minutes.

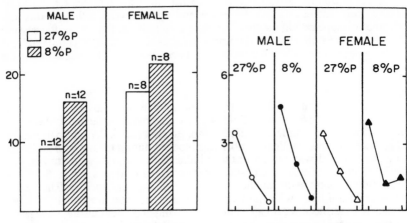

Figure 5. Open field activity at 60 days.

Figure 6. Open field at 109 days:
Activity during 3 periods

During each subinterval, activity (number of squares crossed), defecation and unsupported stand-ups were recorded.

From an initially comparable level of activity in the first interval, all groups tended to suppress activity in the flashing light period (Fig. 6). A further decrease in activity was noted in the third period in all but the female previously malnourished group. This Sex x Diet interaction was statistically significant ($p < 0.05$).

Fixed ratio testing after recovery:

Between 150 and 240 days of age animals were tested on performance under a fixed ratio schedule of reinforcement in fully automated Plexiglas chambers equipped with a bar-press lever activating a 45 mg Noyes pellet dispenser. Rats were food deprived and maintained at 80% of free-feeding body weight. Shaping was conducted on a CRF schedule in daily half-hour sessions until attainment of 60 reinforcements per one session. The day following attainment of the shaping criterion, fixed ratio (FR) testing began with daily 20-minute sessions per animal.

For the first 2 test days, reinforcement was on an FR-1 schedule to determine baseline. During the next 7 consecutive daily sessions, the behavioral output required for a single reinforcement was doubled each day, starting with an FR-1 schedule. Thus on the 7th day subjects needed to press the bar 64 times in order to obtain 1 reinforcement.

For all groups, the average number of reinforcements obtained during the test session decreased rapidly as a function of the increase in FR schedule (Fig 7). Previously well-nourished males obtained significantly more

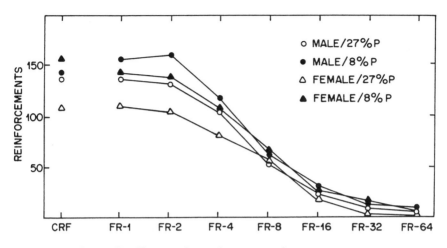

Figure 7. Fixed ratio performance after recovery

reinforcements than female counterparts up until an FR-4 schedule. Thereafter the 2 groups were comparable. A Sex x Diet interaction was also evident in the first 3 testing sessions: previously malnourished rats bar-pressed more than well-nourished ones, and the effect was particularly strong in females.

Passive avoidance after recovery:

Two weeks after completion of FR testing rats were tested on a passive avoidance task previously described in detail (Bengelloun et al., 1976). Briefly, footshock (1 ma for 1.5 seconds) was delivered to the 23.5-hour water-deprived rat each time it licked the water bottle spout in the test chamber during the daily 5-minute test sessions. Acquisition criterion was 2 consecutive days without initiating footshock.

Although they did not differ from controls in terms of number of shocks initiated on Day 1 of testing (Table 5), previously protein-deficient animals

TABLE 5. Passive avoidance performance after recovery

Sex	Diet	n	Shocks initiated		Days to criterion
			Day 1	Total	
Male	27%P	7	2.43 ±0.53	2.86 ± 0.69	3.71 ± 0.95
Male	8%P	6	2.17 ±0.75	3.00 ± 0.63	4.17 ± 0.98
Female	27%P	5	1.80±0.45	1.80 ±0.45	3.00 ± 0.00
Female	8%P	5	1.80 ±0.45	2.60 ±0.27	4.20 ±0.84

initiated a greater number of shocks across days, and therefore required more days to attain criterion (Table 5). This finding was especially pronounced in females.

DISCUSSION

Although protein malnutrition reduced growth to comparable levels in male and female rats, renutrition during a prolonged recovery period allowed these animals to eventually attain control values of body weight, thereby regaining the classic sex difference. Likewise, organ wet weight/body weight ratios reached control levels after renutrition. Our results are by and large in agreement with those reported previously by Winick and Nobel (1965) for animals underfed at weaning, and which were then allowed to recover.

The behavioral tests prior to weaning indicated a generally normal state of affairs; the maternal retrieval test suggested the absence of rejection, whereas the open field yielded the usually observed sex difference in activity. This was important to establish in view of the projected dietary manipulation and the subsequent behavioral tests.

At the end of the diet (60 days), protein malnutrition was found to result in increased levels of open field activity in both males and females. This is in line with previous reports of hyperactivity in the stabilimeter (e.g., Wolf et al., 1986). By 7 weeks after the dietary treatment any open field hyperactivity had disappeared, except perhaps in the previously malnourished female rats, who entered more squares during the final period of testing than any of the other groups.Although no passive avoidance deficit was noted immediately at the end of the dietary period, previously malnourished animals did require more days to attain criterion on a passive avoidance task when tested at the end of the recovery period. Here again, the previously malnourished females appeared to be differentially affected.

In line with the report of Vendite et al. (1985) the behavior of malnourished animals may reflect a memory deficit, since performance on the first day was unaffected. Alternatively, the possibility that these findings reflect an increased disruptive effects of hyperreactivity to electric shock (Vendite et al., 1985; Salbego and Souza, 1986), or even to water deprivation, cannot be ruled out. If this were indeed the case however, the behavioral disruption would be expected from the first day of testing.In the FR task, previously malnourished animals bar-pressed more than control counterparts, and initially obtained more reinforcements. This may be another manifestation of hyperactivity, or it may reflect an acute sensitivity to food deprivation and weight loss in view of their nutritional background. The fact that malnourished females were again more affected than males underlines the apparently differential behavioral vulnerability of females to protein malnutrition.

The present work is important in that it establishes an experimental animal model for kwashiorkor; our rats having exhibited several of the clinical symptoms of the syndrome. We show that when the onset of protein malnutrition begins at weaning, proper nutritional rehabilitation can cause gross morphological parameters to return to control values. Behaviorally, however, lasting effects are noted even after a prolonged recovery period, affecting activity levels and possibly memory and/or sensory reactivity. Perhaps most intriguing are our findings suggesting an increased and differential susceptibility of females to protein malnutrition.

REFERENCES

Aakre B, Strobel DA, Zimmermann RR, Geist CR (1973). Reactions to intrinsic and extrinsic reward in protein malnourished monkeys. Percept Motor Skills, 36:787-790.

Altman J, Das GD, Sudarshan K (1970). The influence of nutrition on neural and behavioral development: I. Critical review of some data on the growth of the body and the brain following dietary deprivation during gestation and lactation. Develop Psychobiol 3: 281.

Bengelloun WA, Burright RG, Donovick PJ (1976). Nutritional experience and spacing of shock opportunities alter the effects of septal lesions on passive avoidance acquisition by male rats. Physiol Behav 16: 583.

Chamove AS (1980). Dietary and metabolic effects on rhesus social behavior: Protein and protein-calorie malnutrition. Develop Psychobiol 13: 287.

Champakam S, Srikantia SG, Gopalan, C. (1968). Kwashiorkor and mental development. Am J Clin Nutr 21: 844.

Cordero ME, Diaz G, Araya J. (1976). Neocortex development during severe malnutrition in the rat. Am J Clin Nutr 29: 358.

Cravioto J, Robles B (1965). Evolution of adaptive and motor behavior during rehabilitation from kwashiorkor. Am J Orthopsychiat 35: 449.

El Khaier A (1986). Etude épidmiologique étiologique clinique biologique évolutive et thérapeutique des malnutritions proteino-caloriques de l'enfant. Doctoral Thesis, Mohamed V University, Rabat.

Geist CR, Zimmermann RR, Strobel DA (1972). Effect of protein-calorie malnutrition on food consumption, weight gain, serum proteins, and activity in the developing rhesus monkey (Macaca mulatta). Lab Anim Sci 22: 369.

Greenough WT, Volkmar FR (1973). Pattern of dendritic branching in occipital cortex of rats reared in complex environments. Exp Neurol 40: 491.

Habicht JP, Yarbrough C, Lechtig A, Klein RE (1974). Relation of maternal supplementary feeding during pregnancy to birth weight. In Winick M (ed.): Current Concepts in Nutrition, Vol 2. New York: John Wiley & Sons, p. 95.

Hall RD (1983) Is hippocampal function in the adult rat impaired by early protein or protein-calorie deficiencies? Develop Psychobiol 16: 395.

Katz HB, Davies CA (1983). The separate and combined effects of early undernutrition and environmental complexity at different ages on cerebral measures in rats. Devel Psychobiol 16: 47.

Khadri N (1987). Malnutrition proteino calorique relevant la tuberculose chez les enfants de moins de 5 ans. Doctoral Thesis, Mohamed V University,

Rabat Lahbabi MS (1987) Profil de la malnutrition proteino-énergétique: Evolution dans la prise en charge nutritionnelle. Doctoral Thesis, Mohamed V University, Rabat.

Levitsky D, Barnes RH (1973). Malnutrition and animal behavior. In Kallen DJ (ed.): Nutrition, Development and Social Behavior. Washington, DC: US Dept HEW Publ No (NIH) 73-242, p. 3.

Lytle LD, Messing RB, Fisher L, Phebus L (1975). Effects of long-term corn consumption on brain serotonin and the response to electric shock. Science 190: 692.

Miller SA (1969). Protein metabolism during growth and development. In Munro HN (ed.): Mammalian Protein Metabolism, Vol 3. New York: Academic Press, p. 189.

Peregoy PL, Zimmermann RR, Strobel DA (1972). Protein preference in protein malnourished monkeys. Percept Motor Skills 35: 495.

Platt BS (1962). Proteins in nutrition. Proc Roy Soc London 156: 337.

Rosso P, Hormazabal J, Winick M (1970). Changes in brain weight, cholesterol, phospholipid and DNA content in marasmic children. Am J Clin Nutr 23: 1275.

Sackett GP (1968). Innate mechanisms, rearing conditions and a theory of early experience effects in primates. In Jones MR (ed.): Miami Symposium on the Prediction of Behavior: Effects of Early Experience. Miami: University of Miami Press, p. 11.

Salbego C, Souza DO (1986). Effects of undernutrition during suckling on phosphoryl-serine levels in brain nuclear proteins of adult rats. J Nutr 116: 2303.

Skiels HM (1966). Adult status of children with contrasting early life experiences. Child Dev Monog Series 31: 3.

Smith CA (1947). Effects of maternal malnutrition upon the newborn infant in Holland (1944-45). Pediat 30: 229.

Vendite D, Wofchuk S, Souza DO (1985). Effects of undernutrition during suckling on footshock escape behavior and on related neurochemical parameters in rats. J Nutr 115: 1418.

Winick M (1976). Malnutrition and Brain Development. New York: Oxford University Press.

Winick M, Nobel A (1965). Quantitative changes in DNA, RNA, and protein during prenatal and postnatal growth. Devel Biol 12: 451.

Winick M, Rosso P (1969). The effect of severe early malnutrition on cellular growth of human brain. Pediat Res 3: 181.

Wolf C, Almli CR, Finger S, Ryan S, Morgane PJ (1986). Behavioral effects of severe and moderate early malnutrition. Physiol Behav 38: 725.

Zimmermann RR, Geist CR, Wise LA (1974). Behavioral development, environmental deprivation, and malnutrition. In Newton G and Riesen AH (eds.): Advances in Psychobiology, Vol 2. New York: John Wiley & Sons, p. 133.

DISCUSSION

Q (van Gelder): There is a major difference between rodents and humans, in that the rodent brain continues to grow, or gains in weight anyway, whereas in human beings, once past the third year or so, there is no change in the weight anymore.

A: Well, that is true. I said that it is an animal model with all the limitations inherent in such model. Whether this is therefore the right model to use, well we use this strategy in the absence, really, of valid controllable experimental conditions in humans. That is one of the major factors.

Comment (Diamond): With regard to the rodent brain continuing to grow, it depends on the parts you are referring to. The cerebral cortex is already going down after one month, i.e. starts to decrease its dimensions, whereas the hippocampus continues to grow throughout the lifetime. So one has to talk about the various parts (and not generalize too much).

Q (S. Hashim): About 20 years ago Dr R Swami from India developed a (Kwashiorkor) model in the monkey. How does that compare with yours.

A: I dealt mostly, with respect to the monkey literature, with the data collected by the Zimmermann group in Geist. Here too there is a suspicion of lasting behavioral effects, in the monkey.

Section II: THE EFFECTS OF (MAL) NUTRITION ON NEUROEMBRYOGENESIS

Understanding the complex process of development of the central nervous system must represent one of the great investigative challenges. In the case of the human brain, several hundred billion cells must develop, differentiate, migrate, seek out often distant target systems, become metabolically active, functionally communicative, suitably insulated, appropriately interconnected and prepared to provide at least the basic behavioral needs for the total living organism, all within a nine month span. Many of the major events in neuroembryogenesis have been described over the past 75 years, but without any appreciation of the mechanisms involved. The beginnings of a more profound understanding of the process have had to await the coming of modern biochemistry and cellular and molecular biology. This cluster of chapters exemplifies some of the approaches currently in use, while providing fascinating glimpses of the forces at work.

My first impression is one of awe, that so many biological processes operating at so many levels of complexity can proceed simultaneously and with so relatively high a degree of accuracy. Although no two brains are genetically alike, nor are the phenotypic expressions of the same set of genetic instructions ever exactly similar (e.g., monozygotic twins), it is still remarkable that clinically recognizable developmental flaws in neural development seldom exceed 2%. There is still almost no understanding of how a set of genes coding for a very large (but not unlimited) array of molecules, can ultimately guide the development of a dense yet precisely interconnected three dimensional matrix. But with this set of papers, we catch a glimpse of these molecules at work during both 'normal' and 'abnormal' circumstances. The latter conditions are interesting, not only for their own sake, but for the insights they provide about normal development. The overall impression is that of Sherrington's "magic shuttle" (1937) magnified many times over, weaving the intricate organic tapestry of brain.

The development of neuronal connectivity is based on a complex set of processes which guide target selection. Jhaveri and colleagues cite approach, waiting period, and terminal arborization as consecutive events in the sequence. During the initial phase of growth, axons follow direct, often stereotypic, routes to their eventual target sites using glial guides. Glial membranes are believed to express a number of molecular species which provide directional guidance and promote axonal growth. Among these, NCAMS seem to inhibit premature arborization while facilitating fasciculation of the growing axons. The matrix protein, heparan sulfate proteoglycan, and possibly Neurofascin, F 11, SNAP/TAG 1, and GAP 43 are similarly believed to assist in encouraging un-branched neurite growth. Progression of such axon bundles is rapid during this generally non-branching, non-arborizing phase and approximates 80 um/hr. Where branching does occur, it develops at the en passant varicosities which stud each axon. The tendency of axons from similar sources to travel en masse, as fascicles or tracts, and the likelihood that specific, recognizable membrane markers facilitate this type of group migration, undoubtedly contribute significantly to path finding and following operations.

However, axonal trajectory is probably not solely the responsibility of membrane bound marker proteins. As-yet-undefined chemotropic agents may also exert potent attractive forces on the migrating growth cones. With a minimum of data, a picture begins to emerge of heterogeneous mechanisms working cooperatively, both locally and remotely, to shape the trajectory and pace of axonal migration.

Pattern and pace of growth change as the target structure is reached. There is perceptible hesitation; the growth cones, for the most part, linger at the nuclear boundary or beneath the cortical plate, awaiting entry cues. It is not clear what these are, nor indeed whether they come primarily from the target (postsynaptic) area or from the source neurons. Furthermore, the same clues do not seem to operate equivalently on all afferent systems awaiting entry. Given two waiting systems, the one may be seen to enter appreciably before the second. We can speculate on the significance of this type of staggered entry, and of the mechanisms which subserve it, but the relevant data still elude us.

Once the growth cones enter the target zone, growth by axon fasciculation is lost and each fiber seems to follow an idiosyncratic course. This may be due to decreasing mutual adhesiveness among the axons and increasing influence of attractants or membrane markers on individual target structures. The terminally arborizing axon advances more slowly (8-10 um/hr) and generates patterns specific to the receptive area it has invaded. There seems to be no question that arbor formation and patterning are influenced jointly by intrinsic properties of the neurons involved and by extrinsic influences from the neuropil field they have invaded. The actual arbor patterns expressed by the terminating axons are likely, also, to depend in part on development and organization of cytoskeleton components.

One final process must be noted; one that provides an enduring theme throughout the remainder of the life of the organism. Plastic restructuring of the axon terminal seems to commence even as the axon arbor reaches full expression. This resculpting undoubtedly reflects changes in both the inner and outer milieux, alterations in usage patterns of the system, etc. One of the most interesting and obvious examples of axonal loss with maturation involves the paring away of major branching systems. Cortical neurons which originally sent multiple branching axon systems into other cortical stations, basal ganglia, descending tracts and corpus callosum, may lose all but one of these axon radicles during the early postnatal period. It is tempting to interpret this initial axonal exuberance and later restriction as another evidence of ontogeny briefly recapitulating more primitive connectional patterns.

The energy to drive these processes seems to come largely from utilization of a combination of glucose and ketone bodies. It is of particular interest that utilization of ketone bodies for metabolic purposes is particularly high in the fetus. Glucose then becomes the principal oxidative fuel as the central nervous system matures and remains so until old age when an increasing proportion of ketone bodies again become used in oxidative metabolism. The significance of these variations is still not entirely clear, but Clark points out that the blood brain barrier is not competent during the fetal period (Cremer, 1982) and it is during this period that the ketone extraction coefficient in the neonatal brain is four times that of the mature adult. Interestingly enough, it now seems likely that the blood brain barrier again loses competence in old age and particularly so in Alzheimer's Disease (Makinodan, 1976). This apparent relationship between ineffective blood brain barrier function and increased utilization at each end of the life cycle could be interpreted as indicating that the well known exclusivity of glucose as the neuronal energy substrate might be more a factor of (non)patency of the cerebrovascular walls than of any intrinsic superiority it may possess as a fuel.

The degree of maturity of the developing nervous system remains closely coupled to the oxidative substrate and to the presence of key enzyme systems like the pyruvate dehydrogenase complex. In non-precocial animals (e.g., rat and man) who are born in relatively immature states, ketone utilization is still relatively high at birth and pyruvate dehydrogenase levels are low. Conversely, in precocial animals (e.g., the guinea pig) the picture is reversed, and pyruvate dehydrogenase has reached 90% of its adult value at birth. The coupling is sufficiently close for Clark to suggest that neurological competence and pyruvate dehydrogenase activity develop and mature together.

A sustained high level of nutritional support is necessary during the formative phases of the central nervous system. As might be expected, significant nutritional deprivation during neuro-embryogenesis is reflected in decreased brain weight and in total numbers of cells. Rather remarkably, malnutrition during the prenatal phase has far less impact (particularly in nonprecocial mammals) than deprivation during the postnatal or suckling period. It is during the latter period (i.e., the first 3 postnatal weeks in rat and the initial 1.5-2 years in man) that the majority of dentate and cerebellar granule cells are formed. Ten to twenty percent decrease in the total cell population and an even more severe deficit in total DNA reflect malnutrition during this epoch. Other effects noted by Lewis in addition to a permanent deficit in numbers of neurons are lasting changes in ratios between various cell types, reduction in numbers of germinal cells postnatally, distortion of the generation cycle (e.g., prolongation of the S phase, and shortening of the G1 phase), increased numbers of degenerate postmitotic cells, prolonged persistence of the cerebellar external granule cell layer, a measurable though reversible diminution in thickness of the cortical plate and an increase (again reversible) of neuronal packing density. The impact of nutritional deprivation on dendritic growth is impressive, but tends to vary somewhat with the type of parent neuron, the latest developing cells showing the most obvious changes. However, even with neurons which appear relatively early in the process of neurogenesis, and where dendrite systems seem most forgiving of nutritional insult when followed by nutritional rehabilitation (e.g., the cerebellar Purkinje cell), structural growth may be recaptured, but topological distortions remain.

Malnutrition may reduce the number of cortical nerve terminals by as much as 60%, thereby contributing significantly to the already-noted cortical thinning. Many investigators have now shown these changes to be reversible, even to the point of "rehabilitation overshoot," (Warren and Bedi, 1984). In the midbrain reticular formation, on the other hand, the direct effect of undernutrition is an apparent 75% increase in synaptic density in the mouse (Cravioto, Hambraeus, Vahlquist, 1974). This phenomenon undoubtedly emphasizes the importance of processes of synapse elimination during normal maturation, and is reminiscent of the equally dramatic loss of dendritic spines from feline reticular neurons during the first 3-4 weeks of postnatal life (Scheibel and Scheibel, 1973).

Neuroglial cells are also significantly affected by nutritional deprivation and in some studies may show a deficit of almost 40%. The later-developing oligodendroglia show appreciably greater loss than astroglia, so it is not unexpected that myelogenesis is also significantly impaired. Structures such as the long ascending and descending tracts, the corpus callosum and the optic tracts show marked retardation of myelin formation, an effect which may or may not be entirely made up through later nutritional rehabilitation. It is clear that much depends on the period and severity of the deprivation, on the cell systems principally affected and, of course, on the organisms in which the effects are observed.

Huether's attempts to tease out the effects of fetal malnutrition on different neurotransmitter systems lead to some surprising findings. Cholinergic and GABAergic transmission are severely depressed in developing organisms, although an appreciable degree of restoration is possible with nutritional rehabilitation. Catecholaminergic and serotonergic systems, on the other hand, seem to proliferate and become more active in the undernourished state, and some of these alterations may persist during subsequent rehabilitation. The key to these anomalous effects appears to lie in the enhanced availability of several precursor amino acids, especially, Tryptophan, Tyrosine and Histidine, which are involved in the synthesis of serotonin, dopamine and norepinephrine, and histamine.

A mechanism putatively responsible for the increased concentration of these aromatic neutral amino acids is thought to be found in the malnutrition induced reduction of serum albumin levels in the circulating blood. Branched chain large neutral amino acids, LNAA's (Val, Leu, Ile) compete with the aromatic neutral amino acids (Trp, Tyr, His) for a common carrier mediated transport system necessary for brain uptake. Huether points out that protein malnutrition "causes a greater depletion of the plasma pool of the LNAA's .... relative to the depletion of Trp (free Trp is actually increased because of the reduced serum albumin level and increased concentrations of free fatty acids which compete with Trp for a common albumin binding site...)." This idiosyncratic effect thereby causes an "increase of the ratio between the concentrations of precursor amino acids for monoamine synthesis and the sum of the concentrations of the competing amino acids for brain uptake...."

There is reason to suspect that, prior to synapse formation, monoamines may be released as hormones to act as morphogenetic or developmental signals helping control neuronal proliferation, migration, outgrowth, synaptogenesis, and cell death. If so, it is clear that the nutritionally deficient fetal brain may undergo profound developmental alterations from deficits (or over abundances) of putative neurotransmitter substances, well before synapses have begun to develop.

One other interesting peculiarity of fetal life is the apparent lack of homeostatic regulation. In the mature organism, if monoamine levels rise, feedback regulatory systems facilitate down-regulation of the appropriate receptors. In the absence of such systems in the fetus, enhanced levels of circulating monoamine leads to increased expression of functional monoamine receptors. This early open loop effect leaves its impress on the entire central nervous system and when the later closed loop systems become functional, the structural pattern already established remains.

In general, the earlier a developing system is exposed to an altered supply of substrate, and the longer the situation persists, the more profound will be the effect. Using only two or three neurotransmitter systems as text, Heuther paints a dramatic picture of the complex and long-term effects of nutritional deprivation during gestation.

The possibilities and limitations of postnatal rehabilitation, both dietary and environmental, have been examined by Diamond and her colleagues using the rat model. Maternal protein deprivation of approximately 50% during the last trimester of pregnancy and during the lactation period result in rat pups with approximately one half the body weight of normally fostered controls and dramatically thinner neocortices. As might be expected, protein rehabilitation partially (though not completely) restores cortical thickness, but the addition of environmental enrichment notably augments the amount of return of cortical thickness toward control values. This report is in essential agreement with previous investigations which noted decreased cortical thickness, and increased cortical cell packing density resulting in part from less dendritic growth. However, failure of dendritic growth in response to nutritional insult turns out to be much more interesting than expected. When the dendrite arbors are analyzed in quantitative fashion, segment order by segment order, it becomes apparent that various parts of the dendrite tree respond idiosyncratically to nutritional deprivation. Lower (first, second and third) order dendrite segments turn out to be much more resistant to protein deprivation than higher (fourth, fifth, and sixth) order systems. The latter are severely affected by nutritional deprivation during third trimester and lactation. Concurrent nutritional and environmental rehabilitation are far more effective in restoring a substantial fraction of the 'lost growth' than nutritional rehabilitation alone. Such studies emphasize the plastic reactivity of outer dendrite segments as well as the subtle but powerful effects of environmental enrichment on brain development.

A remarkable hierarchy of control sequences imposed on neural development is sketched out in this chapter cluster. As fragmentary as the picture still is, one can only be amazed by the diversity and precision of mechanisms simultaneously brought on line by the fertilization of the oocyte. We have already commented on the infrequency with which the processes of neuroembryological development go significantly astray. Almost equally remarkable is the manner in which the effects of severe nutritional deprivation during the developmental period are cushioned and even largely corrected for during early rehabilitation. Truly, Nature looks out after its own.

REFERENCES

Crairoto J, Hambraeus L, Vahlquist B (1974). "Early malnutrition and mental development". Uppsala: Almquist and Wiksell.

Cremer JE (1982). Substrate utilization and brain development. J Cerebr Blood Flow and Metab 2:394-407.

Scheibel ME, Davies TL, Scheibel AB (1973). Maturation of reticular dendrites: Loss of spines and development of bundles. Exp Neurol 38:301-310.

Sherrington CS (1937). "Man on his Nature. The Gifford Lectures." New York: McMillan.

Warren MA, Bedi KS (1984). A quantitative assessment of the development of synapses and neurons in the visual cortex of control and undernourished rats. J Comp Neurol 227:104-108.

Arnold B. Scheibel

(Mal)Nutrition and the Infant Brain, pages 89–109

NUTRITION AND ANATOMICAL DEVELOPMENT OF THE BRAIN

Paul D. Lewis

Department of Histopathology, Charing Cross & Westminster Medical School, University of London, London W6 8RF

In global terms, it is probable that severe childhood undernutrition is one of the most important causes of brain pathology. Yet, because the circumstances that cause major famine and those that permit painstaking scientific medical investigation are mutually exclusive, our direct knowledge of the neuropathology of the undernourished human brain is rudimentary. The encyclopaedic textbook of Dodge, Prensky and Feigin (1975) reviewed abnormalities of brain structure in undernutrition in detail, but alongside a mass of microscopic information obtained from experimental animals the authors could set only meagre human data, principally brain weights. Over the last decade there has been a further and significant increase in the understanding of structural mechanisms of abnormal brain development in laboratory animals, but human neuropathology has stood still in this area. Trowell, Davies and Dean (1954) commented that the changes in the human infant brain in undernutrition had "not been made the subject of special study and it is not known if there is any histological counterpart to the striking mental changes" observed. This state of affairs is unlikely to alter. Reduced head size (Stoch and Smythe, 1963; 1967; 1976), brain weight (Brown, 1966) and brain DNA (cell number; Winick and Rosso, 1969a & b) have been noted in severely undernourished infants, but morphological counterparts to these changes are unknown, apart from what is described in a few published comments (e.g Udani, 1960). Thus in reviewing the effects of nutritional deprivation on the anatomical development of the brain, it is to experimental animal findings rather than to human neuropathology that one must look for a comprehensive body of data.

Some technical considerations

Many experimental techniques have been used to produce undernutrition in laboratory animals. A favoured regime, used in collaborative studies between Dr R Balázs, Dr A J Patel and the author, involves the underfeeding of mother rats by providing about half the normal food supply through pregnancy (from the sixth day) and lactation. Comparing different methods of undernutrition, Altman et al (1971) observed that this treatment produced the most consistent developmental retardation. The fetus is relatively spared under these conditions, at the expense of the mother. The growth of the fetus is also relatively normal when a different experimental procedure is used, aimed at closely simulating the dietary conditions under which malnourished human populations typically exist, i.e. a low protein and high carbohydrate diet from before conception and throughout gestation (Morgane et al, 1978). However, there are limits to the fetal protection possible with such a regime, and more severe nutritional deficiency leads to retarded fetal growth with involvement of the brain (Zamenhof, van Marthens and Grauel, 1971a & b).

Effects of undernutrition on cell acquisition in the brain.

The weight of the brain is significantly decreased in undernutrition; although various anatomical factors are involved, an important part in producing this effect is played by reduction of cell number (Howard, 1965; Winick and Noble, 1966). Undernutrition interferes with cell proliferation in many organs, including the brain. Cell proliferation is vigorous in the mammalian brain not only in fetal life but also in the early postnatal period; almost 50% of forebrain and 97% of cerebellar cells are formed in the rat at this time. It is study of postnatal rat brain cell proliferation that has greatly increased our understanding of major developmental effects of undernutrition.

Cells are mainly formed at circumscribed germinal zones, notably the subependymal layer (SEL) surrounding the forebrain ventricles, the dentate fascia of the hippocampus and the external granular layer (EGL) covering the surface of the cerebellum. In addition, there are numbers of glial precursors scattered throughout the brain. The period of vigorous cell proliferation is also circumscribed; it is largely completed by about 3 weeks after birth in the rat and by 1.5-2 years of age in man (Dobbing and Sands, 1973): germinal zones have disappeared by these times. However, fragments of the SEL persist into later life in both rodents and primates, suggesting that a fraction of the total cell population is renewed from this region even after the early period of high proliferative activity (Smart and Leblond, 1961; Lewis, 1968a &b; Haas, Werner and Fliedner, 1970).

Predominantly glial cells are formed in the forebrain during the postnatal period, but neurogenesis persists in the fascia dentata of the hippocampus and the olfactory lobes (Altman, 1969), while a few neuronal precursors continue to divide in the nucleus septalis accumbens in the first few days after birth (Creps, 1974). Even in adults neurogenesis has been detected in the hippocampus (Kaplan and Hinds, 1977). In the cerebellum most of the nerve cells are formed, nearly all from the EGL, after birth. Only the Purkinje cells and the large neurones in the deep cerebellar nuclei are formed prenatally, while the Golgi cells are generated perinatally. With the exception of the Golgi cells, cerebellar interneurones are produced in the EGL, and this is prominent in man for several months after birth; migrating cells in the cerebellar cortex disappear as late as 18 months (Larroche, 1966). Granule cells, the most abundant interneurones in the cerebellum, have been shown to increase very substantially during the first two years in man (Gadsdon and Emery, 1976), indicating significant postnatal neurogenesis.

Patel, Balázs and Johnson (1973) showed that cell acquisition during gestation, assessed by DNA estimation in the brain of the newborn, was not significantly affected by undernutrition. In contrast, during the suckling period the rate of cell acquisition was depressed thoughout the brain, and although the animals were rehabilitated to a full diet from day 21, moderate depression in cell numbers (10-20% depending on whether forebrain or cerebellum) persisted. Other studies, in which different modes of undernutrition were employed, including food deprivation during the suckling period only and in which rehabilitation after weaning was prolonged, concur in showing that the deficit in brain cell numbers incurred in early life is permanent (Dobbing, 1974; Winick, 1976).

The rate of in vivo DNA synthesis was also studied by Patel and colleagues. The results were unexpected. In contrast to the relatively mild effect on cell number in the brain, undernutrition caused a very severe depression of DNA synthesis rate, which at its lowest was only about 20% (forebrain) to 30% (cerebellum) of control values. It was suggested that a derangement of the replicative cell cycle in the developing brain of undernourished animals could account for the observed discrepancy between the severe depression of DNA synthesis rate and the small decrease of cell acquisition; if the S phase were prolonged by undernutrition to a greater extent than the turnover time, the rate of DNA synthesis would be more depressed than the rate of cell acquisition. This hypothesis was tested by studying cell proliferation kinetics in the germinal zones of undernourished animals, and was supported by the results (Lewis et al, 1975).

Particularly during the first two postnatal weeks, when cell proliferation is most vigorous, the S phase was prolonged much more than the generation time of the germinal cells in the undernourished brain. The relatively small effect of undernutrition on cell cycle time in spite of the marked lengthening of the DNA synthesis phase was a consequence of a severe curtailment of the length of the G1 phase of the cell cycle. This effect appears to be unique for the developing brain. The lengthening of the S phase accompanied by the virtual elimination of the G1 phase has been observed not only in the forebrain SEL and the cerebellar EGL, but in the hippocampal dentate fascia in the developing brain (Lewis, Patel and Balázs, 1979). In contrast, it is not detectable in the residual SEL in food-deprived young adult rats, where both the S phase and the overall cell cycle time are more or less proportionately prolonged (Lewis, Patel and Balázs, 1977). Similarly, in other adult tissues which contain proliferating cells, food deprivation results in a marked lengthening of cell cycle parameters including both the S phase and the G1 phase (Wiebecke et al, 1969; Deo, Bijlani and Ramalingaswami, 1975). These observations suggest that the compensatory reduction of G1 in the face of an extended S phase is characteristic of the developing brain. Table I summarises our findings.

Additional factors may well contribute to the effect of undernutrition on cell formation in the developing brain (Lewis et al, 1975). Thus the effect of

TABLE 1. Effect of Undernutrition on Cell Formation, DNA Synthesis and Cell Cycle Parameters in the Forebrain and the Cerebellum of Developing rat

	Treatment			Age (d)			
		1	6	10	12	14	21
Cell numbers (DNA µg atom-P)							
Forebrain	Control	1.48	1.92	2.20	-	2.56	2.84
	UN(%)[a]	99	90	92	-	88[d]	88[d]
Cerebellum	Control	0.12	0.47	1.99	-	2.64	3.87
	UN(%)	99	98	67[d]	-	85[d]	85[d]
DNA synthesis rate [b]							
Forebrain	Control	755	1052	860	-	722	477
	UN(%)	55[d]	17d	23[d]	-	29[d]	53[d]
Cerebellum	Control	168	806	1504	-	1507	360
	UN(%)	91	30[d]	39	-	51[d]	73
Cell Cycle Parameter (h)[c]							
S-phase	Control	9.6	10.2	-	10.8	-	11.1
	UN(%)	136[d]	138[d]	-	182[d]	-	119
G_1-phase	Conrol	5.7	3.4	-	2.9	-	5.0
	UN(%)	23[d]	6[d]	-	7[d]	-	114
G_2-phase	Control	3.3	2.1	-	1.5	-	2.1
	UN(%)	130	133	-	240[d]	-	114
Total cell cycle	Control	18.7	16.8	-	16.1	-	18.1
	UN(%)	107	104	-	148[d]	-	177

a   The values in the undernourished animals (UN) are expressed as a percentage of controls.

b   DNA synthesis rate was estimated in the terms of the incorporation into DNA per brain part $(\times 10^4)$ corrected for the concentration of acid soluble ^{14}C, 30 mins after the subcutaneous injection of 20 µCi/100g body wt of [2- ^{14}C] thymidine. (From Patel et al., 1973).

c   The estimates of the length of the cell cycle phases were obtained by fitting computer-generated curves to the data representing the percentage labeled mitoses at 1-32 h after injection of [^{3}H]thymidine. Since the estimates in the subependymal layer in the forebrain and the external granular layer in the cerebellum did not differ

→

TABLE 2. Some Reported Effects of Undernutrition and Nutritional Rehabilitation on Morphological aspects of the Central Nervous System (**D**= decrease; **I** = increase; **O** = no change)

Parameter	Undernutrition	Rehabilitation
A. FOREBRAIN		
Weight	**D** 59	**D** 19, 33
Cell number	**D** 46, 65	**D** 19
Cerebrum		
Cortical volume	**D** 38, 59	**O** 5
Cortical thickness	**D**16	**D** 20, **O** 4, 33
Cortical neurones		
Number	**O** 59	**D** 20, **O** 58
Packing density	**I** 16, 24, 28, 40, 59	**O** 28, **D** 20,23, **I** or **O** 38
Fibre density	**D** 22	**O** 28
Fibre growth	**D** 35	**D** 57
Synapse/neurone ratio	**D** 6, 16, 60, 61	**O** 6, **I** 60, 61
Synapse density	**O** 16, 21, 22, 31	**O** 21
Presynaptic thickness	**D** 30	**D** 30
Postsynaptic thickness	**O** 30	**D** 30
Synaptic area	**D** 31	**D** 31
Synaptic curvature maturation	**D** 31	**I** 31
Synaptic vesicle number	**D** 31	**I** 31
Dendritic arborization	**D** 15, 49, 50, 52, 62	**O** 23
Neuroglia		
Numbers	**D** 4, 16, 38	**D** 4, 20, 38, 54, 57, 58
Precursor cell pyknosis	**I** 39, 44	
Astrocytes	**O** 36	
Oligodendrocyte acquisition	**D** 36	**D** 57
Oligodendrocyte maturation	**D** 36	

significantly, the data for the two germinal sites were combined. (From Lewis et al., 1975)

d   Significant differences between control and UN groups: P <0.05

Table 2 (cont'd)

Parameter	Undernutrition	Rehabilitation
Myelination	**D** 4, 7, 35, 64	**D** 4, 7, 64
Distal segment length	**D** 42	
Spine number	**O** 48	
Synaptic density	**O** 47	
Granule cells		
Number	**D** 2, 10	**D** 3, 19
Density	**I** 42, 43, 53	**O** 40, 43
Dendritic number	**O** 62	
Basket cell number	**D** 10	
Stellate cell number	**O** 10	
Golgi cell number	**O** 10	
Granule: Purkinje cell ratio	**D** 5	**D** 5, **O** 3
Climbing fibre: Purkinje cell circuit	**O** 26	
Granular layer synapses/neurones	**D** 6	**O** 6
Mossy fibre-granule cell- Purkinje cell circuit	**O** 26, 37, 45	
External granular layer		
Pyknotic index	**I** 39	
Pyknotic clearance	**D** 34	
Postnatal persistance	**I** 40, 53	
Neuroglia		
Bergmann glia		
Number	**D** 10, 13	
Development	**I** 11, 13	
Molecular layer number	**D** 10	
Internal granular layer number	**D** 10	
Profiles in molecular layer	**D** 9	
Oligodendrocyte development	**D** 12	
Thalamus		
Dendritic arborisation	**D** and **O** 51	
Hippocampus		
Dimensions		**O** 33
Granule cell layer thickness	**D** 41	
Granule cell density	**D** 32	
Pyramidal cell number	**D** 32	
Synapses per granule cell	**D** 1	**I** 1
Optic nerve		
Fibre number	**D** 7, 56, 63	**O** 7, 63
Fibre diameter	**D** 7, **O** 7	**O** 7

Table 2 (cont'd)

Parameter	Undernutrition	Rehabilitation
Myelin lamellae	D 63	O 63

B. HINDBRAIN

Cerebellum

Weight	D 2, 19, 42, 46	D 3, 19
Cell number	D 46	D 19
Cortical area	D 2, 10	D 3, 20
Foliar development	D 14, 25	

Nerve cells
  Purkinje cells

Number	O 10, D 3	O20, D 3
Density	I 6, 42, 43	O43, I 6
Dendritic network		
Size/complexity	D 42, 48, 55	O 3, 43, 47
Segment number	D 42	

Brainstem

Reticular formation		
Synaptic density		I 17
Dendritic development	I or D 27	
Lateral vestibular nuclei		
Neuronal density	I 29	
Nucleus raphe dorsalis		
Dendritic development	I or D 18	

Most of these data come from rats undernourished during brain development, i.e. in gestation and the suckling period, although in some experiments the food restriction was continued into the post-weaning period. The reversibility of some effects of undernutrition was studied in animals fed normally after weaning.

Key: reduction or slowing: D
       increase: I
       no change: O
       in comparison with controls

1. Ahmed et al., 1987; 2. Barnes and Altman (1973a); 3. Barnes and Altman (1973b); 4. Bass et al. (1970a); 5. Bedi et al. (1980a); 6. Bedi et al. (1980b) ; 7. Bedi and Warren 91983); 8. Benton et al. (1966); 9. Clos et al. (1973); 10. Clos et al. (1977); 11. Clos et al. (19779); 12. Clos et al. (1982a); 13. Clos et al. (1982b); 14. Conradi and Muentzing (1985); 15. Cordero et al. (1985); 16. Cragg (1972); 17. Cravioto et al. (1976); 18. Diaz-Cintra et al. (1974); 19. Dobbing (1974); 20. Dobbing et al. (1971); 21. Dyson and Jones 91976); 22. Eayrs and Horn (1955); 23. Escobar 91974); 24.

                                                    ⟶

undernutrition on cell acquisition in the developing brain so far identified include (1) distortion of the generation cycle, the S phase being prolonged and the G1 phase severely curtailed; (2) reduction of germinal cell numbers postnatally; (3) increase in numbers of degenerate postmitotic cells in germinal zones, possibly resulting from delayed clearance; (4) slightly prolonged persistence of the cerebellar external granular layer; (5) a permanent deficit in brain cell numbers; and (6) lasting changes in the cellular composition of the brain, affecting ratios of different cell types (Balázs, Jordan, Lewis and Patel, 1986).

The observed cell cycle changes are of great interest. The significant and selective prolongation of the S phase in undernutrition is particularly intriguing as the length of this phase of the cell cycle has been generally found to be remarkably constant. In contrast, the G1 phase usually shows the greatest variation in length (Cleaver, 1967). During early embryogenesis the G1 period is very short and even virtually absent, and it tends to lengthen with advancing age (Prescott, 1976; Lewis; 1978). It would appears therefore that the germinal cells in the developing brain of undernourished rats in the postnatal period reverted, at least in this respect, to a more primitive pattern of replication. Although the G1 phase may be an expendable period in the cell cycle, there are indications that certain processes occurring during a limited period in the G1 phase are critical in terms of the full expression of the normal differentiated function of some cells (Vonderhaar and Topper, 1974). Thus, while the virtual elimination of the G1 phase may be an effective means of compensating for the prolongation of the S phase of the germinal cells in the undernourished brain, it might have adverse effects on the progeny of cells which are near to their terminal division in the postnatal period.

Undernutrition and the structural development of neurones.

The earliest observation suggesting the possibility of impaired structural development of neurones in the undernourished brain was that of Sugita (1918), who showed that undernutrition in early life resulted in deficit in brain weight and a reduction in the thickness of the cerebral cortex in young rats.

Gambetti et al. (1974); 25. Gopinath et al. (1976); 22. Eayrs and Horn 91955); 23. Escobar (1974); 24. Gambetti et al. (1974); 25. Gopinath et al. (1976); 26. Hajos et al. (unpublished); 27. Hammer (1981); 28. Horn (1955); 29. Johnson and Yoesle (1975); 30. Jones and Dyson (1976); 31. Jones and Dyson 91981); 32. Jordan et al. (1982); 33. Katz and Davies (1982); 34. Koppel et al. (1983); 35. Lai and Lewis (1980); 36. Lai et al. (1980); 37. Legrand (1967); 38. Leuba and Rabinowicz (1979); 39. Lewis (1975); 40. Lewis et al. (1975); 41. Lewis et al. (1979); 42. McConnell and Berry (1978a); 43. McConnell and Berry (1978b) 44. Nazarevskaya et al. (1982); 45. Neville and Chase (1971); 46. Patel et al. (1973); 47. Rebière (1973); 48. Rebière and Legrand (1972); 49. Salas (1980); 50. Salas et al. (1974); 51. Salas et al. (1986); 52. Schoenheit (1982); 53. Sharma et al. (1987); 54. Siassi and Siassi (1973); 55. Sima and Persson (1975); 56. Sima and Sourander (1974); 57. Sturrock et al. 91976); 58. Sturrock et al. (1977); 59. Sugita (1918); 60. Warren and Bedi (1982); 61. Warren and Bedi (1984); 62. West and Kemper (1976); 63. Wiggins et al. (1984); 64. Wiggins et al. (1985); 65. Winick (1976).

Cragg (1972) found that the cortex (about 1.5 mm thick) was slightly thinner (0.2 mm) in rats undernourished through 50 days of life, an effect that can be reversed by nutritional rehabilitation (Katz and Davies, 1982). During the period of undernutrition, the packing density of neurones in cerebral and cerebellar cortex and brainstem nuclei was found to be higher that in controls, indicating slowing or reduction of development of neuropil and\or glia (Cragg, 1972; Stewart, Merat & Dickerson; 1974; Gambetti et al, 1974; Johnson and Yoesle, 1974; McConnell and Berry, 1978a & b). However, in nutritionally rehabilitated rats high neuronal packing density was shown to decrease and disappear (Leuba and Rabinowicz, 1979) or even reverse (Dobbing, Hopewell and Lynch, 1971) with time. Decrease in nerve cell density, particularly in deeper cortical layers, was found to be more marked than for glial cells, suggesting a selective neuronal loss under these conditions. Nerve cell loss, especially in cortical layer VI, has also been reported (Escobar, 1974). Since the full neuronal complement of the cerebral neocortex is believed to be generated in the rat before birth, i.e. before the major impact of the nutritional insult on the developing brain, such findings would suggest that normal food supply is required not only for the formation of cells, but also for their maintenance.

Reduction in neuropil, implicit in the finding of increased nerve cell packing density, has been studied in the cerebral cortex, and the lessening or disappearance of some effects following nutritional rehabilitation has been confirmed. Indeed, the emphasis of neuroanatomical research on undernutrition over the past decade has been on the reversibility of induced changes (see Table 2).

Many investigators have concentrated on the influence of nutritional deprivation while it is in effect, often during the suckling period and before the development of neuronal processes has been completed. It has been established that the area occupied in the cerebral cortex by the neuropil is decreased in undernourished animals (Gambetti et al, 1974). In developing experimental animals all components of the neuropil seem to be affected. Fibre density is markedly reduced at 24 days (Eayrs and Horn, 1955), as is the basilar dendritic network of the large pyramidal cells in 7-15 day old undernourished rats (Salas, Diaz and Nieto, 1974). However, the length of oblique and basal dendrites of pyramidal cells in layer IIIb is normal in the 30 day old progeny of protein-deficient mother rats (West and Kemper, 1976). The development of neuronal interconnections appears to be retarded. Although the distribution of various forms of spines on the dendrites of pyramidal cells is normal, their number and density are significantly reduced in undernutrition (Salas, Diaz and Nieto, 1974; West and Kemper, 1976; Salas, 1980; Schonheit, 1982). Further, the calculated value of the number of nerve terminals per nerve cell in the cerebral cortex is severely depressed to about 60% of the control level (Cragg, 1972). This observation indicates a severe interference with the development of neuronal connectivity.

Alterations in the packing density of neurones (Horn, 1955) and synapse number per unit area (Dyson and Jones, 1976) during undernutrition were found to be reversed by nutritional rehabilitation, and other studies have confirmed that the number of synapses per cortical neurone can be restored to normal by rehabilitating 30 day old undernourished animals for 130 days (Bedi et al, 1980). It may be that the effect of previous undernutrition is to reduce the extent of normal elimination of otherwise redundant synapses, allowing restoration of the control synapse to neurone ratio.

It is now clear that nutritional rehabilitation may reverse neuropil changes induced by undernutrition. A reduction in synapse to nerve cell ratio in visual and frontal cortex was found not only to disappear (Bedi et al, 1980b), but even to show a reversal or rehabilitation overshoot (Warren and Bedi, 1984). A similar finding was obtained for the hippocampal dentate gyrus (Ahmed et al, 1987), a brain region susceptible to impairment of postnatal cell acquisition and believed to be important in spatial memory function. Thus, there is accumulating evidence that even severe changes in neural network formation induced by undernutrition appear to be potentially reversible with time and full dietary intake. The reversibility of the reduced or retarded forebrain axonal growth implicit in the findings of several authors (Sima and Sourander, 1974; Lai and Lewis, 1980), is probable in view of this evidence and may ultimately be complete. Synaptic development in the occipital cortex in protein-deprived and rehabilitated rats has been investigated in detail using quantitative ultrastructural techniques (Dyson and Jones, 1976; Jones and Dyson, 1981). The findings suggested altered functional development in the undernourished cortex. Adaptive changes occurred in conditions of nutritional restriction, and near-control status was ultimately reached with subsequent dietary rehabilitation.

It was noted earlier that undernutrition interfered with cell proliferation in the developing brain. Although effects on nerve cells in the forebrain due to restricted cell acquisition appear small and limited to regions with prolonged neurogenesis, such as the hippocampus and presumably the olfactory lobes, this is not the case with the cerebellum. Here, a large fraction of the total nerve cell population is acquired in the early postnatal period, and nutritional deficit may have repercussions on cellular composition and organisation.

Purkinje cells, formed exclusively before birth, may be affected by undernutrition. Dobbing, Hopewell and Lynch (1971) reported a mean decrease of about 20% in Purkinje cell numbers and a 12% reduction in the ratio of granule to Purkinje cells in the vermis of undernourished rats. Barnes and Altman (1973b) observed a persistent deficit in Purkinje cells over the period from 30 to 120 days in animals rehabilitated after severe gestational-lactational undernutrition. At 120 days the deficit was only 12% and the granule cel\Purkinje cell ratio was normal. Milder undernutrition has no influence on the final number of Purkinje cells. Clos et al (1971) observed no change in Purkinje cell numbers at 35 days in severely undernourished rats, while McConnell and Berry (1978a & b) also found no marked effect on Purkinje cell numbers, there being a 24% increase in numerical density at 30 days and no change in this measure in rats rehabilitated to 80 days. The other cerebellar neurones for which estimates from several laboratories are available are the granule cells. These are the most abundant and the only excitatory interneurones in the cerebellar cortex, and about half their total number is generated after 10 days of age.

All observations (Dobbing, Hopewell and Lynch, 1971; Barnes and Altman, 1973; Clos et al , 1977; McConnell and Berry, 1978b; Bedi et al, 1980b) have showing that undernutrition decreases granule cell numbers, with a degree of recovery occurring with rehabilitation after weaning, possibly due to the persistence of the EGL in the cerebellum of undernourished rats (Rebiere and Legrand, 1972; Lewis et al, 1975). Such restoration is incomplete, for rehabilitation fails to reverse a 25-30% deficit in estimated total granule cell number (McConnell and Berry, 1978) or a comparable deficit in granule to Purkinje cell ratio (Bedi et al, 1980). Undernutrition has no significant effect on the number of either the perinatally formed Golgi cells or the stellate cells ("birthday" in the second week of life), in contrast to a marked deficit, about 35%, in the number of basket cells, formed in the first postnatal week (Clos et al, 1977).

Undernutrition has only a minor adverse influence on the development of neuronal circuits in the cerebellum. The maturation of Purkinje cells is somewhat delayed (Rebière and Legrand, 1972). Some observations have suggested that in previously undernourished animals, the Purkinje cell domain, a measure of dendritic arborization, is grossly unaffected (Neville and Chase, 1971; Barnes and Altman, 1973). However, at 30 days the area of the molecular layer is markedly reduced; since the dendritic tree of the Purkinje cells and the ascending and descending vertical dendrites of the basket cells extend across the entire thicknesss of this layer, these structures are reduced in proportion to the decrease in its width. The length of the dendrites of the granule cells and the oblique branches of the basket cells are also reduced, but the number of the granule cell dendrites is normal (West and Kemper, 1976). McConnell and Berry (1978a) observed that while the overall size of the Purkinje cell dendritic tree is depressed, it develops as in controls by terminal branching with only minor deviation from the usual purely random branching pattern. These authors looked at the reversibility of undernutrition effects on Purkinje cell dendritic growth. Nutritional rehabilitation, implemented at days 10 and 15, completely restored to normal both the Purkinje cell network size and granule cell numbers, but in animals fed ad libitum after day 20 deficits in both estimates persisted. The topology of the dendritic network after rehabilitation was different from controls (McConnell and Berry, 1978a and b; 1981).

Electron microscopy has been of limited value in identifying changes in neuronal circuits in the undernourished brain. However, quantitative ultrastructural studies have revealed a 30% reduction of synapse to neurone ratio in the internal granular layer at 30 days, an effect that disappears with prolonged rehabilitation (Bedi et al, 1980a).

Positive as well as negative structural on neurones and neuronal circuits may be seen in the undernourished brain. Thus Cravioto, Hambraeus and Vahlquist (1974) observed a persistent 75% increase in synaptic density in the midbrain reticular formation of previously undernourished mice. It was suggested that the morphological changes might be the structural correlates of the functional alterations in arousal previously observed in undernourished and rehabilitated animals (Dobbing and Smart, 1973; Randt and Derby, 1973). Studies reported by Diaz-Cintra et al (1981) also raise the possibility that the effect of undernutrition is not always manifested as retarded development of nerve cells. In the nucleus raphe dorsalis of protein restricted animals there was a general lag in the linear development of secondary dendrites and absence of a normal transient increase in synaptic spines on primary and secondary dendrites of the nerve cells, suggesting a curtailment of the normal process of elimination of redundant synapses.

Effects of undernutrition on neuroglia and myelin

A number of studies have shown effects of undernutrition on glia within the brain. Bass, Netsky and Young (1970a and b) reported that both the formation of glial cells and their migration to the cerebral cortex were severely retarded, producing decreased numbers of mature oligodendroglia and poorly stained myelin. Dobbing, Hopewell and Lynch (1971) also observed a significant reduction in glial cell numbers throughout the cerebral cortex of undernourished rats rehabilitated after weaning. Quantitative histological studies on cerebral cortex of rats undernourished to 35 days of age have shown that the deficit in total number of neurones is only about 10% while that of glial cells is approximately 40%, glial cell size also being reduced (Clos et al, 1977).

Undernutrition may have different effects on the various neuroglial subpopulations. In rats and mice the formation of astrocytes begins in late fetal life and precedes that of oligodendroglia, the generation of which only gets under way towards the end of the first week after birth (Skoff, Price and Stocks, 1976; Lewis et al, 1977a). Undernutrition, unless it is so severe as to interfere with the survival of both fetus and mother, will have its main effect on cell proliferation in the early postnatal period and after a significant proportion of the astrocyte subpopulation has been acquired. The studies of Sturrock, Smart and Dobbing (1976; 1977) showed a reduction in the number of oligodendroglia in the white matter of mice undernourished during the suckling period and subsequently rehabilitated, without diminution of astrocyte numbers in a grey region. Robain and Ponsot (1978) examined the neuroglial population both in spinal cord and in brain. They found impairment of glial development in undernourished rats. Glial proliferation and cell number were reduced by 50% in cuneate and gracile tracts at day 10. A similar reduction was found in glial density in the corpus callosum at day 19. Maturation of neuroglia was also markedly affected. In general abnormalities and deficiencies in myelination were more prominent in regions which mature relatively late, such as the corpus callosum.

Retarded myelination was also indicated by the reduction in the calibre of the spinal tracts. Lai, Lewis and Patel (1980) confirmed effects on the maturation of corpus callosal neuroglia, oligodendrocytes showing major changes. At day 15 the proportion of astroglia relative to oligodendroglia was increased in undernourished rats, indicating a delay in the acquisition of the later developing cells. The differentiation of oligodendroglia was retarded. Clos et al also showed impaired maturation of oligodendrocytes in undernourished cerebellum up to 40 days. In contrast, the early morphological stages of the maturation of Bergmann astocytes were advanced in undernutrition, but the cells stayed in an intermediate stage of differentiation longer than controls (Clos, Legrand and Legrand, 1979).

Retardation of proliferation and maturation of oligodendroglia partly explains the vulnerability of myelination in the brain to nutritional deficiency. That undernutrition affected myelin products was originally inferred from studies on the cholesterol content of the brain (Dobbing, 1964). Fishman, Madyastha and Prensky (1971) isolated myelin and reported that in 21 and 53 day old undernourished animals its weight was respectively 87% and 71% of that obtained from control brains. Morphological investigations confirm that neonatal undernutrition results in retarded myelination. The observations of Clos and Legrand (1969; 1970) suggest that myelination is defective; in 12 day old undernourished rats the normal relationship between axon diameter and number of myelin lamellae deposited is distorted and in peripheral nerve, Schwann cell differentiation is impaired ultrastructurally. Hedley-Whyte (1973) confirmed that in the sciatic nerve undernutrition during the suckling period slowed down the acquisition of myelin sheath more than it retarded axonal expansion, but she did not observe structural abnormalities in Schwann cells. She also noticed that the effect of food deprivation limited to the early part of the suckling period was reversed after three weeks of rehabilitation, but effects brought about by prolonging undernutrition were only partially reversed by optimal feeding up to 46 days of age.

Sturrock, Smart and Dobbing (1976) studied the effect of neonatal undernutrition on mouse anterior commissure after 19 weeks of rehabilitation and observed a normal relationship between axon diameter and number of myelin lamellae. A detailed light and electron microscopic study by Lai and Lewis (1980) produced further findings on axon-myelin sheath relationships in undernutrition. In the corpus callosum, the percentage of axons myelinated at 15, 21 and 48 days in undernourished rats was lower than in controls. The number of lamellae constituting the myelin sheath was also reduced at 15 and 21 days, but at 48 days no difference was evident between control and experimental groups, suggesting that a catch-up in myelination had occurred. A linear relationship between myelin sheath thickness and axonal diameter was observed in both groups of animals; however, a long-term effect on axonal growth was suggested by the observation that in 48 day old undernourished animals axonal diameter was reduced relative to myelin sheath thickness. The major effect of undernutrition in fibre tracts nevertheless seems to be retardation in myelination. Myelin initiation appears normal, yet the progress of myelination is so impeded that at 30 days promyelinating fibres are increased fifteen fold in pyramidal tracts. Wiggins and colleagues (1984, 1985, 1986) have confirmed that undernutrition retards the acquisition of myelin lamellae in optic nerve, corpus callosum and pyramidal tracts, an effect which is probably incompletely removed with time and nutritional rehabilitation.

Conclusions

Although undernutrition during development produces a vast array of neuroanatomical changes, evidence accumulating over the past decade points encouragingly to the reversibility of many of these. The present state of knowledge suggests that irreversible neuropathological alterations due to early undernutrition are few, and restricted to deficits in cell number in brain regions where neurogenesis is prolonged. Lasting alterations have been detected in the undernutrition are few, and restricted to deficits in cell number in brain regions where neurogenesis is prolonged. Lasting alterations have been detected in the neuronal composition of such regions where normal connections of nerve cells may be affected. Although restitution of synapse: neuron ratio is seen with subsequent rehabilitation, it may well be a functionally important fact that the number of synapses per nerve cell appears significantly depressed in the cerebral cortex during postnatal undernutrition. This suggests that undernutrition imposes a limitation on the complexity of neuronal circuits, and thus of the functional capabilities of the brain. Neuroglial cells also seem to be sensitive to nutritional deficiency during development, and impairment of the capacity of oligodendrocytes to myelinate normally may be a factor of functional significance as well as one contributing to permanent reduction in brain weight.

REFERENCES

Ahmed MGE, Bedi KS, Warren MA, Kamel MM (1987). Effect of a lengthy period of undernutrition from birth and subsequent nutritional rehabilitation on the synapse: granule cell neuron ratio in the rat dentate gyrus. J Com. Neurol 263:146-158.

Altman J, (1969). DNA metabolism and cell proliferation. In Lajtha A (ed): "Handbook of Neurochemistry", New York: Plenum Press, Vol 2, pp 137-182,

Altman J, Das GD, Sudarshan K, Anderson JB (1971). The influence of nutrition on neural and behavioral development. II. Growth of body and brain in infant rats using different techniques of undernutrition. Dev Psychobiol 4:55-70.

Balázs R, Jordan T, Lewis PD, Patel AJ (1986). Undernutrition and brain development. In Falkner F, Tanner JM (eds): "Human Growth", second edition. New York: Plenum Press, Vol 3, pp 415-473, .

Barnes D, Altman J (1973a). Effects of different schedules of early undernutrition on the preweaning growth of the rat cerebellum. Exp Neurol 38:406-409.

Barnes D, Altman J, (1973b). Effects of two levels of gestational-lactational undernutrition on the postweaning growth of the rat cerebellum. Exp Neurol 38: 420-428.

Bass NH, Netsky MG, Young E (1970a). Effect of neonatal malnutrition on developing cerebrum. I. Microchemical and histologic study of cellular differentiation in the rat. Arch Neurol 23:289-302.

Bass NH, Netsky MG , Young E (1970b). Effect of neonatal malnutrition on developing cerebrum. II. Microchemical and histologic study of myelin formation in the rat. Arch Neurol 23:303-313.

Bedi KS, Warren MA (1983). The effects of undernutrition during early life on the rat optic fibre number and size-frequency distribution. J Comp Neurol 219: 125-132.

Bedi KS, Thomas YM, Davies CA, Dobbing J (1980a). Synapse to neuron ratios of the frontal and cerebellar cortex of 30 day old and adult rats undernourished during early postnatal life. J Comp Neurol 193:49-56.

Bedi KS, Hall R, Davies CA, Dobbing J (1980b). A stereological analysis of the cerebellar granule and Purkinje cells of 30 day old and adult rats undernourished during early postnatal life. J Comp Neurol 193:863-870.

Benton JW, Moser HW, Dodge PR, Carr S (1966). Modification of the schedule of myelination in the rat by early nutritional deprivation. Pediatrics 38:801-807.

Brown RE (1966). Organ weight in malnutrition with special reference to brain weight, Dev Med Child Neurol 8:512-522.

Cleaver JE (1967). Thymidine Metabolism and Cell Kinetics, North-Holland, Amsterdam.

Clos J, Rebière A, Legrand J (1973). Differential effects of hypothyroidism and undernutrition on the development of glia in the rat cerebellum, Brain Res 63:445-449.

Clos J, Favre C, Selme-Matrat M, Legrand J (1977). Effects of undernutrition on cell formation in the rat brain and specially on cellular composition of the cerebellum. Brain Res 123:13-26.

Clos J, Legrand C, Legrand J (1979). Early effects of undernutrition on the development of cerebellar Bergmann glia. Ann Biol Anim Biochim Biophys 19:167-172.

Clos J, Legrand MC, Legrand J, Ghandour MS, Labourdette G, Vincendon G, Gombos G (1982a). Effects of thyroid state and undernutrition on S100 protein and astroglia development in rat cerebellum. Dev Neurosci 5:285-292.

Clos J, Legrand J, Limozin N, Dalmasso C, Laurent G (1982b). Effects of abnormal thyroid state and undernutrition on carbonic anhydrase and oligodendroglia development in the rat cerebellum. Dev Neurosci 5:243-251.

Conradi NG, Muntzing K (1985). Cerebellar foliation in rats. 2. Effects of maternal malnutrition on the formation of fissures in female rats. Acta Path Microbiol Immunol Scand A 93:391-395.

Cragg BG (1972). The development of cortical synapses during starvation in the rat. Brain 95:143-150.

Cravioto J, Hambraeus L, Vahlquist B (1974). "Early Malnutrition and Mental Development". Uppsala: Almqvist & Wiksell.

Cravioto HM, Randt CT, Derby BM, Diaz, A (1976). A quantitative ultrastructural study of synapses in the brains of mice following early life undernutrition. Brain Res 118:304- 306.

Creps ES (1974). Time of neuron origin in preoptic and septal areas of the mouse: An autoradiographic study. J Comp Neurol 157:161-243.

Deo MG, Bijlani V, Ramalingaswami V (1975). Nutrition and cellular growth and differentiation. In Brazier MAB (ed): "Growth and Development of the Brain" IBRO Monograph Series, Vol 1, New York: Raven Press, pp 1-6.

Diaz-Cintra S, Cintra L, Kemper T, Resnick O, Morgane PJ (1981). The effects of protein deprivation on the nucleus raphe dorsalis: A morphometric Golgi study in rats of three age groups. Brain Res 221:243-255.

Dobbing J (1974). The later development of the brain and its vulnerability. In Davies JA, Dobbing J (eds): "Scientific Foundations of Pediatrics", London: Heinemann, pp 565-577

Dobbing J, Sands J (1973). The quantitative growth and development of human brain. Arch Dis Child 48: 757-767.

Dobbing J, Smart JL, (1973). Early undernutrition, brain development and behaviour. In Barnet SA (ed): "Ethology and Development." London: Heinemann pp 16-37.

Dobbing J, Smart JL (1974). Vulnerability of developing brain and behaviour. Br Med Bull 30:164-168.

Dobbing J, Hopewell JW, Lynch A (1971). Vulnerability of developing brain: VII. Permanent deficit of neurons in cerebral and cerebellar cortex following early mild undernutrition. Exp Neurol 32: 439-447.

Dodge PR, Prensky AL, Feigin RD (1975). "Nutrition and the Developing Nervous System". St. Louis: Mosby.

Dyson SE, Jones DG (1976). Some effects undernutrition of synaptic development - A quantitative ultrastructural study. Brain Res 114:365-378.

Eayrs JT, Horn G (1955). The development of cerebral cortex in hypothyroid and starved rats. Anat Rec 121:53-61.

Escobar A (1974). Cytoarchitectonic derangement in the cerebral cortex of the undernourished rat. In Cravioto J, Hambraeus L, Vahlquist B (eds): "Early Malnutrition and Mental Development". Uppsala: Almquist & Wiksell, pp 55-59

Fishman MA, Madyastha P, Prensky AL, (1971). The effect of undernutrition on the development of myelin in the rat central nervous system. Lipids 6:458-465.

Gadsdon DR, Emery JL(1976). Some quantitative morphological aspects of post-natal human cerebellar growth. J Neurol Sci 29:137-148.

Gambetti P, Autilio-Gambetti L, Rizzzuto N, Shafer B, Pfaff, L (1974) Synapses and malnutrition: Quantitative ultrastructural study of rat cerebral cortex. Exp Neurol 43:464-473.

Gopinath G, Bijlani V, Deo MG (1976). Undernutrition and the developing cerebellar cortex in the rat. J Neuropathol Exp Neurol 35:125-135.

Haas RJ, Werner J, Fliedner TM (1970). Cytokinetics of neonatal brain cell development in rats as studied by the "complete 3H-thymidine labelling" method. J Anat 107:421-437.

Hammer RPJr (1981). The influence of pre- and postnatal undernutrition on the developing brain stem reticular core: A quantitative Golgi study. Dev Brain Res 1:191-201.

Hedley-Whyte ET(1973). Myelination of rat sciatic nerve: Comparison of undernutrition and cholesterol biosynthesis inhibition. J Neuropathol Exp Neurol 32:284-302.

Horn G (1955). Thyroid deficiency and inanition: The effects of replacement therapy on the development of the cerebral cortex of young albino rats. Anat Rec 121:63-79.

Howard E (1965). Effects of corticosterone and food restriction on growth and on DNA, RNA and cholesterol contents of the brain and liver in infant mice. J Neurochem 12:181-191.

Johnson JE, Yoesle RA (1975) The effects of malnutrition on the developing brain stem of the rat: A preliminary experiment using the lateral vestibular nuclei. Brain Res 89:170-174.

Jones DG, Dyson SE (1976). Synaptic junctions in undernourished rat brain - An ultrastructural investigation. Exp Neurol 51:529-535.

Jones DG, Dyson SE (1981). Influence of protein restriction, rehabilitation and changing nutritional states on synaptic development: A quantitative study in rat brain. Brain Res 208:97-112.

Jordan TC , Howells KF, McNaughton N, Heatlie PL (1982). Effects of early undernutrition on hippocampal development and function. Res Exp Med (Berlin) 180:201-207.

Kaplan MS, Hinds JW (1977). Neurogenesis in the adult rat: Electron microscopic analysis of light radioautographs. Science 197:1092-1094.

Katz HB, Davies CA(1982) Effects of early life undernutrition and subsequent environment on morphological parameters of the brain. Behav Brain Res 5:53-64.

Koppel H, Lewis PD , Patel AJ (1983). Cell death in the external granular layer of normal and undernourished rats: further observations, including estimates of rate of cell loss. Cell Tissue Kinet 16:99-106.

Lai M , Lewis PD (1980). Effects on undernutrition on myelination in rat corpus callosum. J Comp Neurol 193:973-982.

Lai M, Lewis PD , Patel, AJ (1980). Effects of undernutrition on gliogenesis and glial maturation in rat corpus callosum. J Comp Neurol 193:965-972.

Larroche JC (1966). The development of the central nervous system during intrauterine life. In Falkner F (ed): "Human Development". Philadelphia: Saunders, pp 257-276.

Legrand J (1967). Analyse de l'action morphogénétique des hormones thyroïdiennes sur le cervelet du jeune rat. Arch Anat Microsc. Morphol Exp.56:205-244.

Leuba G, Rabinowicz T (1979). Long term effects of postnatal undernutrition and maternal malnutrition on mouse cerebral cortex, I. Cellular densities, cortical volume and total numbers of cells. Exp Brain Res 37:283-298.

Lewis PD (1968a). The fate of the subependymal cell in the adult rat brain, with a note on the origin of microglia. Brain 91:721-736.

Lewis PD (1968b). Mitotic activity in the primate subependymal layer and the genesis of gliomas. Nature (London) 217:974-975.

Lewis PD (1975). Cell death in the germinal layers of the postnatal rat brain. Neuropathol Appl Neurobiol 1:1-9.

Lewis PD (1978). The application of cell turnover studies to neuropathology. In Smith WT, Cavanag JB (eds): "Recent Advances in Neuropathology". London: Churchill Livingstone, pp 41-65.

Lewis PD, Balázs R, Patel AJ, Johnson AL (1975). The effect of undernutrition in early life on cell generation in the rat brain. Brain Res 83:235-247.

Lewis PD, Patel AJ, Balázs R (1977b). Effect of undernutrition on cell generation in the adult rat brain. Brain Res 138:511-519.

Lewis PD, Patel AJ, Balázs R (1979). Effect of undernutrition on cell generation in the rat hippocampus. Brain Res 168:186-189.

McConnell P, Berry M (1978a). The effects of undernutrition on Purkinje cell dendritic growth in the rat. J Comp Neurol 177:159-171.

McConnell P, Berry M (1978b). The effect of refeeding after neonatal starvation on Purkinje cell dendritic growth in rat. J Comp Neurol 178:759-772.

McConnell P, Berry M (1981). The effects of refeeding after varying periods of neonatal undernutrition on the morphology of Purkinje cells in the cerebellum of the rat. J Comp Neurol 200:463-479.

Morgane PJ, Miller M, Kemper T, Stern W, Forbes W, Hall R, Bronzino J, Kissane J, Hawrylewicz E, Resnick O (1978). The effects of protein malnutrition on the developing central nervous system in the rat. Neurosci Biobehav Rev 2:137-230.

Nazarevskaya GD, Savrova OB , Medvedev DI, Reznikov K Yu (1982). (Analysis of proliferation and death of cells in the subependymal and subgranular germinative brain zones of mice subjected to the effect of malnutrition in early postnatal ontogenesis). Ontogenez 13:589-595.

Neville HE, Chase HP (1971). Undernutrition and cerebellar development. Exp Neurol 33:485-497.

Patel AJ, Balázs R, Johnson AL (1973). Effect of undernutrition on cell formation in the rat brain. J Neurochem 20:1151-1165.

Prescott DM (1976). The cell cycle and the control of cellular replication. Adv Genet 18:100-177.

Randt CT , Derby BM (1973). Behavioral and brain correlations in early nutritional deprivation. Arch Neurol (Chicago) 28:167-172.

Rebière A (1973). Aspects quantitatifs de la synaptogénèse dans le cervelet du rat sous-alimente des la naissance. Comparaison avec l'animal hypothyroïdien. CR Acad Sci (Paris) 276:2317-2320.

Rebière A, Legrand J (1972). Effets comparés de la sous-alimentation, de l'hypothyroïdisme et de l'hyperthyroïdisme sur la maturation histologique de la zone moléculaire de cortex cérébelleux chez le jeune rat. Arch Anat Microsc Morphol Exp 61:105-106.

Robain O, Ponsot G (1978). Effects of undernutrition on glial maturation. Brain Res 149:379-397.

Salas M (1980). Effect of early undernutrition on dendritic spines of cortical pyramidal cells in the rat. Dev Neurosci 3:190-117.

Salas M, Diaz S, Nieto A (1974) Effects of neonatal food deprivation on cortical spines and dendritic developemnt of the rat. Brain Res 73:139-144.

Salas M, Torrero C, Pulido S (1986). Undernutrition induced by early pup separation delays the development of the thalamic reticular nucleus in rats. Exp Neurol 93:447-455.

Schonheit B (1982). Uber den Einfluss einer frühen postnatalen Mangelernährung auf die Reifung Kortikale Neurone bei der Ratte. J Hirnforsch 23:681-692.

Sharma SK, Nayar U, Maheshwari MC, Singh B (1987). Effects of undernutrition on developing rat cerebellum. Some electrophysiological and neuromorphological correlates. J Neurol Sci 78:261-272.

Siassi F, Siassi B (1973). Differential effects of protein-calorie restriction and subsequent repletion on neuronal and nonneuronal components of cerebral cortex in newborn rats. J Nutr 103:1625-1633.

Sima A, Persson L (1975). The effect of pre- and postnatal undernutrition on the development of the rat cerebellar cortex. I. Morphological observations, Neurobiology 5:23-34.

Sima A, Sourander P (1974). The effect of early undernutrition on the calibre spectrum of the rat optic nerve, Acta Neuropath. (Berlin) 28:151-160.

Skoff RP, Price DL, Stocks A (1976). Electron microscopic autoradiographic studies of gliogenesis in rat optic nerve. II. Time of origin. J Comp Neurol 169:313-333.

Smart I, Leblond CP (1961). Evidence for division and transformations of neuroglia cells in the mouse brain, as derived from radioautography after injection of thymidine-H3. J Comp Neurol 116:349-367.

Stoch MB, Smythe PM (1963). Does undernutrition during infancy inhibit brain growth and subsequent intellectual development? Arch Dis Child 38:546-552.

Stoch MB, Smythe PM (1967). The effect of undernutrition during infancy on subsequent brain growth and intellectual development. S Afr Med J 41:1027-1030.

Stoch MB, Smythe PM (1976). 15 year developmental study on effects of severe undernutrition during infancy on subsequent physical growth and intellectual functioning. Arch Dis Child 51:327-336.

Sturrock RR, Smart JL, Dobbing J (1976). Effects of undernutrition during the suckling period on growth of the anterior and posterior limbs of the mouse anterior commissure. Neuropathol Appl Neurobiol 2:411-419.

Sturrock RR, Smart JL, Dobbing J (1977). Effect of undernutrition during the suckling period on the indusium griseum and rostral part of the mouse anterior commissure. Neuropath Appl Neurobiol 3:369-375.

Sugita N (1918). Comparative studies on the growth of the cerebral cortex. VII. On the influence of starvation at an early age upon the development of the cerebral cortex. Albino rat. J Comp Neurol 29:177-240.

Trowell HC, Davies JNP, Dean, FRA. (1954). Kwashiorkor, Arnold, London.

Udani PM (1960). Neurological manifestations of kwashiorkor, Indian J Child Health 9:103-112.

Vonderhaar BK, Topper YJ (1974). A role of the cell cycle in hormone-dependent differentiation. J Cell Biol 63:707-712.

Warren MA, Bedi KS (1982). Synapse-to-neuron ratios in the visual cortex of adult rats undernourished from about birth until 100 days of age. J Comp Neurol 2 10:59-64.

Warren MA, Bedi KS (1984). A quantitative assessment of the development of synapses and neurons in the visual cortex of control and undernourished rats. J Comp Neurol 227:104-108.

West CD, Kemper TL (1976). The effect of a low protein diet on the anatomical development of the rat brain. Brain Res 107:221-237.

Wiebecke B, Heybowitz R, Lohrs U, Eder M (1969). The effect of starvation on the proliferation kinetics of the mucosa of the small and large bowel of the mouse. Virchows Arch (Cell Pathol) 4:164-175.

Wiggins RC, Fuller GN, Brizzee L, Bissel AC, Samorajski T (1984). Myelination of the rat optic nerve during postnatal undernourishment and recovery: a morphometric analysis. Brain Res 308:263-272.

Wiggins RC, Bissel AC, Durham L, Samorajski T (1985). The corpus callosum during postnatal undernourishment and recovery: a morphometric analysis of myelin and axon relationships. Brain Res 328:51-57.

Wiggins RC, Delaney AC, Samorajski T (1986). A morphometric analysis of pyramidal tracts structures during postnatal undernourishment and recovery. Brain Res 368:277-286.

Winick M (1976). Malnutrition and Brain Development, Oxford University Press, London.

Winick M, Noble A (1966). Cellular response in rats during malnutrition at various ages. J Nutr 89:300-306.

Winick M, Rosso P (1969a). The effect of severe early malnutrition on cellular growth of human brain. Pediatr Res 3:181-184.

Winick M, Rosso P (1969b). Head circumference and cellular growth of the brain in normal and marasmic children. J Pediatr 74:774-778.

Zamenhof S, van Marthens E, Grauel L (1971a). Prenatal cerebral development: Effect of restricted diet, reversal by growth hormone. Science 174:954-955.

Zamenhof S, van Marthens E, Grauel L (1971b). DNA (cell number) and protein in neonatal rat brain: Alteration by timing of maternal dietary protein restriction. J Nutr 101:1265-1270.

DISCUSSION

Q (G. Hashim): I want to ask you a very simple question. Do you think that undernutrition, as opposed to malnutrition, is something that slows brain development (but in fact) is later on (in life) reversible?

A: I am not sure. Simple questions are always in fact unanswerable, of course. You see, undernutrition may (also) be malnutrition, or not. Simply because one does not know between species what the differing dietary requirements are.

Given that protein-calorie malnutrition, in whatever form, is a constant in the disadvantaged child populations we are talking about. Also, given that by simple reduction of protein and (or?) calories in the diet of experimental animals you can bring about reproducible changes in the nervous system, I prefer to think that undernutrition is the critical issue. Whether there are selective problems that are produced through deficiencies of this or that (specific nutritional) factors, I am not in a position to say.

Q (G. Hashim): I do gather from your presentation that those early changes which you have seen during development, have proven to be reversible. I am not now referring to quantitative (DNA) reverses.

A: Reversibility implies plasticity whithin the system, for whatever reason. Whether this represents the formation of new circuits, whether it is a reduction in elimination of otherwise redundant circuits, I am not sure whether the quality of nutrition is relevant to that. As far as I can see, severe metabolic disturbances induced by undernutrition affect cell proliferation. The chronology of cell proliferation is such that it may be difficult or impossible for the brain to catch up with this. Now, the severe metabolic disturbances we are talking about also produce effects on differentiating cell populations which may have the capacity, one way or another, to restore the deficit when the metabolic disturbance is reversed.

Q (G. Hashim): Certainly this is true of oligodendrocytes. You mention that there is a reduction in myelination, and therefore brain weight, and essentially what that means is that this whole thing may be reversible. I mean, oligos can be cued to make more myelin, right?

A: Well, there are permanent problems with oligodendrocytes although they are not major problems. If their maturation is affected you may be left with axons which are of a disproportionate size, and which have got internodal myelin segments which are inappropriate to their size. I assume this will have repercussions on conduction and, therefore, on synchrony; it must have significant functional repercussions.

Q (Lajtha): Just to follow this up. If you have a low protein (5%) diet or you have normal protein and faulty metabolities, can you single out one cell population that will be particularly vulnerable?

A: I can't . Can you suggest any.

Q **(Lajtha):** I guess the most rapidly growing.
A: Perhaps those formed for the shortest period?

Q **(Scheibel):** May I ask you a question. In your experimental paradigm do you start the delay in nutrition or starvation conditions before conception? I missed that.
A: No, no, this is post-conception. It is a much used model. You want the animal to conceive, but once it has conceived you want to try to restrict the development while letting the pregnancy to continue.

Q **(Scheibel):** The reason why I ask Dr. Lewis that question: I was quite fascinated by the steadfastness with which it is the late or later, or longer, developing cell groups that are most affected and perhaps also show that they can be changed when you replace the nutrition. We have been looking at some other syndromes in the human, particularly things like schizophrenia and autism, and there it seems to be some of the very early developing cells which show the differences: hippocampal pyramidal cells and the cerebellar Purkinje cells. So (in these conditions) quite clearly (certain factors) interfere very early on in the process of neurogenesis.
A: Yes, plainly one can have timed insults throughout pregnancy. These may be viral infections or toxic exposure(s) and which can knock out, even when these (exposure) occurs over a restricted period, one of these susceptible large bodied - long axons cell populations.

(Mal)Nutrition and the Infant Brain, pages 111–125
© 1990 Wiley-Liss, Inc.

ELONGATION AND ARBORIZATION OF CNS AXONS

Sonal Jhaveri, Michael A. Edwards, Reha S. Erzurumlu, Gerald E. Schneider

Department of Brain & Cognitive Sciences, M.I.T., Cambridge, MA 02139, and Department of Developmental Neurobiology, E.K. Shriver Center, Waltham, MA 02154.

The intricate network of vast numbers of neurons in the mammalian brain is assembled in a relatively short period of time during prenatal and early postnatal life. Within this period, millions of differentiating cells elaborate axonal processes which navigate through a changing environment to arrive at terminal regions where they select specific cells on which to synapse. Accordingly, axonogenesis in developing vertebrates exhibits two major stages: **target approach** and **target invasion**. The two stages are separated by a waiting period during which axons are present in the vicinity of target zones but do not approach postsynaptic cells. Here we review studies on axon maturation within the framework of this two-stage sequence. We argue that growth characteristics of axons are qualitatively different in each stage. The susceptibility of immature cells to extrinsic influences differs significantly during the two phases.

AXON ELONGATION

Elongating Axons Follow Stereotypic Routes.

Elongating axons take the most direct routes, without significant exploratory wandering, to reach their destinations. In the Syrian hamster, retinal axons emerge from the eye on embryonic day 11 (E11) and elongate in a nearly linear path through the optic stalk and chiasm and over the surface of the diencephalon to reach the midbrain tectum (Jhaveri et al, 1983a). Anterograde HRP labeling of the developing retinofugal pathway reveals little indication of deviations from this simple, stereotypic route (see also, Reh & Kalil, 1981; Schreyer & Jones, 1982; Bunt et al. 1983; Harris et al., 1987).

The role of glia in defining pathways for elongating axons, especially those that grow subpially, has been indicated: Preformed glial channels precede the outgrowth of retinal axons into the optic stalk (Silver & Sidman, 1980) and longitudinal axons in the dorsolateral spinal cord (Nordlander & Singer, 1982). Fibers elongating along superficial routes associate closely with end-feet of radial glial cells (Silver & Rutishauser, 1984; Morris et al., 1988; Vanselow et al., 1989) whereas for deeper-running axon systems, immature astrocytes could direct elongation (Noble et al., 1984), analogous to guidepost cells used by insect pioneering axons (Caudy & Bentley, 1986). In the region of the future callosum, an astrocytic bridge develops **prior to** the arrival of crossing axons (Silver et al., 1982) and in genetically acallosal animals, artificial bridges coated with immature astrocytes provide a permissive substrate for cortical axons to cross (Silver & Ogawa, 1983).

In contrast to passive guidance along preformed pathways, recent studies have revived the classical hypothesis that elongation of axons to their targets may depend upon chemotropic cues. In *Xenopus* embryos, axons from ectopically transplanted eyes head directly for the tectum, without seeking out normal trajectories of retinotectal axons (Harris, 1986). Similarly, axons from fetal mouse retina transplanted ectopically beneath the superior colliculus (SC) of neonatal rats exhibit oriented growth toward their target (Hankin & Lund, 1987), suggesting a relatively broad distribution within the developing brain of cues that influence the direction of growth by particular CNS axons.

Elongating Axons Fasciculate

The large majority of axons elongating toward their targets grow in fascicles confined within discrete tracts. Recent tissue culture studies indicate that such homotypic fasciculation may be implemented by a contact-mediated, cell-surface recognition process. Retinal neurites fasciculate preferentially with axons of other retinal cells (Bray et al., 1980), whereas their growth cones collapse, with a concomitant cessation of motility and neurite withdrawal, upon contact with non-retinal processes (Kapfhammer & Raper, 1987)

Elongating Axons Grow At A Relatively Rapid Rate

In the hamster visual system, retinal axons grow from the chiasm (where they are present by E11.5) to the caudal end of the SC (arriving there by E13.5), having traveled a distance of approximately 4 mm in 2 days (Jhaveri et al., 1983a, Schneider et al., 1985). This rate of about 80 μm/hr is comparable to previous estimates for axon elongation *in vivo* (range, 20-80 μm/hr; Lund & Bunt, 1976; Bunt et al., 1983; Huang & Jacobson, 1986; Harris et al., 1987; Davies, 1987). Substrate adhesivity is critical in determining rates of neurite extension (rev. Letourneau, 1985), although variations in this rate may also be intrinsically determined (Davies, 1989).

Elongating Axons Show Minimal Branching

During target approach, CNS axons are thin, have relatively linear trajectories and show no major branching except for occasional forking (Morest, 1968; Schneider et al. 1985; Sachs et al., 1986; Harris et al., 1987; Morris et al., 1988; Naegele et al., 1988). Optic tract axons in embryonic hamsters exhibit only occasional short filopodial extensions from *en passant* varicosities, a morphology consistent with features of relatively rapid and direct growth (Jhaveri et al., 1983a; Schneider et al., 1985).

Axon Order Is Established During Target Approach.

A significant degree of topographic organization has been documented within the optic nerve and tract (Horder & Martin, 1978; Bunt and Horder, 1983; Walsh & Guillery, 1985; Fujisawa, 1987), within geniculocortical radiations (Nelson & LeVay, 1985), and within somatosensory tracts (Whitsel et al., 1970; Erzurumlu and Killackey, 1983). Such organization does not depend on the presence of a target (Reh et al., 1983) but may be determined by a spatiotemporal order of outgrowth (Schreyer & Jones, 1988) or selective fiber-fiber interactions (Scholes, 1979; Fujisawa, 1987; Rager et al., 1988). Although strict neighbourhood relations of individual fibers are not maintained (Williams & Rakic, 1985) the coarse global organization may be sufficient to contribute significantly to establishment of topographic connections.

Elongating Axons Are Exuberant In Their Projections.

In kittens and neonatal rodents, neurons that project contralaterally via the corpus callosum arise from large areas of neocortex which are acallosal in maturity (Innocenti, 1981; Ivy & Killackey, 1982). Occipital cortical neurons send axons to the spinal cord and cerebellum which are collaterals of corticotectal and corticopontine fibers; as the animal develops, only projections to the colliculus and the pontine gray are maintained (Stanfield & O'Leary, 1985). Retinal axons in neonatal rodents project over the inferior colliculus and caudally as far as the cerebellar peduncle; over time, the "anomalous" axons are withdrawn (Frost, 1984; Edwards et al., 1986b). These examples have some common characteristics: the projections are not random but are directed along restricted pathways, they involve axons which approach but do not invade targets, and they are removed by a process of collateral elimination rather than cell death (O'Leary et al., 1981; Schneider et al., 1987).

Why elongating axons should have exuberant projections remains a mystery. The transience may represent a recapitulation of the evolutionary history of the species in which they occur (Ebbesson, 1984), or it could reflect a developmental strategy employed by the growing axon: inappropriate signals from incorrect targets may influence the forging of regionally specific neuronal projections.

THE WAITING PERIOD

Growing afferents do not immediately commence arborization upon arriving at the target but remain at the target threshold for some time before invading terminal regions and selecting postsynaptic partners. This pre-invasion stage has been referred to as the waiting period (Lund & Mustari, 1977; Rakic, 1977; Distel & Holländer, 1980; Schreyer & Jones, 1982; Shatz & Luskin, 1986; O'Leary & Terashima, 1988). In the hamster, retinal axons grow past the lateral geniculate body on E13, but do not send collaterals into the nucleus for another three days (Jhaveri et al., 1983a; Schneider et al., 1985). Further caudally the early retinofugal axons do not form a well-defined "tract" outside the SC, but course within the undifferentiated superficial gray and optic fiber layers. Yet, terminal ramification is delayed for 3 days after the first wave of retinal axons reach the tectum (see Edwards et al., 1986b; Sachs et al., 1986; rev., Schneider et al., 1987). That axons can form some synapses immediately upon arrival at their targets (e.g. McGraw & McLaughlin, 1980; Shatz & Kirkwood, 1984) does not contradict the generality of the phenomenon of a delay between stages of axon elongation and arborization.

It is unclear whether this delay reflects maturational processes within afferent neurons or within the target. In some systems, the end of the waiting period coincides with the completion of target neuron migration (Morest, 1968; Rakic, 1977; Jhaveri et al., 1983b; Edwards et al., 1986a; Shatz & Luskin, 1986). In the cat geniculocortical system, the waiting period involves establishment of primitive connectivity with a population of transient neurons in the intermediate zone under the cortical plate (Chun et al., 1987). Arguments for a dominant role of target maturation, however, are weakened by evidence of waiting periods in the development of **later-arriving** axon populations: Corticotectal fibers arrive in the hamster SC on P5, after retinotectal axons begin to elaborate terminal arbors and establish a topographically ordered projection; yet they wait for three more days in the optic fiber layer before entering the superficial gray layer (Ramirez et al., 1990). Advances in our understanding of molecules which regulate successive stages of growth should elucidate this issue.

AXON ARBORIZATION

Once inside the target, the task of developing axons is significantly different. Instead of rapid elongation across vast territories to reach a specific region, axons must cover shorter distances, select a group of neurons, and weave an arbor containing the appropriate cellular machinery to enable them to communicate with this subset of cells.

Arborizing Axons Have Non-Stereotyped Trajectories

It is common for certain classes of axon arbor, for example type L1 (Y-like) retinotectal afferents in rodents (Sachs & Schneider, 1984), to exhibit a convergence of several meandering collateral branches upon a focal zone of termination, suggesting a diffuse exploratory growth quite different from the pattern evident during axon elongation. Such trajectories are also commonly seen for Type R1 axons in the LGBd (unpubl. data). (Nevertheless, regularities do exist in patterns of axonal branching, suggesting that the non-stereotyped trajectories may represent a special axon class, perhaps originating from early born cells). Gierer (1987) has proposed a model to show that meandering fiber pathways may reflect the response of axons to graded distributions of guidance cues.

Arborizing Axons Are Not Fasciculated.

An obvious difference between elongating and arborizing axons is the absence of fasciculation exhibited by the latter. It is clear from tissue culture studies that axonal growth cones preferentially advance and show increased branching on substrates to which they adhere best (Letourneau, 1985). Thus, transitions from fasciculated elongation to collateral branching and target invasion might arise from an increased adhesiveness of axons for target structures rather than for each other. However, in culture, axonal branching occurs exclusively by bifurcation of a terminal growth cone; whether the same substrate influences apply to such branching as to the "interstitial" collateralization often observed *in vivo* remains to be determined (Schneider et al., 1987; O'Leary & Terashima, 1988).

Arborizing Axons Advance At A Slow Net Rate.

As noted, retinofugal fibers advance at a rate of about 80 μm/hr while approaching central target nuclei. However, once collateral branching is initiated within the LGBd the front of retinogeniculate fibers traverses the lateral-to-medial extent of the nucleus (a distance of 120 μm) at a slower rate - about 8-10 μm/hr (Jhaveri et al., 1983a). This may result from a decreased growth rate for collateralizing axons or it may reflect an increased turnover associated with cycles of extension and retraction. Observations of axons in living *Xenopus* embryos support the former possibility (Harris et al., 1987).

Axonal Arborization is Associated with Remodeling.

Regressive events which occur during axonal arborization and synaptogenesis are not characteristic of the elongation stage: early stages of terminal branching concur with the period of cell death among afferent populations (Cowan et al., 1984; Finlay & Pallas, 1989), whereas more subtle forms of remodelling are associated with sculpting of axonal ramifications as they establish topographic and laminar distributions (Shatz & Sretavan, 1986; Schneider et al., 1987). During early stages of arbor focalization, numerous short collaterals present on immature afferents are lost, along with the progressive elaboration of one or a few branches (Jhaveri & Morest, 1982; Jackson & Parks, 1982; Schneider et al., 1985; Sachs et al., 1986; Shatz & Sretavan, 1987; Naegele et al., 1988; Udin, 1989) resulting in the formation of a topographically organized map. The establishment of eye-specific lamination by retinogeniculate axons in cats is another form of selectivity implemented by loss of sprouts from inappropriate layers (Shatz & Sretavan, 1987). Cell death is also implicated in the refinement of topographic connections (Fawcett & O'Leary, 1985; Finlay & Pallas, 1989) but the degree to which axons so eliminated form arbors before cell death occurs has not been established (Edwards et al., 1986b).

Such remodelling associated with early stages of arborization is hindered in one way or another by the blockade of neural activity achieved with TTX application (Fawcett & O'Leary, 1985; Schmidt, 1985; Stryker & Harris, 1986). It is as yet unclear whether influences of neural activity are mediated via direct effects on axon growth or regression, or instead via disturbances of some form of trophic communication between axons and target cells (e.g. activity-related uptake or secretion of trophic factors).

During later stages of arborization, after significant numbers of synapses have formed, competition between adjacent axons can play an important role in shaping the mature arbor size (Hubel et al., 1977; Garraghty, et al., 1986; Shatz & Sretavan, 1986; Stryker and Harris, 1986). The pivotal role of neural activity in influencing these competitive interactions is underscored by recent studies in the visual system (rev. Udin & Fawcett, 1988), where the NMDA class of glutamate receptors has been implicated (Cline et al., 1987).

The Role of the Target Neuropil in Arbor Formation .

Examination of mature arbors in various CNS sites suggests that the form of terminal ramifications arises as a function of both intrinsic properties of the neurons of origin and extrinsic influences from the target neuropil (Mugnaini, 1970). A classic example is the cerebellar climbing fiber, the unmistakable appearance of which correlates both with its unique source from the inferior olivary complex and with the configuration of the Purkinje cell dendrites with which it intertwines. A more dominant influence from the neuropil on arbor form is seen on mossy fibers innervating the cerebellar granule cell layer: all mossy fibers have large varicosities and show a distinctive branching pattern despite their origin from diverse regions (Palay & Chan-Palay, 1974). During postnatal development in mice, individual climbing or mossy fibers may transiently form branches in the inappropriate layer, nevertheless they exhibit termination patterns characteristic of that layer (Mason & Gregory, 1984). Similarly, retinogeniculate axons in rodents are collaterals of retinotectal fibers (Dreher et al., 1985), yet optic arbors within the lateral geniculate are strikingly different from those within the superior colliculus (Sachs & Schneider, 1984; Erzurumlu et al., 1988).

MOLECULAR DIFFERENTIATION AND AXONAL GROWTH MODES

Molecular changes which might regulate the transition between the two modes of growth could theoretically involve a decreased expression of molecules which promote fasciculation, or expression of new ones which stimulate arborization.

The best candidate for a molecule involved in axon fasciculation is the set of cell adhesion molecules termed variously as NgCAM/NILE/L1/G4: its expression is virtually restricted to fasciculated axons during fetal and neonatal development, is largely lost during arborization, and is strongly implicated in axon-axon adhesion in tissue culture studies (Stallcup et al., 1985; Dodd et al., 1988; Rutishauser & Jessell, 1988). Application of antibodies against L1 to developing limb nerves induces collateral branching, suggesting that loss of its expression during normal development might promote onset of arborization (Landmesser et al.,1988).

The adhesion molecule NCAM is also present on growing axons during elongation and later is expressed at reduced levels in neuropil regions (rev.

Rutishauser & Jessell, 1988). However, a more general function for NCAM, other than just involvement in axon fasciculation, is suggested from effects of anti-NCAM antibodies applied *in vivo*: elongating axons in the chick optic stalk lose their preference for growing along radial glial endfeet (Silver & Rutishauser, 1984) and arborizing optic axons regress from antibody-treated regions of the frog tectum (Fraser et al., 1988). The presence of NCAM on elongating axons is complemented by expression of the protein on radial glial endfeet during optic axon elongation and on neuropil elements at later stages (rev. Rutishauser & Jessell, 1988).

Other molecules which have a potent influence on neurite outgrowth *in vitro*, e.g., certain proteins of the extracellular matrix and diffusible molecules from astroglial or neuronal sources (revs. Lander, 1987; Sanes, 1989) can serve as external cues to regulate growth patterns of axons. As a specific example, a laminin-like molecule is localized on the surface of radial glia early on, and on immature astrocytes of the rodent optic nerve (McLoon et al., 1986; Liesi & Silver, 1988), suggesting that it may be involved in the elongation of growing axons. However, in tissue culture, laminin is particularly potent in inducing neuritic **branching**, as opposed to axon **extension** (rev. Lander, 1987). Interestingly, another extracellular matrix protein, heparan sulfate proteoglycan, promotes unbranched neurite outgrowth (Hantaz-Ambroise et al., 1987). Both unbranched and branched patterns of neurite outgrowth from ciliary ganglion neurons have also been induced with different protein factors extracted from fetal calf muscle (Vaca et al., 1985). And finally, growth-inhibiting proteins present in the plasma membrane of oligodendrocytes (Caroni & Schwab, 1988) might act to promote nonfasciculated growth and slow the net advance of arborizing axons. The presence of such factors on oligodendrocytes in the mature CNS may be a reason why regenerating axons fail to elongate for substantial distances in the adult brain and only form short terminal branches (Aguayo, et al., 1982).

Other candidates for promotion of axonal fasciculation include F11, neurofascin (Rathjen et al., 1987) and SNAP/TAG-1 (Yamamoto et al., 1986; Dodd et al., 1988). Age-dependent changes in the responsiveness of CNS neurons to the neurite-promoting effects of laminin, reflecting changes in the expression of the extracellular matrix-binding protein integrin, have been documented *in vitro* (Hall et al., 1987; Neugebauer et al., 1988), though it is unclear to what extent such altered integrin expression would influence growth patterns at the end of the elongation period or during the arborization stage.

Finally, the membrane phosphoprotein GAP-43 has received much attention recently (rev. Benowitz & Routtenberg, 1987). In the primary visual system GAP-43 is present at high levels along the entire axon during elongation and early arborization, becomes progressively more restricted to the terminal neuropil during later stages of arbor elaboration and is negligible by the time of eye opening (Moya et al., 1989). Thus, activity-dependent down-regulation of GAP-43 is suggested. Although GAP-43 is undoubtedly involved in early stages of axon growth, its contribution may relate to membrane turnover rather than to determining patterns of growth.

Aside from membrane proteins, developmental changes in the cytoskeleton are potentially significant for regulating growth modes. Thus, the branching of cultured neurites is inhibited by treatment with taxol, a microtubule stabilizing agent (Letourneau et al., 1986), indicating that the cytoskeleton may be critically involved in the **initiation** of branch formation.

PERIODS OF VULNERABILITY DURING AXON GROWTH AND IMPLICATIONS FOR MALNUTRITION

Responses of cells to axonal damage differ markedly during the periods of axon elongation and axon arborization (rev. Schneider et al., 1987). Subsequent to optic tract transection during the elongation or waiting periods, retinal ganglion cells do not die but rather preserve the capability to regenerate across the cut (So et al., 1981). However, as arborization progresses, the trophic dependence of cells upon their targets seems to increase: later transections result in retinal ganglion cell death, which reaches a peak and then decreases again, presumably as sustaining collaterals become established (Perry & Cowey, 1982). During normal development, major influences of spontaneous neural activity are exerted on remodelling processes associated with shaping of focal end-arbors, establishment of precise topographic maps, and the segregation of axonal fields related to functional units. It is the later stages of these processes, the final elaboration of CNS circuitry, that are most influenced by sensory deprivation. Structural deficits caused by developmental undernutrition as studied in animal models, appear to be of a similar nature. Thus, reductions in numbers of synapses per neuron, dendritic spine densities, cortical thickness, and glia-to-neuron ratios measured in malnourished animals (rev. Bedi & Warren, 1988) closely resemble deficiencies produced by sensory deprivation or an "impoverished" environment during development (see Diamond, this volume). Although it is hopeful for prospects of recovery from malnutrition that drastic alterations in the developmental program are not evident, it is unfortunate that more sophisticated studies of nutritional deprivation effects on axonal morphologies and patterns of connectivity have not been undertaken. Moreover, long-range prospects for devising means to induce re-expression of growth-regulatory proteins might be relevant for interventions to facilitate recovery from undernourishment.

Acknowledgements: Supported by NIH Grants EY05504 (S.J.), EY06080 & NCH21018 (M.A.E.), EY00126 (G.E.S.).

REFERENCES

Aguayo AJ, Richardson PM, David S, Benfey M (1982). Transplantation of neurons and sheath cells - a tool for the study of regeneration. In Nicholls JG (ed): "Repair and Regeneration of the Nervous System". Berlin: Springer-Verlag, pp 94-105.
Bedi KS, Warren MA (1988). Effects of nutrition on cortical development. In Peters A, Jones EG (eds): "Development and Maturation of Cerebral Cortex". New York: Plenum, pp 441-478.

Benowitz LI, Routtenberg A (1987). A membrane phosphoprotein associated with neural development, axonal regeneration, phospholipid metabolism, and synaptic plasticity. Trends Neurosci 10:527-532.

Bray D, Wood P, Bunge RP (1980). Selective fasciculation of nerve fibers in culture. Exp Cell Res 130:241-25.

Bunt SM, Horder TJ (1983). Evidence for an orderly arrangement of optic axons within the optic nerve of the major non-mammalian vertebrate classes. J Comp Neurol 213:94-114.

Bunt SM, Lund RD, Land PW (1983). Prenatal development of the optic projection in albino and hooded rats. Dev Brain Res 6:149-168.

Caroni P, Schwab ME (1988). Two membrane protein fractions from rat central myelin with inhibitory properties for neurite growth and fibroblast spreading. J Cell Biol 106:1281-1288.

Caudy M, Bentley D (1986). Pioneer growth cone steering along a series of neuronal and non-neuronal cues of different affinities. J Neurosci 6:1781-1795.

Chun JJM, Nakamura MJ, Shatz CJ (1987). Transient cells of the developing mammalian telencephalon are peptide immunoreactive neurons. Nature 325:617-620.

Cline HT, Debski EA, Constantine-Paton M (1987). N-methyl-D-aspartate receptor antagonist desegregates eye-specific stripes. Proc Nat Acad Sci 84:4342-4345.

Cowan WM, Fawcett JW, O'Leary DDM, Stanfield BB (1984). Regressive events in neurogenesis. Science 225:1258-1265.

Davies AM, (1987). The growth rate of sensory nerve fibres in the mammalian embryo. Development 100 307-311.

Davies AM (1989). Intrinsic differences in the growth rate of early nerve fibres related to target distance. Nature 337:553-555.

Distel H, Holländer H (1980). Autoradiographic tracing of developing subcortical projections of the occipital region in fetal rabbits. J Comp Neurol 192:505-518.

Dodd J, Morton SB, Karagogeos D, Yamamoto M, Jessell TM (1988). Spatial regulation of axonal glycoprotein expression on subsets of embryonic spinal neurons. Neuron 1 105-116.

Dreher B, Sefton AJ, Ni SYK, Nisbett, G (1985). The morphology, number, distribution and central projections of class I retinal ganglion cells in albino and hooded rats. Brain, Behav Evol 26:10-48.

Edwards MA, Caviness VS Jr, Schneider GE (1986a). Development of cell and fiber lamination in the mouse superior colliculus. J Comp Neurol 248:395-409.

Edwards MA, Schneider GE, Caviness VS Jr (1986b). Development of the crossed retinocollicular projection in the mouse. J Comp Neurol 248:410-421.

Ebbesson SOE (1984). Evolution and ontogeny of neural circuits. Behav Brain Sci 7:321-366.

Erzurumlu RS, Killackey HP (1983). Development of order in the rat trigeminal system. J Comp Neurol 213:365-380.

Erzurumlu RS, Jhaveri S, Schneider GE (1988). Distribution of morphologically different retinal axon terminals in the hamster dorsal lateral geniculate nucleus. Brain Res 461:175-181.

Fawcett JW and O'Leary DDM (1985) The role of electrical activity in the formation of topographic maps in the nervous system. TINS 8:201-206.

Finlay BL, Pallas SL (1989). Control of cell number in the developing mammalian visual system. Prog Neurobiol 32:207-234.

Fraser SE, Carhart MS, Murray BA, Chuong C-M, Edelman GM (1988). Alterations in the Xenopus retinotectal projection by antibodies to Xenopus N-CAM. Devel Biol 129:217-230.

Frost DO (1984). Axonal growth and target selection during development:retinal projections to the ventrobasal complex and other 'nonvisual' structures in neonatal Syrian hamsters. J Comp Neurol 230:575-592.

Fujisawa H (1987). Mode of growth of retinal axons within the tectum of Xenopus tadpoles, and implications in the ordered neuronal connection between the retina and the tectum. J Comp Neurol 260:127-139.

Garraghty PE, Sur M, Sherman SM (1986). Role of competitive interactions in the postnatal development of X and Y retinogeniculate axons. J Comp Neurol 251:216-239.

Gierer A (1987). Directional cues for growing axons forming the retinotectal projection. Development 101:479-489.

Hall DE, Neugebauer KM, Reichardt LF (1987). Embryonic neural retinal cell response to extracellular matrix proteins: developmental changes and effects of the cell substratum attachment antibody (CSAT). J Cell Biol 104:623-634.

Hankin MH, Lund RD (1987). Role of the target in directing the outgrowth of retinal axons: transplants reveal surface-related and surface-independent cues. J Comp Neurol 263:455-466.

Hantaz-Ambroise D, Vigny M, Koenig J (1987). Heparan sulfate proteoglycan and laminin mediate two different types of neurite outgrowth. J Neurosci 7:2293-2304.

Harris WA (1986). Homing behaviour of axons in the embryonic vertebrate brain. Nature 320:266-269.

Harris WA, Holt CE, Bonhoeffer F (1987). Retinal axons with and without their somata, growing to and arborizing in the tectum of Xenopus embryos: A time-lapse video study of single fibres in vivo. Development 101:123-133.

Horder TJ, Martin KAC (1978). Morphogenetics as an alternative to chemospecificity in the formation of nerve connections. In Curtis ASG: (ed) Cell-cell Recognition, Soc Exp Biol Symp 32: pp 275-358.

Huang S, Jacobson M (1986). Neurites show pathway specificity but lack directional specificity or predetermined lengths in Xenopus embryos. J Neurobiol 17:593-604.

Hubel DH, Wiesel TN, LeVay S, (1977). Plasticity of ocular dominance columns in monkey striate cortex. Phil Trans R Soc Lond B 278:377-409.

Innocenti G (1981). Growth and reshaping of axons in the establishment of visual callosal connections. Science 212:824-827.

Ivy GO, Killackey HP (1982). Ontogenetic changes in the projection of neocortical neurons. J Neurosci 2:735-743.

Jackson H, Parks TN (1982). Functional synapse elimination in the developing avian cochlear nucleus with simultaneous reduction in cochlear nerve axon branching. J Neurosci 12:1736-1743.

Jhaveri S, Edwards MA, Schneider GE (1983a). Two stages of growth during development of the hamster's optic tract. Anat Rec 205: 225.

Jhaveri S, Edwards MA, Schneider GE (1983b). Relationship of lateral geniculate neuron migration to stages of optic tract growth in the hamster. Soc Neurosci Abs 9: 702.

Jhaveri S, Morest DKM (1984). Sequential alterations of neuronal architecture in nucleus magnocellularis of the developing chicken: a Golgi study. Neuroscience 7:837-853.

Kapfhammer JP, Raper JA (1987). Collapse of growth cone structure on contact with specific neurites in culture. J Neurosci 7:201-212.

Lander AD (1987). Molecules that make axons grow. Molec Neurobiol 1: 213-245.

Landmesser L, Dahm L, Schultz K, Rutishauser U (1988). Distinct roles for adhesion molecules during innervation of embryonic chick muscle. Devel Biol 130:645-670.

Letourneau PC (1985). Axonal growth and guidance. In Edelman GM, Gall WE, Cowan WM (eds): "Molecular Bases of Neural Development". New York: Wiley, pp 269-294.

Letourneau PC, Shattuck TA, Ressler AH (1986). Branching of sensory and sympathetic neurites in vitro is inhibited by treatment with taxol. J Neurosci 6:1912-1917.

Liesi P, Silver J (1988). Is astrocyte laminin involved in axon guidance in the mammalian CNS? Devel Biol 130:774-785.

Lund RD, Bunt AH (1976). Prenatal development of the central optic pathways in the albino rats. J Comp Neurol 165:247-274.

Lund RD, Mustari MJ (1977). Development of the geniculo cortical pathway in rats. J Comp Neurol 173:289-306.

Mason CA, Gregory E (1984). Postnatal maturation of cerebellar mossy and climbing fibers: transient expression of dual features on single axons. J Neurosci 4:1715-1735.

McGraw CF, McLaughlin BJ (1980). Fine structural studies of synaptogenesis in the superficial layers of the chick optic tectum. J Neurocytol 9:79-93.

McLoon SC, McLoon LK, Palm SL, Furcht LT (1986). Transient expression of laminin in the optic nerve of the developing rat. J Neurosci 8: 1990.

Morest DK, (1968). The growth of synaptic endings in the mammalian brain: A study of the calyces of the trapezooid body. Z fur Anat Entw 127:201-220.

Morris RJ, Beech JN, Heizmann CW (1988). Two distinct phases and mechanisms of axonal growth shown by primary vestibular fibres in the brain, demonstrated by parvalbumin immunohistochemistry. Neurosci 27:571-596.

Moya KL, Jhaveri S, Schneider GE, Benowitz LI (1989). Immunohistochemical localization of GAP-43 in the developing hamster retinofugal pathway. J Comp Neurol 288:51-58.

Mugnaini E (1970). Neurones as synaptic targets. In Anderson P, Jansen JKS (eds): "Excitatory synaptic mechanisms". Oslo: Universitesvorlatget, 146-169.

Naegele JR, Jhaveri S, Schneider GE (1988). Sharpening of topographical projections and maturation of geniculocortical axon arbors in the hamster. J Comp Neurol 277:593-607.

Nelson SB, LeVay S. (1985). Topographic organization of the optic radiation of the cat. J Comp Neurol 240:322-330.

Neugebauer KM, Tomaselli KJ, Lilien J, Reichardt LF (1988). N-cadherin, NCAM, and integrins promote retinal neurite outgrowth on astrocytes in vitro . J Cell Biol 107:1177-1187.

Noble M, Fok-Seang J, Cohen J (1984). Glia are a unique substrate for the in vitro growth of central nervous system neurons. J Neurosci 4:1892-1903.

Nordlander RH, Singer M (1982). Spaces precede axons in Xenopus embryonic spinal cord. Exp Neurol 75:221-228.

O'Leary DDM, Stanfield BB, Cowan WM (1981). Evidence that the early postnatal restriction of the cells of origin of the callosal projection is due to the elimination of axonal collaterals rather than to the death of neurons. Dev Brain Res 1:607-617.

O'Leary DDM, Terashima T (1988). Cortical axons branch to multiple subcortical targets by interstitial axon budding: Implications for target recognition and 'waiting periods'. Neuron 1:901-910.

Palay SL, Chan-Palay V (1974). "Cerebellar Cortex: Cytology and organization" Berlin: Springer.

Perry VH, Cowey A (1982). A sensitive period for ganglion cell degeneration and the formation of aberrant retinofugal connections following tectal lesions in rats. Neurosci 7:583-594.

Rager U, Rager G, Kabiersch A (1988). Transformations of the retinal topography along the visual pathway of the chicken. Anat Embryol 179:135-148.

Rakic P (1977). Prenatal development of the visual system in rhesus monkey. Phil Trans Roy Soc Lond B 278:245-260.

Ramirez JJ, Jhaveri S, Hahm J-O, Schneider GE (1990). Maturation of projections from occipital cortex to the ventral lateral geniculate and superior colliculus in postnatal hamsters. Dev. Brain Res. - in press.

Rathjen FG, Wolff JM, Frank R, Bonhoeffer F, Rutishauser U (1987). Membrane glycoproteins involved in neurite fasciculation. J Cell Biol 104:343-353.

Reh T, Kalil K (1981). Development of the pyramidal tract in the hamster. I. A light microscopic study. J Comp Neurol 200:55-67.

Reh TA, Pitts E, Constantine-Paton M (1983). The organization of fibers in the optic nerve of normal and tectumless Rana pipiens. J Comp Neurol 218:282-296.

Rutishauser U, Jessell TM (1988). Cell adhesion molecules in vertebrate neural development. Physiol Rev 68 819-857.

Sachs GM, Jacobson M, Caviness VS Jr (1986). Postnatal changes in the pattern of arborization of murine retinocollicular axons. J Comp Neurol 246: 395-408.

Sachs GM, Schneider GE (1984). Morphology of optic tract axons arborizing in the superior colliculus of the hamster. J Comp Neurol 230:155-167.

Sanes JR (1989). Extracellular matrix molecules that influence neural development. Ann Rev Neurosci 12:491-516.

Schmidt JT (1985). Formation of retinotopic connections: Selective stabilization by an activity-dependent mechanism. Cell Molec Neurobiol 5:65-84.

Schneider GE, Jhaveri S, Edwards MA, So K-F (1985) Regeneration, rerouting and redistribution of axons after early lesions: changes with age and functional impact. In Dimitrijevic M, Eccles JC (eds): "Recent Advances in

Restorative Neurology, Upper Motoneuron Function and Dysfunction". Basel: Karger, pp 291-310.

Schneider GE, Jhaveri S, Davis W (1987). On the development of Neuronal arbors. In Chagas C, Linden R (eds): "Developmental Neurobiology of Mammals". Vatican City, Pontifical Academy of Sciences, pp 31-64.

Scholes JH (1979). Nerve fibre topography in the retinal projection to the tectum. Nature 278:620-624.

Schreyer DJ, Jones EG (1982). Growth and target finding by axons of the corticospinal tract in prenatal and postnatal rats. Neurosci 8:1837-1853.

Schreyer DJ, Jones EG (1988). Topographic sequence of outgrowth of corticospinal axons in the rat: a study using retrograde axonal labeling with Fast blue. Dev Brain Res 38:89-101.

Shatz CJ, Kirkwood P (1984). Prenatal development of functional connections in the cat's retinogeniculate pathway. J Neurosci 4:1378-1397.

Shatz CJ, Luskin MB (1986). The relationship between the geniculocortical afferents and their cortical target cells during development of the cat's primary visual cortex. J Neurosci 6:3655-3668.

Shatz CJ, Sretavan DW (1986). Interactions between retinal ganglion cells during the development of the mammalian visual system. Ann Rev Neurosci 9:171-207.

Silver J, Lorenz SE, Wahlsten D, Coughlin J (1982). Axonal guidance during development of the great cerebral commissures: descriptive and experimental studies, *in vivo*, on the role of preformed glial pathways. J Comp Neurol 210:10-29.

Silver J, Ogawa M (1983). Postnatally induced formation of the corpus callosum in acallosal mice and glia-coated cellulose bridges. Science 220:1067-1069.

Silver J, Rutishauser U (1984). Guidance of optic axons *in vivo* by a preformed adhesive pathway on neuroepithelial endfeet. Devel Biol 106:485-499.

Silver J, Sidman RL (1980). A mechanism for the guidance and topographic patterning of retinal ganglion cell axons. J Comp Neurol 189:101-111.

So K-F, Schneider GE, Ayres SA (1981). Lesions of the brachium of the superior colliculus in neonate hamsters: Correlation of anatomy with behavior. Exp Neurol 72:379-40.

Stallcup WB, Beasley LL, Levine JM (1985). Antibody against nerve growth factor-inducible large external (NILE) glycoprotein labels nerve fiber tracts in the developing rat nervous system. J Neurosci 5:1090-1101.

Stanfield BB, O'Leary DDM (1985). The transient corticospinal projection from the occipital cortex during postnatal development of the rat. J Comp Neurol 238:236-248.

Stryker MP, Harris WA (1986). Binocular impulse blockade prevents the formation of ocular dominance columns in cat visual cortex. J Neurosci 6:2117-2133.

Udin SB (1989). Development of the nucleus isthmi in Xenopus. II: Branching patterns of contralaterally projecting isthmotectal axons during maturation of binocular maps. Visual Neurosci 2:153-163.

Udin SB, Fawcett JW (1988). Formation of topographic maps. Ann Rev Neurosci 11:289-328.

Vaca K, McManaman J, Bursztajn S, Appel SH (1985). Differential effects of two fractions from fetal calf muscle on cultured chick ciliary ganglion cells. Dev Brain Res 19:37-46.

Vanselow J, Thanos S, Godement P, Henke-Fahle S, Bonhoeffer F (1989). Spatial arrangement of radial glia and ingrowing retinal axons in the chick optic tectum during development. Dev Brain Res 45:15-27.

Walsh C, Guillery RW (1985). Age-related fiber order in the optic tract of the ferret. J Neurosci 5:3061-3069.

Whitsel BL, Petrucelli LM, Sapiro G, Ha H (1970). Fiber sorting in the fasciculus gracilis of squirrel monkeys. Exp Neurol 29:227-242.

Williams RW, Rakic P (1985). Dispersion of growing axons within the optic nerve of the embryonic monkey. Proc Nat Acad Sci 82:3906-3910.

Yamamoto M, Boyer AM, Crandall JM, Edwards MA, Tanaka H (1986). The expression of stage-specific neurite-associated proteins in the murine central and peripheral nervous system recognized by a monoclonal antibody. J Neurosci 6:3576-3594.

DISCUSSION

Q (G. Hashim): Considering that axon elongation (and myelin) itself, and also considering that the oligos produce a factor which arrests the axon, do you think this is a trophic factor or factors, and is it produced by the target cell(s)?

A: The oligos are usually not in the target area. It is something which has been investigated along the elongation pathway. For example in the optic nerve, there are certain types of oligos that have been identified, which secrete this inhibitory factor; it is not trophic, well, it is anti-trophic, negative tropism and they (the factors) only seem to occur (appear) after a certain stage of development. So that the axons have already (grown) past this area, in normal development, by the time these oligos begin to secrete the factor. What happens after the optic nerve has been cut is that axons will not regenerate to the region where these oligos are present and are secreting this factor. M. Schwartz studies involve (reacting) an antibody to this particular protein that is secreted on the surface of the oligos. He finds that if he puts in this antibody he can get axons to go past the region of the cut.

Q (G. Hashim): Well, I am more concerned with the axon itself e.g. the retinal axon and the target cell. You think the target cell is calling.

A: Yes, there is considerable evidence that there are certain types of diffusible factors. How specific they are just for the retinal ganglion cells is another question. But there is certainly a lot of evidence that nerve growth factor, for example, is a chemotrophic factor and very much atttracts axons to grow.

Q (van Gelder): I just want to follow this up. I will be showing a series of slides tomorrow which may be relevant to this question; it is not my work. If you take glial cells from the same region of the axon, you get very good interaction, strong differentiation of the neuronal perikaryum. If instead of a mesencephalic glia and a mesencephalic neuron, you take a striatal glia and you put it with the mesencephalic neuron, the neuron will not differentiate at all. And there are some beautiful illustrations demonstrating this. Which seems to strongly indicate that it is the glia which can only direct the proper cell in the proper area.

A: So you are saying that if the trophic factors exist, that they are specific for certain sets of axons.

Q (van Gelder): It has to be, this in itself is evidence that it has to be a trophic factor.

A: That is right. But my feeling is, if you are saying that the glial cells are the ones that are attracting specific axons, then I have trouble, especially with the pathway guidance function of glial cells. It ends up with the glial cells being inherently more intelligent then the neurons. And I have trouble with that hypothesis.

Q (S. Hashim): In traveling a distance during its elongation the axon can grow 200 mm/day, 80 μm/hr. This area, if you square or cube it in a three-dimensional manner would contain how many other cells?

A: Oh, millions of other cells.

Q (S. Hashim): Right. So how does this darn neuron, this intelligent axon, negociate itself out of this mass of cells?

A: Well, it obviously is following very specific cues, not only on other axons which have pioneered the way for it, but also cues coming from the target. What I am saying is, if there are no cues from other neurons and if it is the glial cells, than you are just pushing the (problem) a little further down and you are saying that the glial cells now have decided where the axon is going to grow.

And that is a little more difficult for me to accept. If only because there is a lot more variety in neuronal cells and you expect that the specificity comes from this variety, rather than just from ten different kinds of glial cells that exist.

Q (S. Hashim): Well maybe there are helper neurons or whatever for this system to go. It is like being squished in a crowd and it has to negociate itself out.

A: Absolutely, and this has been shown in the insect nervous system very elegantly by Bentley and his co-workers, that there are what they call guide post cells. They refer to them as non-neuronal cells but whether they are glial cells or not is still controversial.

Q (Diamond): I am just curious. If we have the radial glia in the cortex to help the neurons migrate, that is very nice, these turn into astroglia supposedly. But when you see these (immages) that show the syncitium formed by astrocyte, maybe they form a connection that allow then these fibers to grow. Is there any evidence that these (guide cells) are present in syncitium.

A: Well, only in what Gerry Silver and Sidman and Jake Shapiro have shown in reconstructing the holes in this syncitium. They find that, if they reconstruct that in three dimensions, you actually get tunnels, what looks like tunnels. And this has also been shown in the spinal cord, that there are tunnels.

Comment (Scheibel): With Dr. Jasper here, I have to mention one observation if I may. As I look at the beautiful orchestration of the arborizations Dr Jhaveri shows, I go back to some work I did some years ago. We did developmental studies of the Ventral-Basal Nucleus in the kitten thalamus, starting at day 1 and going up to about 35 days.

We did Golgi studies and we also did in situ microelectrode studies. Put these together temporally and what you find is that the arbors, just as the speaker showed, come in and just sort of wave around. You have this array of thalamic cells waiting, as it were waiting breathlessly, but when you sample this population with a microelectrode there is no electrical activity at all from them. Then at the time some few days after birth, when the arbors make a decision, then for the first time you get spiking activity. Very beautiful orchestration.

(Mal)Nutrition and the Infant Brain, pages 127–139
© 1990 Wiley-Liss, Inc.

THE DEVELOPING CEREBRAL CORTEX: NUTRITIONAL AND ENVIRONMENTAL INFLUENCES

Arianna Carughi, Kenneth J. Carpenter, Marian C. Diamond

Departments of Nutrition (A.C., K.J.C) and Physiology-Anatomy (M.C.D.), University of California, Berkeley, California 94720, USA

One of us (MCD) has been studying the impact of the environment on the anatomy of the cerebral cortex for over a quarter of a century. For most of this time it was the interaction between the normal, healthy, laboratory rat brain and the external, and some facets of the internal, environment that attracted our curiosity. Now since we have accumulated a good deal of information on how the anatomy of the normal male and female forebrain develops and ages and how enriched and improverished experiential environments can alter cortical structure (Diamond, 1988), we can use these data to study other variables that might change cortical morphology. In the present or recent experiments in our laboratory these variable features include magnetic field effects created by superconductor magnets, opiate blockers, aromatase blockers, electrolytic lesions, and nutritional deficiencies. It is the latter that will be presented here.

A brief review of the effects of environmental enrichment and impoverishment on cortical morphology might be of use before introducing the most recent work on nutritional deficiencies and rehabilitation combined with environmental experiments. The fact that the structure of the cerebral cortex could change in response to environmental factors was first published in 1964 (Diamond et al., 1964). In this report we presented data that illustrated statistically significant 6% differences in the cerebral cortical thickness between enriched and impoverished rats, particularly in the occipital cortex. Cell counts revealed that in the enriched rats there were fewer neurons per microscopic field compared with counts in similar cortical areas in the impoverished rats' cortices. Such a finding suggested that the enriched rats had more dendritic branching to account for the greater distance between the neuronal soma. That this was actually the case, i.e. more dendrites in the enriched brains than in the impoverished brains, was later shown by Holloway working in our laboratory (Holloway, 1966). Later, other investigators confirmed these findings in other cortical areas (Greenough et al., 1973).

Over the years, the following parameters were measured: the area of the neuronal soma and nuclei, the number of dendritic spines, the length of the post synaptic thicknening, the number of glial cells and capillary dimensions (Diamond, 1988). We found that in these measurements there were significant differences between the enriched and nonenriched animals. Furthermore, we could measure these cortical changes at any age, from preweaned, to young adults, to middle-aged, and also, most importantly, to extremely old-aged rats. In other words, the plasticity of the cortex was evident at any age (Diamond, 1988). As mentioned for previous data, in the ensuing years these findings have been supported by other laboratories (Walsh et al., 1973).

The role of the environment in compensating for some nutritional deficits have been demonstrated in children as well. Significant progress in tests of mental development can be seen if environmental modification is added to child rehabilitation/supplementation dietary programs (Graham-McGregor et al., 1983). Thus, environmental enrichment appears to aid the recovery from some of the behavioral deficits due to malnutrition.

To study the effects of environmental enrichment on brain structure of protein deprived and then protein rehabilitated rats, a graduate student from our Berkeley Department of Nutrition, Arianna Carughi, inquired about a cooperative effort under the guidance of Professors Kenneth J. Carpenter and Marian C. Diamond. The results of these studies satisfied the requirements for her PhD thesis and are the foundation for this report.

METHODS

Dietary and Behavioral Condition

Twenty-one Sprague-Dawley rats, 12 days pregnant, were ordered from outside distributors and offered a 17% protein diet upon arrival at the Department of Physiology-Anatomy animal laboratory. On the 17th day of pregnancy, the rats were separated into two groups: controls and protein restricted. The six controls continued on the 17% protein diet for the remainder of pregnancy and during lactation for 21 days. The fifteen protein restricted rats were given a diet containing 8% protein for the remainder of pregnancy and during lactation.

At parturition all the litters were culled to 8 pups. At weaning, 21 days of age, 24 male pups were randomly assigned from the controls to two environmental conditions: standard (SC CONT) or enriched (EC CONT). The standard condition consisted of four cages (32x32x20 cm) with three pups per cage having access to 17% protein diets. On the other hand, the enriched condition consisted of 1 large cage (70x70x45 cm) with twelve pups and "toys", objects for the animals to explore and climb upon. These animals were also maintained on the 17% protein diet. In summary, the controls lived in standard or enriched conditions with 17% protein diets.

At weaning pups from mothers on restricted diets (8% protein) were assigned to one of four groups: standard environment, 17% protein rehabilitated diet (SC REHAB); enriched environment, 17% protein rehabilitated diet (EC REHAB); standard environment, 6% protein diet (SC LOPRO); enriched environment, 6% protein diet (EC LOPRO). There were twelve animals in each of the four groups, and the standard and enriched environments were the same as those for the controls. The animals lived in their respective environments for 30 days, with the toys in the enriched environments being changed daily from a common pool. The animal room was kept at $72 \pm 2°$ F, a relative humidity of 50 $\pm 5\%$ and a 12 hour light period, from 6 am to 6 pm. After 30 days, the animals were anesthetized with sodium phenobarbital and sacrificed by decapitation.

Histological Procedures and Brain Measurements

The brains were removed from the skull and processed according to the Golgi-Cox method of Ramon-Moliner. Coronal sections 50 micra and 150 micra thick were cut from Cedukol embedded material. Subcortical landmarks were utilized to insure uniform sampling: immediately anterior to the crossing of the corpus callosum=frontal cortical sample; immediately anterior to the crossing of the anterior commissure=parietal cortex; at the crossing of the posterior commissure=occipital cortex. The 50 micra sections were stained with cresylechtviolet and used for cortical thickness and subcortical measures. The 150 micra sections were used for dendritic branching studies.

With the aid of a microslide projector, images of the sections were projected and measurements were taken of the various outlined areas, cerebral cortex, hippocampus, and diencephalon (Some details are presented in Diamond et al., 1975).

RESULTS

Body weights: At weaning, 21 days of age, there was a 50% difference in body weights between the protein restricted pups (8%) and the control pups (17%) (Fig 1).

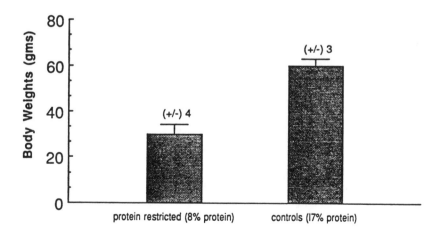

Fig. 1. Body Weights at Weaning: 21 days of age (N = 12/group)

There were no significant differences in final body weights between the standard and enriched pairs, but between the different dietary groups there were marked differences. When the rats' final body weights were taken at 51 days of age, the standard and enriched rehabilitated rats' weight was 25% less than the standard and enriched controls; whereas, the standard and enriched low protein rats' body weight was 65% less than the standard and enriched rehabilitated rats (Fig. 2). It is important to keep in mind these final body weight differences when the brain and dendritic measurements of the various groups will be mentioned later in the paper.

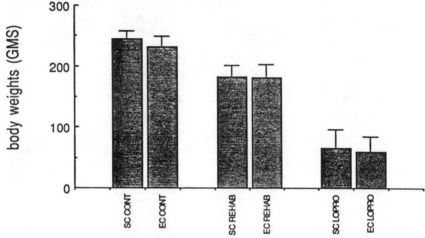

Fig. 2. Final Body Weights: 51 days of age (N = 9-12/group)

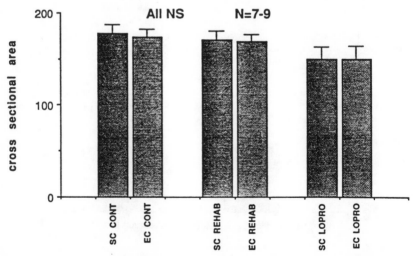

Fig. 3. Dimensions of diencephalon: estimated cross-sectional area (N = 7-9/group)

Brain Measurement:

Diecephalon: The dimensions of the diencephalons (HxW) from the enriched rats were not significantly different from the standard in any of the experimental conditions (Fig. 3). This finding, showing the stability of the dimensions of the diencephalon as a consequence of differential environmental living conditions, has been reported previously (Diamond et al., 1966).

However, the dimensions of the diencephalon from the protein rehabilitated animals were 13% greater than those from the animals on the low protein diets. These results show that protein deficiency will alter the dimensions of the diencephalon; whereas, the environmental living conditions used in these experiments do not.

Hippocampus: In general, the enriched living conditions produced a thicker hippocampus than did the control conditions, but the differences were not statistically significant (Fig. 4). There were no significant differences between right and left hemispheres, and no significant interactions between side and diet, side and environment or diet and environment. In other experiments, we had shown that there were no significant right-left differences in the thickness of the hippocampus from control animals at 90 days of age so that these data showing no differences at 41 days add support to the earlier findings. The major right-left differences in this area of the brain were seen at 21 days of age and before (Diamond, 1982).

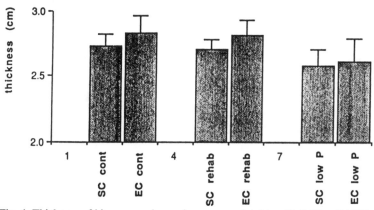

Fig. 4. Thickness of hippocampal complex: mean of right and left (N = 8P-10/group)

Cerebral cortex: Since there were six different conditions including the controls and experimental groups and nine cortical areas were measured in each brain, not all of the cortical data will be presented here. A few examples will be offered to note some of the effects. For all three dietary treatments, the frontal cortex was significantly thicker in the animals housed in the enriched conditions than in those housed in the standard conditions, averaging 4% (p<0.05) between enriched and standard controls and 6% (p<0.05) between enriched and standard

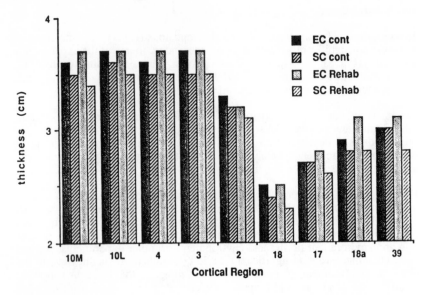

Fig. 5. Cortical thickness: rehabilitation

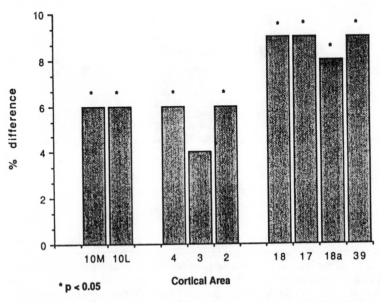

Fig. 6. Percent difference in cortical thickness: standard rehabilitation vs enriched rehabilitation (N = 5-10/group).

rehabilitated animals. In the occipital cortex, these differences averaged 3% (p<0.05) between the enriched and standard controls animals. And 9% (p<0.05) differences were noted in the occipital cortex between the enriched rehabilitated animals and that of the standard rehabilitated animals (Figs. 5 & 6). It is interesting to note that the differences between the enriched and standard were even greater in the rehabilitated animal's brains than in the enriched and standard control animals' brains.

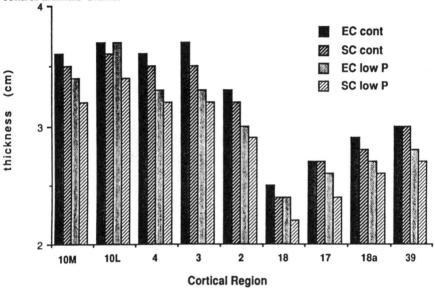

Fig. 7. Cortical thickness: Standard protein versus low protein.

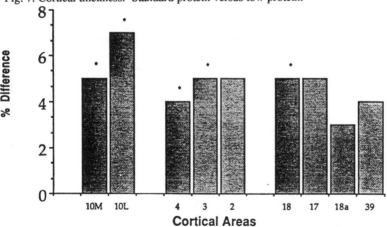

Fig.8. Percent difference in cortical thickness between standard low protein and enriched low protein (N = 5-11/group).

As might be predicted, the animals living in standard conditions on low protein diets had the thinnest cortices in all areas measured compared with animals in all the other groups (Fig. 7.). Yes, the enriched condition, low protein animals did have thicker cortices than the standard condition, low protein animals, though the differences were nonsignificant (Fig. 8.).

In measuring the basal dendrites of pyramidal cells in layers II and III of area 18 in the cerebral cortex, it was noted that there were more stained neurons in the right hemisphere than in the left. This finding supports previous results indicating that in the male cerebral cortex more neurons per unit area (area 39) are found in the right side than in the left (McShane et al., 1988).

By grouping the dendritic orders into the low orders: including the first, second, and third, and the high orders, including the fourth, fifth, and sixth, very interesting results were obtained. In spite of the fact that there were marked body weight differences among the controls, rehabilitated, and low protein animals, the low order dendrites were all identical in number (Fig. 9). The stability of these first three orders under such vastly different conditions was amazing.

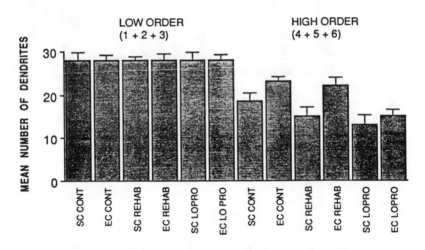

Fig. 9. Effect of environmental enrichment and nutritional rehabilitation on dendritic branching number (N = 9-12/condition).

However, the high order dendrites showed a great deal of variability. Most importantly, in our opinion, was the 44% greater number of dendrites in the protein rehabilitated enriched animals's brains than in the protein rehabilitated control brains. Though the number of 4th, 5th, and 6th order dendrites in the rehabilitated animals did not reach the number in the standard and enriched controls, the difference in higher order dendrites between the enriched and standard rehabilitated animals was greater than that in the enriched and standard controls (21%). Even the enriched low protein animals had 11% (NS) more high order dendrites than the standard low protein animals.

As stated earlier, enriched living conditions can benefit normal cortical structure at any age. And as we can see from these experiments, enriched living conditions are beneficial for brain development even in protein deprived and protein rehabilitated animals.

CONCLUSIONS

Body weights:

1. Protein deprivation during the last trimester of pregnancy and lactation reduced the body weights of the offspring by 50% at weaning (21 days of age) compared to controls.

2. The final body weights at 51 days of age were not significantly different between those rats living in enriched versus those living in standard conditions in spite of their diets. However, the body weights of the low protein recipients were 74% and 65% lower than the controls or rehabilitated animals, respectively.

Diencephalon:

3. The dimensions of the diencephalon in the enriched animals were not significantly different from those in the standard conditions. Both the control rats and the rehabilitated rats had significantly larger diencephalons than the low protein rats. Again as with the body weights, there were no statistically significant environmental effects, but there were significant dietary effects.

Hippocampus:

4. In general, the enriched condition produced a thicker hippocampus than did the control condition, but the differences were not significant. There were no significant differences in hippocampal thickness between animals in the various dietary groups.

Cerebral cortex:

5. Animals on low protein diets in standard colony conditions had the thinnest cortices compared to the other groups.

6. Animals subjected to diets low in protein during pregnancy and lactation and then rehabilitated to 17% protein diets had on the average thicker cortices than either the controls or the low protein animals.

7. Occipital cortical pyramidal cell basal dendrites in the first three orders are amazingly consistent irrespective of diet and housing conditions.

8. Occipital cortical pyramidal cell basal dendrites in the last three orders are altered by both dietary and environmental conditions. The protein rehabilitated

and environmentally enriched animals' dendrites showed statistically significant differences compared to their controls.

These results demonstrate the plasticity of the cerebral cortex as a consequence of dietary and environmental interactions and offer optimism with regard to cortical morphological growth after dietary protein rehabilitation and enriched environments following protein deprivation during development.

REFERENCES

Diamond MC, Krech D, Rosenzweig MR (1964). The effects of an enriched environment on the histology of the rat cerebral cortex. J. Comp. Neurol. 123:111-120.

Diamond MC, Law F, Rhodes H, Lindner B, Rosenzweig MR, Krech D, Bennett EL (1966). Increases in cortical depth and glia numbers in rats subjected to enriched environment. J. Comp. Neurol. 128:117-126.

Diamond MC, Johnson RE, Ingham CA (1975). Morphological changes in the young, adult and aging rat cerebral cortex, hippocampus and diencephalon. Behav. Biol. 14:163-174.

Diamond MC, Murphy GM, Akiyama K, Johnson RE (1982). Morphologic hippocampal asymmetry in male and female rats. Exp. Neurol. 73:553-566.

Diamond MC (1988). Enriching Heredity. The Free Press, New York, New York.

Graham-McGregor S, Schofield W, Harris L (1983). Effect of psychosocial stimulation on mental development of severely malnourished children; an interim report. Pediatrics 72:239-243.

Greenough WT, Volkman F, Juraska JM (1973). Effects of rearing complexity on dendritic branching in frontolateral and temporal cortex of the rat. Exp Neurol 41:371-378.

Holloway RL (1966). Dendritic branching: some preliminary results of training and complexity in rat visual cortex. Brain Res 2:393-396.

McShane S, Glaser L, Greer ER, Houtz J, Tong MF, Diamond MC (1988). Cortical asymmetry -- neurons-glia, female-male: A preliminary study. Exp Neurol 99:353-361.

Walsh R, Cummins RA, Budtz-Olsen OE (1973). Environmentally induced changes in the dimensions of the rat cerebrum: A replication and extension. Dev Psychobiol 6:3-8.

DISCUSSION

Q (Audience): What is the meaning of the enriched environment. Is it the grouping of the animals together , (or) is it the presence of toys?

A: It is both. If one has just 12 rats living in a large cage together, one can change the cortex slightly. If one has just one rat in the cage with all the toys, the cortex does not change at all; he does not play with those toys when he lives there by himself.

Q (Audience): What about sex as a factor.

A: If we have males and females living together in the enriched environment, the females become pregnant. And that pregnancy affects that cortex, right. When we do these experiments we just measure the male cortex to see the effect of him living with the female. So since we have the 30 day paradigm, we leave the male and females together for 15 days, then take those females out and put some other females in; so males will go for 30 days. And their corticis do get larger.

Q (S. Hashim): What about music.
A: We have not studied music. One laboratory did study music with the rat. Instead of showing primarily the occipital cortex having the greatest changes, they showed that the auditory cortex did.

One other thing with this. People always ask us, will we get the changes if the rat just watches the others play with the toys. And the answer is no. They need to participate actively.

Q (Jhaveri): Have you any comment why the occipital cortex is so susceptible to such changes and not the somato-sensory area.
A: Let me say that we are dealing with male rats here. If we look at their corticis - male right and left cortex - we find a significant differences on the right side in the visual - spatial area, in the occipital cortex. We can reverse these right - left differences with stress, there are all sorts of different ways, and we have done so in the past to show how readily one can change the right - left pattern. But to continue answering your question.

When we put the females in the enriched environment alone, we change her visual - spatial cortex by only 4%, not as much as we changed the male. However, we change her somato-sensory cortex more; the differences there become significant.

So the male is a visual-spatial animal while - as my former professor, a male, used to say - females are more feeling than the male.

Q (G. Hashim): When you are talking about thickness, changes in thickness, you are implying changes in function. Could you expand on that ?
A: As I said earlier, the changes in thickness show that we have increased the dimensions of the nerve cell, every one we have measured: soma, dendrites, spines, postsynaptic thickening, and an increase in glial cells. These rats in an enriched environment have a thicker cortex. We have not yet studied the protein-deficient ones for learning, that is a new investigation But with long-time enriched environments, those rats with a thicker cortex ran a better maze than those with a thinner one.

Q (Reader): Do these changes in the visual cortex involve a specific layer?
A: We find that it is layers II and III which show the greatest changes, but then we find the other changes occur as well (in other layers?).

Q (Reader): Do you count the spines?
A: The spines have been counted. These were counted by another group. We prepared the animals at Berkeley and then send the brains on down to Professor A Globus who was counting spines at the time. Yes, he found there were more spines per unit area on the dendrite in the enriched animal than in the non-enriched.

Q (Rassin): What did the food-intake in these different groups look like?

A: The problem is that we are dealing with 12 animals in a cage and we have not actually worked with food intake for that reason. This was one of the first questions we were asked, but you noticed, the body weights did not differ when we keep them in for 30 days. In our first experiments we kept them in for 80 days, and in those experiments the body weights of the (environmentally) impoverished were 8% greater than those in the enriched. I mean, they just sat by the food cup, that is all they had to do, and they ate.

Q (Rassin): You have not made any effort to regulate the food, i.e. not allow the animals to eat as much as they want?

A: We have not, so far. If you have a good idea how we can, that is our problem. We would have to isolate the animals to measure the food, but once you isolate the animals, that cortex goes down. And it goes down much more readily than it goes up with enrichment.

Q (Huether): Maybe I missed the point but if you put 12 male rats in a cage, how do you deal with the hierarchy. This may also influence cortical development.

A: Well, we pay no attention to the hierarchy when we do our sampling. We take all 12 brains and the Standard Deviation is very small with this. We can change the cortex in 4 days and have a significant $p < 0.001$ level. I mean, (it is) a very small S.D.

Hiearachy is not showing up in this case. What we would have to do sometime, which would be nice since our conversation earlier, is to look at the serotonin levels amongst these. Mark them (rats), take video pictures of them, and see who the active dominant ones are, then look (at serotonin in the cortex).

Q (S. Hashim): Excuse me, but is it not true that in the absence of females there is no hierarchy, it does not mean anything.

A: Well, we even went so far, because we wanted to see the effect of crowding, to put 24 animals in a cage. The students decided they still did not look crowded so we put 36 animals in the cage. At 36 it was decided that they were crowded, and I called up the next morning to find out whether they survived the night, with 36 males living in this space. They got along beautifully, in fact their cortex changed even more when we looked at them after 30 days.

Q (Audience): Did you look at the metabolic rate of the enriched animals and impoverished rats.

A: No, we have not done that as yet.

Q: (Dr H. Jasper): I am interested in your *old* rats.

A: We are *all* interested in the old rats.

Q (Jasper): Did you find that the old rats had a diminished thickness compared to their controls.

A: No we did not. I did not bring that slide today. But we have the data showing that we actually increase the cortex as much in our old rats as we did in our young rats. We can increase it as much as 10% in the old rats. Admittedly we had them in for three times as long. We don't know over the short term whether they would change as much.

Q (Jasper): Is this really an increase or is this merely a decrease in atrophy.

A: That is actually a good question. We think that it is an increase because when we did the 112 days old animals, we had three groups. We had a baseline i.e. we took the animals before they went in, and then we had the enriched, and finally, the control group. Both the enriched and the controls (112 days) were above the baseline, so it truly was an enrichment, it was not just maintaining a decrease. It is true that the cortex grows for the first month in the rat and than goes down (like so), but what we have been able to show is that we can change the slope of that curve at any age.

Q (Jasper): *Very* encouraging.

A: It is *very* encouraging. We are very optimistic, all of us. Right!

(Mal)Nutrition and the Infant Brain, pages 141–156
© 1990 Wiley-Liss, Inc.

MALNUTRITION AND DEVELOPING SYNAPTIC TRANSMITTER SYSTEMS: LASTING EFFECTS, FUNCTIONAL IMPLICATIONS

Gerald Huether

Max-Planck-Institut für experimentelle Medizin, Forschungsstelle Neurochemie, Hermann-Rein-Str. 3, 3400 Göttingen, FRG

Even though the brain is protected by various homeostatic mechanisms against wide fluctuations in the availability of essential nutrients, food deprivation is known to affect the metabolic state of the brain. Because many feedback regulatory loops for substrate acquisition are not yet elaborated and because the requirements of essential substrates are particularly high during brain growth and maturation, the developing brain is especially vulnerable to an inadequate supply of nutrients. Given the fact that infant malnutrition is a world wide problem currently affecting an estimated 300 million infants, numerous studies have been conducted to define the consequences of an inadequate dietary food supply on the growth and the functional maturation of the developing brain. Up to now most of the work in this area has been primarily descriptive. Given these data, however, it would appear that in particular the altered amino acid supply in protein malnutrition affects normal brain development through its interference with either protein accretion or transmitter formation. The most pressing question is now: How can we exactly assess, identify and prevent the circumstances under which an inadequate amino acid supply will cause irreversible alterations of normal brain development? There is no simple answer to this question. It took us quite a while to realize that one and the same nutritional imbalance may have rather different consequences, that its outcome will depend on several other factors.

The first factor is the state of maturity of the developing brain when it is confronted with a deficient nutritional supply. There are certain periods during brain development when the brain, or better: the developmental processes that take place in certain areas of the brain are particularily vulnerable to changes of their nutritional supply. We have learned a lot about the role of the time of onset of the nutritional insult on the developing brain in animal models of pre- peri- and postnatal protein malnutrition.

The second factor interfering with the outcome of nutritional deficits during brain development is already much less understood: It is the interaction normal brain development. Some of these extrinsic factors can be other nutrients which may enhance or suppress the effects of an inadequate supply of certain nutrients on the developing brain, but they can also be other environmental factors, reaching from external temperature and daylight exposure to the intoxication by environmental noxes or the kind and degree of emotional and sensory stimulation or stress. Intrinsic factors which may enhance or suppress the consequences of nutritional imbalances on the developing brain may be individual variations in the efficiency and the state of maturation of the peripheral metabolic pathways and mechanisms involved in the control of the brain`s nutrient supply.

And, as if this would make the picture not yet sufficiently complicated a third factor additionally contributes to the outcome of nutritional imbalances on the developing brain. The role of this important factor is even less understood, because it acts not prior to, not together with, but after the nutritionally caused defect of the developing brain. It is the plasticity which occurs during nutritional rehabilitation. Only in rare, exceptional cases do we get an impression of the tremendous plasticity exerted by a damaged developing brain. In all other cases we have no idea to what extent plasticity, by means of structural and functional rearrangements does contribute to remodel and to rearrange the brain`s connectivity, and to make the original defect vanish - at least in terms of subsequent brain function.

The brain's plasticity to compensate for certain developmental defects creates an additional problem which is of equal theoretical and practical importance, and which is related to the reversibility and irreversibility of developmental processes in general, and of developmental failures in particular: If the proper formation of a certain structure or a specific neuronal pathway is disturbed, we end up with structural aberrations, such as deficits in cell number and connectivity. All structural deficits of the developing brain are irreversible in later life. If, however, other neurons, by increasing their dendritic arborization or by additional axonal sprouting and synapse formation will compensate for the original defects we may not see any functional deficit in later life. The conclusion that the consequence of early nutritional deprivation, for example, can be reversed in later life, is wrong. There is no way to reverse any process during brain development, once it became manifested in terms of structural changes. It is the change of structure that, on the one hand, represents an irreversible final stage of any developmental process and that, on the other hand, becomes the starting point - the basis of all future developmental events.

In order to differentiate between primary causes and secondary consequences of nutritionally induced developmental failures, one has to extrapolate from findings that have been made in animal models designed to investigate the effects of well defined, nutritional inadequacies on the developing brain. Nevertheless, one has to be aware that these extrapolations may easily overemphasize the actual contribution of an individual factor, in particular, if the original findings were obtained under well defined experimental conditions which exaggerate the role of specific factors, and which may not apply to other, more complex situations.

Phenomenology of the effects of experimental malnutrition on developing transmitter systems

Given the number of possible variables with respect to the kinds and degrees of malnutrition, the species and the age of the animals studied, or the area of the brain investigated, it is not surprising that a review of the published literature reveals rather conflicting data as to the type of the neurochemical changes which may occur (see Table 1). What is certain, however, is that under

TABLE 1. Survey of Published Findings on the Effect of Experimental Malnutrition on Developing Transmitter Systems.

Transmitter system studied:	Effect caused by experimental malnutrition on:					
	Synthezizing enzyme	Transmitter level	Degrading enzyme	Metabolite level	Transmitter turnover	Receptor density
Ach	± 3 ↓ 1,2	± 5 ↓ 4,5	± 11-13 ↑ 6-11	. . .	. . .	±↓↑ 14
GABA	↓ 15-20	?	± 21	. . .	. . .	↑ 22,23
Asp, Glu	. . .	↓ 24	. . .	. . .	. . .	. . .
Tau	. . .	↑ 24	. . .	. . .	. . .	. . .
HA	. . .	↑ 25,26	. . .	. . .	. . .	. . .
DA	↓ 45,46 ↑ 27-30	↓ 21-36 ↑ 37	. . .	. . .	. . .	↓ 38
NA	↓ 45,46 ↑ 27-30	± 39 ±↓ 40 ↓ 41-46 ↑ 47,48	. . .	. . .	↓ 45,46,49	↓ 50
HT	↓ 52,53 ↑ 51	± 52 ±↓ 54-56 ±↑ 57,58 ↓ 59-61 ↑ 62-71	. . .	↑ 62-66, 72,73	±↑ 75	. . .

Many of the published findings are conflicting and depend on the species, the kind of malnutrition, its onset and duration, and the age of the animals when the measurements were made. In all these studies it is difficult to distinguish between those changes which are due to and which merely reflect the structural abnormalities (loss of certain cell types and synapses) and the direct effects of malnutrition on individual transmitter systems.

Abbreviations:

Ach=acetylcholine   GABA=γ-aminobutyric acid   Asp=aspartate
Glu=glutamate   Tau=taurine   HA=histamine
DA=dopamine   NA=norepinephrine   HT=5-hydroxytryptamine, serotonin
↓ = decrease, ↑ = increase, ± = no effect; numbers refer to original publications (available from the author on request). Most effects are reviewed in Stern et al. (1973), Hawrylewicz and Kissane (1980), Wiggins et al. (1984) and Enwonwu (1988).

nutrition can alter the neurochemical balance in the developing brain. It is interesting that not all transmitter systems appear to be similarly affected. In general, the published data suggest that cholinergic and GABAergic transmission may be reduced in the developing brain, but these effects seem to be rapidly restored upon nutritional rehabilitation. In contrast, catecholaminergic and serotoninergic systems would seem to be more active in the undernourished state than in controls, and at least some of the changes seem to persist during nutritional rehabilitation. There are undoubtedly many additional effects of malnutrition on the maturation of other, e.g. the various peptidergic transmitter systems that have yet to be characterized. Because some of the effects on individual transmitter systems may be restricted to discrete areas of the malnourished brain, a more regional analysis may uncover much more dramatic changes than most of the currently available data would suggest. Hence, a substantial amount of descriptive work has yet to be done until a more complete picture of the phenomenology of the changes of developing transmitter systems in the malnourished brain can be drawn.

On the other hand, substantial progress has been made in recent years towards a better understanding of the role of nutritional factors on the maturation and functional activity of one group of transmitters, i.e. monoaminergic transmitter systems. Based on this knowledge, a causal relationship between the altered availability of individual precursor amino acids in the malnourished brain and its effect on the formation of the respective monoamines and on the maturation of monoaminergic transmitter systems is about to emerge. At least some of the mental and cognitive defects seen in humans suffering from undernutrition during early infancy seem to be related to lasting consequences of the altered precursor availability on the proper function and maturation of monoaminergic transmitter systems.

Protein malnutrition precursor availability and monoamine synthesis in the developing brain.

The rate limiting step of the synthesis of monoamines is not saturated in vivo. Therefore, an altered availability of the individual precursor amino acids, Trp, Tyr (Phe) and His can affect the rate by which the respective transmitter amines, serotonin (5-HT), catecholamines (dopamine, DA, norepinephrine, NE) and histamine (HA) can be formed. This dependency exists not only in the adult (Wurtmann, et al., 1980; Fernstrom, 1983; Enwonwu, 1988), but also in the developing brain (Huether, 1984, 1988; Garabal, et al., 1988). The availability of precursor amino acids in the brain is not only gouverned by their blood supply (the actual concentration of free circulating Trp, Tyr or His), actual concentration of free circulating Trp, Tyr or His), but additionally affected by the blood concentrations of, in particular, the branched chain large neutral amino acids (LNAA) which compete with the aromatic neutral amino acids for a common carrier-mediated active transport system forbrain uptake (see Fig. 1). Protein malnutrition causes a greater depletion of the plasma pool of the LNAA`s (Val, Leu, Ile) relative to the depletion of Trp (free Trp is actually increased because of the reduced serum albumin level and the increased concentrations of free fatty acids which compete with Trp for a common albumin binding site (Pardridge, 1979)), of Tyr (the depletion of which can to some extent be counteracted by an increased rate of Phe-hydroxylation by Phe-hydroxylase in the liver or by Tyr-hydroxylase in the brain (Maher, 1988)) and of His (the plasma concentration of His actually increases when the dietary protein intake is reduced (Enwonwu, 1988)). Consequently, protein malnutrition under most circumstances causes an increase of the ratio between the concentrations of precursor amino acids for monoamine synthesis and the sum of the concentrations of the competing amino acids for brain uptake (see insertion in Fig. 1). Most likely this increased precursor availability is the cause of the unexpected elevation of monoamines and their metabolites found by several authors in the brain of malnourished animals. (for ref. see Table 1)

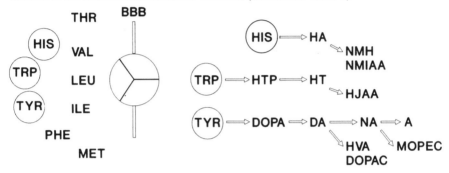

PLASMA LEVELS	CONTROL	MALNOURISHED
$\sum$ VAL, LEU, ILE (Mμ)	346 ± 56	149 ± 61
HIS / LNAA	0.123	0.333
TRP / LNAA	0.015	0.031
TYR / LNAA	0.083	0.120

Fig. 1. Availability of the precursor amino acids for the synthesis of their respective monoamines and metabolites in the malnourished brain.

The synthesizing enzymes of all three pathways are not saturated in vivo, the rate of amine formation is limited by the availability of their individual substrates. Brain uptake of precursor amino acids is dependent on the blood concentration of other large neutral amino acids competing for a common binding site at the L-transport system of the blood brain barrier (BBB).

In 60 days old guinea pigs, malnourished from weaning by reducing the dayly ration to half the normal intake, a preferential depletion of the branched chain amino acids in the plasma is seen. Consequently, the ratio between the individual precursor amino acids (histidine increased, tryptophan and tyrosine slightly decreased) and their competitors for brain entry is significantly elevated.

Abbreviations:

HIS=histidine	TRP=tryptophan	TYR=tyrosine
HA=histamine	HT=5-hydroxytryptamine	DA=dopamine
NA=norepinephrine	A=epinephrine	VAL=valine
LEU=leucine	ILE=isoleucine	LNAA=large neutral amino acids

Peculiarities of monoamine synthesis and monoamine functions during brain development.

Apart from the unexpected dependency of monoamine formation on precursor availability, research in recent years has uncovered some additional peculiarities of the regulation and the role of monoamines in the developing brain.

At rather early developmental stages, before functional monoaminergic synapses are formed, monoamines seem to be released in a hormone like manner and to act as morphogenetic or developmental signals. In particular serotonin and norepinephrine have been shown to be involved in the regulation of neuronal proliferation, migration, outgrowth of processes, synaptogenesis and cell death (for ref. see Table 2). Interestingly enough, each one of these individual processes has also been found to be affected in the undernourished brain long before an involvement of monoamines in the regulation of these developmental events was demonstrated. It had been suggested that amino acid starvation must initiate an intercellular regulatory response which results in the cessation of growth and the initiation of cell differentiation (Marin, 1976, 1977). The increased formation of monoamines in the malnourished brain may represent at least one part of this response since the overall effect of monoamines during brain development is a promotion of differentiation processes (Oey, 1975; Chubakov et al., 1986). Because an acceleration of individual steps of brain morphogenesis will easily disrupt the tight sequential timing between the various interdependent events, the structural development would proceed in a much less elaborated manner, with reduced cell numbers and decreased synaptic connectivity.

Another peculiarity of monoaminergic signalling in the developing brain that may also affect certain brain functions in later life comes into play after functional monoaminergic synapses have been formed. It is the autoregulation of monoamine receptor expression by synaptic monoamine release. Whereas in the adult brain receptor density is up and down regulated by a feedback mechanism if less, respectively more monoamines are released, the reverse is seen in the developing brain: An increased release of monoamines leads to an increased expression of functional momoamine receptors and vice versa (Devitry et al., 1986; Whitaker-Azmitia and Azmitia, 1986; Miller and Friedhoff, 1988; Garabal et al., 1988). This open loop regulatory system is later transferred into a closed feedback regulatory loop. The altered receptor expression established during the open loop phase by an altered monoamine release seems to become permanently stabilized during subsequent loop closure. Therefore, experimental manipulations of developing monoaminergic systems can result in an altered responsiveness of monoaminergic systems in later life (for references see Miller and Friedhoff, 1988).

Permanent changes of monoaminergic systems can additionally be brought about by adaptive responses of the pathways involved in the metabolism of monoamines and their precursor amino acids to long lasting changes of the amino acid supply. The biochemical basis of this phenomenon is still poorly understood: If an adult organism is confronted with an increased

TABLE 2. A Survey of Published Data on the Involvement of Monoamines in the Regulation of Individual Events During Brain Development. Each One of these Events is also Affected by Malnutrition.

DEVELOPMENTAL EVENT	CONROLLED BY		AFFECTED BY MALNUTRITION
	SEROTONIN	CATECHOLAMINES	
Receptor expression	1,2	3-6	7
△			
Synaptogenesis	8	9-11	12
△			
Outgrowth of processes	8,13,14	15-16	17-19
△			
Migration	20	21,22	23
△			
Proliferation	8,24-26	27-29	30-32

Numbers refer to following references:
1) Devitry et al. 1986; 2) Whitaker-Azmitia and Azmitia 1986;
3) Rosengarten and Friedhoff 1979; 4) Moon 1984;
5) Miller and Friedhoff 1988; 6) Garabal et al. 1988;
7) see Table 1, 8) Chubakov et al. 1986;
9) Kasamatsu and Pettigrew 1979; 10) Parnavelas and Blue 1982;
11) Zecevic and Rakic 1982; 12) Gundappa and Desiraju 1988;
13) Haydon et al. 1984; 14) Whitaker-Azmitia and Azmitia 1986;
15) Berry et al. 1980; 16) Felten et al. 1982;
17) Cordero et al. 1985; 18) Salas et al. 1986;
19) Adaro et al. 1986; 20) Wallace 1988;
21) Lidov and Molliver 1979; 22) Rosenstein and Brightman 1981;
23) Debassio and Kemper 1985; 24) Lauder and Krebs 1978;
25) Lauder et al. 1982; 26) Lauder 1983;
27) Patel et al. 1977; 28) Lewis et al. 1977;
29) Bendek and Hahn 1982; 30) Winick and Noble 1966;
31) Howard and Granoff 1968; 32) Dobbing et al. 1971.

supply of, e.g. Trp, the altered brain Trp supply is readily counterregulated by an increased expression of liver Trp-pyrrolase, and accelerated Trp-degradation. This adaptive response is completely reversed if the normal Trp-supply is restored. During embryogenesis and early life, such feedback mechanisms for the regulation of nutrient supply are not yet operating with the same efficiency. Therefore subsequent pathways, e.g. serotonin synthesizing and degrading enzymes in the developing brain, become additionally affected and can adapt to the altered substrate supply. It seems that the earlier and the longer a developing system is confronted with an altered substrate supply the greater is the number of metabolic pathways affected downstream from its metabolism and the more unlikely is a rapid and complete restoration of the original balance when the dietary intake is normalized. This situation can be illustrated experimentally by the changes seen in steady state levels of serotonin and hydroxyindoleacetic acid

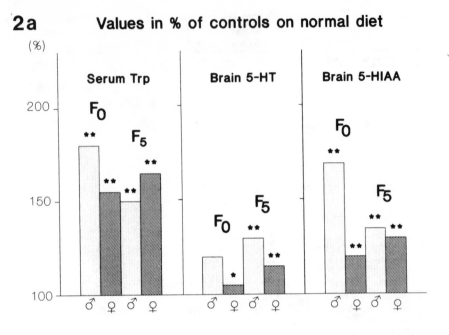

2a   Values in % of controls on normal diet

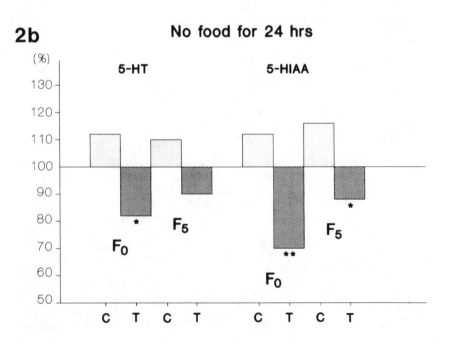

2b   No food for 24 hrs

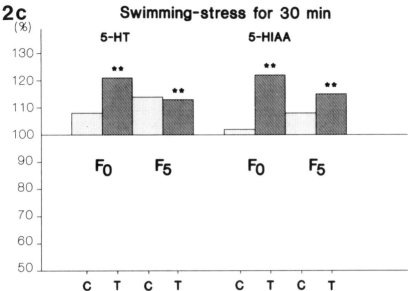

Fig. 2a.   Effect of the consumption of tryptophan enriched diets (3.7fold higher than normal rat chow) either from weaning (F0) or throughout five generations (F5) on brain serotonin (5-HT) and 5-hydroxyindoleacetic acid (5HIAA) of 60 day old rats. One resp, two asterisks indicate significant differences from control values (p<0.05; p<0.01).
Fig. 2b.   Steady state levels: Effect of fasting (C=control diet, T=Trp- enriched diets.
Fig. 2c.   Effect of swimming-stress in a water basin 30°C (C=control diet, T=Trp-enriched diet).

and in the responses of both indoles towards a challenge in chicks which were exposed to an increased Trp-availability during embryogenesis (see Huether, 1988) or in rats which were reared for several generations on Trp-enriched diets (Fig. 2). Such long lasting changes may be of particular importance if the effects of malnutrition on the developing human brain are discussed. In most underdeveloped countries, malnutrition lasts for more than only one generation. Apart from some preliminary studies (Cowley and Griesel, 1966; Zamenhof et al., 1971; Bresler et al., 1975; Salas and Torrero, 1979; Galler and Manes, 1980; Galler and Propert, 1981; Zamenhof and van Marthens, 1982; Resnick and Morgane, 1984) the possible generational effects of malnutrition on the developing brain have not found much attention until now.

Conclusions and perspectives

The findings summarized in this short review clearly document that developing transmitter systems can be affected my malnutrition during early infancy. The current knowledge of the courses of these changes and their consequences for later brain function is most advanced with respect to monoamines. In the mature brain, serotonin and catecholamines are involved in the regulation of various rather basic brain functions (see Fig. 3). The synthesis and therefore the ability to release certain amounts of these

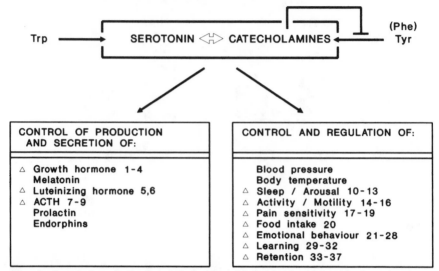

Fig. 3. Serotoninergic and catecholaminergic mechanisms are involved in the regulation of many physiologic and behavioural reactions. This figure summarizes only those functions which have been shown to be affected by an altered availability of either Trp or Tyr. Triangles mark those functions which have been shown to be affected by malnutrition too, numbers indicate references

1 - 4) Pimstone et al. 1973, 1975a, 1975b; 5) Pimstone et al. 1974; 6) Becker 1983; 7) Smith et al. 1975; 8) Dörner 1982; 9) Adlard and Smart 1972; 10) Wiener and Levine 1982; 11) Wiener et al. 1983; 12) Levine 1983; 13) Levine et al. (1982);14) Simonson et al. 1968; 15) Smart and Dobbing 1971; 16) Jordan et al. 1980; 17) Levitsky and Barnes 1970; 18) Smart et al. 1975; 19) Lynch 1976; 20) Katz et al. 1979; 21) Hanson and Simonson 1971; 22) Sobotka et al. 1974; 23) Smart et al. 1976; 29) Goodlett et al. 1986; 30) Klein et al. 1972; 31) Katz et al. 1979; 32) Leathwood 1978; 33) Frankova and Barnes 1968; 34) Frankova 1973; 35) Simonson and Chow 1970; 36) Peters 1979; 37) Halas et al. 1983.

transmitters upon stimulation is dependent on the availability of the respective precursor amino acids. Because the availability of Trp, Tyr and especially His is increased by malnutrition, brain functions controlled by monoaminergic mechanisms are most likely affected as long as the altered substrate supply persists. Because at least serotonin and norepinephrine play a particular role as developmental signals during brain morphogenesis, the increased formation of these modulators during early brain development may additionally and permanently affect the structural development of the brain. Because many feedback regulatory loops for the control of substrate supply and receptor expression are not yet elaborated during early brain development the increased availability of precursor amino acids may cause long lasting changes of the expression of enzymes and receptors involved in the control of later monoaminergic activity. Based on these different pieces of evidence at least some of the structural and functional changes observed in the brains of experimental animals and human subjects which suffered from undernutrition during early life can be explained.

REFERENCES

Adaro L, Fernandes V, Kaufmann W (1986). Effects of nutritional-environmental interactions upon body-weight, body size and development of cortical pyramids. Nutr Rep 33:1013-1020.

Adlard BPF, Smart JL (1972). Adrenocortical function in rats subjected to nutritional deprivation in early life. J Endocrinol 54:99-105.

Balazs R, Jordan T, Lewis PD, Patel AJ (1986). Under nutrition and brain development. In Falkner F, Tanner JM (eds): "Human Growth" Vol. 3, Plenum, pp 415-473.

Becker DJ (1983). The endocrine responses to proteincalorie malnutrition. Ann Rev Nutr 3:187-212.

Bendek G, Hahn Z (1982). Effect of amphetamine on the metabolism and incorporation of (3-H)-thymidine into DNA of developing rat brain. Dev Neurosci 4:55-65.

Berry M, McConell P, Sievers J (1980). Dendritic growth and the control of neuronal form. In Hunt RK, Monroy A, Moscana AA (eds): "Current Topics in Developmental Biology," New York: Academic Press, pp 67-101.

Bresler DE, Ellison GE, Zamenhof S (1975). Learning deficits in rats with malnourished grandmothers. Develop Psychobiol 8:315-323.

Chubakov AR, Gromova EA, Konovalo GV, Sarkisov EF, Chumasov EI (1986). The effects of serotonin on the morphofunctional development of rat cerebral neocortex in tissue-culture. Brain Res 369: 285-297.

Cordero ME, Trejo M, Garcia E, Barros T, Colombo M (1985). Dendritic development in the neocortex of adult rats subjected to postnatal malnutrition. Early Human Dev 12: 309-321.

Cowley JJ, Griesel RD (1966). The effect on growth and behavior of rehabilitating first and second generation low protein rats. Animal Behav 14:506-517.

Debassio WA, Kemper TL (1985). The effects of protein derivation on neuronal migration in rats. Dev Brain Res 20:191-196.

Devitry F, Hamon M, Catelon J, Dubois M, Thibault J (1986). Serotonin inhitiates and autoamplifies its own synthesis during mouse central nervous system development. P.N.A.S. 83:8629-8633.

Dobbing J, Hopewell JW, Lynch A (1971). Vulnerability of the developing brain:VII Permanent deficit of neurons in cerebral and cerebellar cortex following early mild undernutrition. Exp Neurol 32:439-447.

Dörner G (1982). Hormones, nutrition and brain development. Bibliotheca Nutr Dieta 31:19-31.

Enwonwu CO (1988). Amino acid availability and control of histaminergic systems in the brain. In Huether G (ed): "Amino Acid Availability and Brain Function in Health and Disease", Nato ASI Series Vol. H20, Heidelberg: Springer-Verlag, pp 167-174.

Felten DL, Hallman H, Jonsson G (1982). Evidence for a neurotrophic role of noradrenaline neurons in the postnatal development of rat cerebral cortex. J Neurocytol 11:119-135.

Fernstrom JD (1983). Role of percursor availability in control of monoamine biosynthesis in brain. Physiol Reviews 63:484-546.

Frankova S (1973). Influence of the familiarity with the environment and early malnutrition on the avoidance learning and behaviour in rats. Activ Nerv Suppl 15:207-216.

Frankova S, Barnes RH (1968). Influence of malnutrition in early life on exploratory behaviour in rats. J Nutr 96:477-484.

Frankova S and Barnes RH (1968b). Effect of malnutrition in early life on avoidance conditioning and behaviour of adult rats. J Nutr 96:485-493.

Galler JR and Manes M (1980). Gender differences in visual discrimination by rats in response to malnutrition of varying durations. Dev Psychobiol 13:409-416.

Garabal MV, Arevalo RM, Diazpalarea MD, Castro R, Rodriguez M (1988). Tyrosine availability and brain noradrenaline synthesis in the fetus - control by maternal tyrosine ingestion. Brain Research 457:330-337.

Goodlett CH R, Valentino ML, Morgrawe PJ, Resnick O (1986). Spatial cue utilization in chronically malnourished rats: task-specific learning deficits. Dev Psychobiol 19:1-15.

Gundappa G, Desiraju T (1988). Deviations in brain development of F2 generation on caloric undernutrition and scope of their prevention. Brain Research 456: 205-223.

Halas ES, Eberhardt MJ, Diers MA, Sanstead HN (1983). Learning and memory impairment in adult rats due to severe zinc deficiency during lactation. Physiol Behav 30:371-381.

Hanson HM, Simonson M (1971). Effects of fetal under nourishment on experimental anxiety. Nutr Rep Int 4:307-314.

Hawrylewicz EJ, Kissane JQ (1980). The effect of protein restriction on brain biogenic amines. In Parvez H, Parvez S (eds): "Biogenic Amines in Development", Elsevier/North-Holland: Biomedical Press, pp 493-517.

Haydon PG, MC Cobb DP, Kater SB (1984). Serotonin selectively inhibits growth cone motility an synaptogene sis of specific identified neurons. Science 226:561-564.

Howard E, Granoff DM (1968). Effect of neonatal food restriction in mice on brain growth, DNA and cholesterol, and on adult delayed response learning. J Nutr 95:111-121.

Huether G (1984). The influence of increased availability of tryptophan on the formation of tryptamine and serotonin during early ontogenesis. In Schlossberger HG, Kochen W, Linzen B & Steinhart H (eds): "Progress in Tryptophan Research", Berlin, New York: Walter de Gruyter & Co, pp 613-622.

Huether G (1988). Consequences of experimental modulations of amino acid availability during brain development. In Huether G (ed): "Amino Acid Availability and Brain Function in Health and Disease" Nato-ASI Series, Vol. H20, Heidelberg: Springer-Verlag, pp 421-429.

Jordan TC, Heatlie PL, Howells KF, Hughes DA (1980). Brain and behavioural correlates of early undernutrition. Presented at the Twenty-Second International Congress of Psychology, Leipzig.

Kasamatsu T, Pettigrew JD (1979). Preservation of linocularity after monocular deprivation in the striate cortex of kittens treated with 6-Hydroxydopamine. J Comp Neurol 185:139-162.

Katz HB, Ostwald R, Rosett RE (1979). The compensatory role of food motivation in the maze learning performance of lactationally undernourished rats. Develop Psychobiol 12:305.

Klein RE, Lester BM, Yarbrough C, Habicht J-P ((1972). Cross cultural evaluation of human intelligence. In: "Ciba Fdn Symp.on Lipids, Malnutrition and the Developing Brain." Amsterdam: Elsevier, pp 249-265.

Lauder JM (1983). Hormonal and humoral influences on brain development. Psychoneuro 8:121-155.

Lauder JM, Krebs H (1978). Serotonin as a differentiation signal in early neurogenesis. Develop Neurosci 1: 15-30.

Lauder JM, Wallace JA, Krebs H, Petrusz R, McCarthy K (1982). In vivo and in vitro development of serotonergic neurons. Brain Res 9 605-625.

Leathwood P (1978). Influence of early undernutrition on behavioural development and learning in rodents. In Gottlieb G (ed): "Studies on the Development of Behaviour and the Nervous System; Early Influences" Vol 4, New York: Academic Press, p 187.

Levine S (1983). A psychological approach to the ontogeny of coping. In Germezy N, and Rutter M (eds): "Stress, Coping and Development in Children", New York: McGraw-Hill, pp 241-257.

Levine S, Coe C, Wiener SG (1982). Mother-infant relationships and the development of coping. Baroda J Nutr 9:116-122.

Levitsky DA, Barnes RH (1970). Effect of early malnutrition on the reaction of adult rats to aversive stimuli. Nature 225:468-469.

Lewis PD, Patel AJ, Bender G, Balazs R (1977). Effect of reserpine on cell proliferation in the developing rat brain: a quantitative histological study. Brain Res 129: 299-308.

Lidov HGW, Molliver ME (1979). Neocortical development after prenatal lesions of noradrenergic projections. Neurosci Abst 5:341.

Lynch A (1976). Passive avoidance behavior and response thresholds in adult male rats after early postnatal undernutrition. Physiol Behav 16:27-32.

Maher TJ (1988). Modification of synthesis, release, and function of catecholaminergic systems by phenylalanine. In Huether G (ed): "Amino Acid Availability and Brain Function in Health and Disease", Nato ASI Series, Vol H 20, Heidelberg: Springer Verlag, pp 201-206.

Marin FT (1976). Regulation of development in Dictystelium discoideum: I. Initiation of the growth to development transition by amino acid starvation. Dev Biol 48:110-160.

Marin FT (1977). Regulation of development in Dictyostelium discoideum: II. Regulation of early cell differentiation by amino acid starvation and intercellular interaction. Dev Biol 60 389-395.

Miller JC, Friedhoff AJ (1988). Prenatal neurotransmitter programming of postnatal receptor function. Prog Brain Res 73:509-522.

Moon SL (1984) Prenatal haloperidol alters striatal dopamine and opiate receptors. Brain Research 323:109-113.

Oey J (1975). Noradrenaline induces morphological alterations in nucleated and enucleated rat C6 glioma cells. Nature 257:317-319.

Pardridge WM (1979). Tryptophan transport through the blood-brain barrier: in vivo measurement of free and albumin bound amino acids. Life Sci 25:1519-1528.

Parnavelas JG, Blue, ME (1982). The role of the noradrenergic system on the formation of synapses in the visual cortex of the rat. Devl Brain Res 3:140-144.

Patel AJ, Bender G, Balazs R, Lewis PD (1977). Effect of reserpine on cell proliferation in the developing rat brain: a biochemical study. Brain Res 129:283-297.

Peters DP (1979). Effects of prenatal nutrition on learning and motivation in rats. Physiol Behav 22:1067-1071.

Pimstone BL, Becker DJ, Hausen JDL (1973). Human growth hormone and sulphation factor in protein-calorie malnutrition. In Gardner LI, Amacher, P (eds): "Endrocrine Aspects of Malnutrition", The Croc Foundation, Santa Ynez, California pp. 73-90.

Pimstone BL, Becker DJ, Kronheim S (1974). LH and FSH response to gonadotrophin releasing hormone in normal and malnourished infants. Horm Metab Res (Suppl) 5:179-183.

Pimstone BL, Becker DJ, Kronheim S (1975a). Serum growth hormone responses to thryptotropine releasing hormone in children with protein calorie malnutrition. Horm Metab Res 7:358-360

Pimstone BL, Becker DJ, Kronheim S (1975b). Disappearance of plasma growth hormone in acromegaly and protein-calorie malnutrition after somatostatin. J Clin Endocrinol 40:168-171.

Resnick O, Morgane PJ (1984). Generational effects of protein malnutrition in the rat. Dev Brain Res 15:219-227.

Rosengarten H, Friedhoff AS (1979). Enduring changes in dopamine receptor cells of pups from drug administration to pregnant and nursing rats. Science 203:1133-1135.

Rosenstein JM, Brightman MW (1981). Anomalous migration of central nervous tissue to transplanted autonomic ganglia. J Neurocytol 10:387-409.

Salas M, Torrero C (1979). Maternal behavior of rats undernourished in the early postnatal period. Bol Estud Med Biol Mex 30:237-244.

Salas M, Torrero C, Pulido S (1986). Undernutrition induced by early pup separation delays the development of the thalamic reticular neurons in rats. Exp Neurol 93:447-455.

Simonson M, Chow BF (1970). Maze studies on progeny of underfed mother rats. J Nutr 100:685-690.

Simonson M, Sherwin RW, Kanilane JK, Yu WY, Chow BF (1968). Neuromotor development in progeny of underfed mother rats. J Nutr 98:18-24.

Smart JL, Dobbing J (1971). Vulnerability of developing brain. VI. Relative effects of foetal and early postnatal undernutrition on reflex ontogeny and development of behaviour in the rat. Brain Res 33:303-314.

Smart JL, Whatson TS, Dobbing J (1975). Thresholds of response to electric shock in previously undernourished rats. Br J Nutr 34:511-516.

Smart JL, Tricklebank MD, Adlard BPF, Dobbing J (1976). Nutritionally small-for-date rats:Their subsequent growth, regional brain 5-hydroxytryptamine turnover, and behaviour. Pediatr Res 10:807-811.

Smith SR, Bledsoe T, Chhetri MK (1975). Cortisol metabolism and the pituitary-adrenal axis in adults with protein-calorie malnutrition, J Clin Endocrinol Metab 40: 43-52.

Sobotka TJ, Cook MP, and Brodie RE (1974). Neonatal malnutrition: Neurochemical, hormonal and behavioural manifestations. Brain Res 65:443-457.

Stern WC, Miller M, Forbes WB, Morgane PJ, Resnick O (1973). Ontogeny of the levels of biogenic amines in various parts of the brain and peripheral tissues in normal and protein malnourished rats. Expt Neurol 49: 314-326.

Wallace J (1988). Neurotransmitters and early embryogenesis. In Huether G (ed): "Amino Acid Availability and Brain Function in Health and Disease" Nato-ASI Series, Vol. H20, Heidelberg: Springer-Verlag, pp 431-440.

Whitaker-Azmitia PM, Azmitia AC (1986). Auto-regulation of fetal serotonergic neuronal development - role of high affinity serotonin receptors. Neurosci L 67:307-312.

Wiener S, Robinson L, Levine S (1983). Influence of perinatal malnutrition on adult physiological and behavioral reactivity in rats. Physiol Behav 30:41-50.

Wiener SG, Levine S (1982). Effects of malnutrition in early life on modification of stress induced rise in plasma corticosterone level by consummatory behaviour in adult rats. Baroda J Nutr 9:123-128.

Wiggins RC, Fuller G, Enna SJ (1984). Undernutrition and the development of brain neurotransmitter systems. Life Sci. 35:2085-2094.

Winick M, Noble A, (1966). Cellular response in rats during malnutrition at various ages. J Nutr 89:300-306.

Wurtman RJ, Heftt F, Melamed E (1980). Precursor control of neurotransmitter synthesis. Pharmacol Rev 32:315-335.

Zamenhof S, van Marthens E (1982). Chronic undernutrition for 10 generations:differential effects on brain and body development among neonatal rats. Nutr Rep Int 26: 703-709.

Zamenhof S, van Marthens E, Grauel L (1971). DNA (cell number) in neonatal brain: second generation (F+40V2-40V) alterations by maternal (F+40Vo-40V) dietary protein restriction. Science 172:850-851.

Zecevic N, Rakic L (1982). Development of the rat neocortex-potential role of mono-aminergic input. Per Biol 84:297-304.

DISCUSSION

Q (Reader): In the (one before last) slide you showed the variations between 5-HT and hydroxyindole-acetic acid (5-HIAA); there was an increase of about 6.5. Now, if you look at the ratio of 5-HIAA and serotonin, it (seems that) demonstrates a reduction in the turnover rate. My question is, do you have a reduction of the hydroxylase activity, or is the expression of the enzyme reduced?

A: This is exactly what we are doing at the moment. These are just the first preliminary data showing that there is something changed in the system and that these rats respond differently to the same stimulus. This is not only true for the injection of, lets say, a challenge of tryptophan. You can also stimulate the system in other ways and you will always see that these rats show other changes. For instance, 24 hrs fasting affects serotonin and 5-HIAA levels in the rats which have been on the tryphophan enriched diet for several generations, in a different manner than rats on the same diet for only one generation. But you are right, we now have to measure enzymes and the level of expression of enzymes and receptors.

Q (G. Hashim): Gerald, how do you envisage this generational effect: is it mainly genetic or acquired.

A: It is very difficult to say. Actually I just can guess, give my own impression and my own feeling or intuition. We know of a number of biochemical pathways, the expression of which is dependent on precursor supply. So, the earlier during development the supply is altered, the earlier and the more massive is the change of the respective enzyme. Because, biochemical pathways are interrelated, they stabilise each other, and it might be that the earlier you change one thing, the more you get a sort of network which stabilises the situation. Of course, in that case there must be a difference if the rat is placed for just one generation on such a diet than when the diet persists through more than one generation. The pup, through the mother, is affected earlier and earlier by the modifications.

Q (G. Hashim): You envision this as a sort of challenge of the environment on the development of the embryo.

A: Yes, this is exactly what I mean. Although it is difficult to put it into terms of biochemical mechanisms.

Q (Diamond): I just want to say that we see the same phenomenon with our enriched rats. We can get incremental increases in the cortex over several generations of enriched rats. You do not stand alone.

A: This is beautiful, because I really feel somewhat isolated. As a biochemist one seems to be standing alone with such generational effects. It is nice to see that structural and morphological changes can also occur over several generations. This is beautiful!

Section III: NEUROCHEMICAL INTEGRATION DURING BRAIN
MATURATION

The human genome ensures that following fertilization, the ovum will invariably develop into a human being. However, there still exists a large difference between the brain of a newborn, with close (cognitive) similarities to an infant ape brain, and that of a four years old child or an adult. Beginning at birth with a brain suitable to a sensorially sheltered, aquatic organism, the organ after birth must yet undergo enormous structural and cognitive expansion to assure survival in practically any natural or, even, artificial ecosystem and psychological stress condition. Conversely, it is the nature of a particular ecosystem and psycho-social experiences which will determine the final outcome of brain development, both in terms of biological as well as intellectual maturation.

Until just before birth, much of the CNS represents mostly a network of primary neuronal connections; only when non-neuronal cell populations become integrated within this network can one begin to discern the unique properties which sets the human brain apart from any other species. Together with the onset of bipedal locomotion, speech and (with it?) cognitive powers begin to far outdistance the communication and learning skills of sub-human primates. Since during evolution bipedalism preceded by far the increase in brain size and its associated abilities, the evolutionary limits set by a compromise between cranial circumference and the width of the birth canal infers that much of what typifies the human brain only develops after birth. Infant brain development is anatomically defined by increased aborization and connectivity between neurons, the marked accelleration in myelination by the oligodendrocytes, and the establishment of the astroglial network in close apposition to neuronal structures as well as to the physical limits of the central nervous system: blood vessels, ventricular spaces and the meninges (blood-brain barrier systems).

Within the context of this developmental period, van Gelder reviews the specific importance of the (astro)glia in forming anatomical substrates for axonal growth, and the mutual influence on neuronal network expansion of cytokines derived from neurons and glia. The emphasis that brain function depends on the interdependent integration of neurochemical processes, with component metabolic events divided between neurons and glia, is further discussed in terms of intracranial water homeostasis and the inhibition-excitation balance in cerebral regions. The author proposes that taurine is an amino acid needed to regulate the interstitial water balance, whereas the compartmentation between neurons and astrocytes of glutamic acid metabolism regulates the extracellular actions of excitatory glutamate and inhibitory GABA, as well as providing a mechanism by which water influx into the cranium can be balanced by intracranial water outflux. Astrogliosis in the human brain being primarily a post-natal development, it is evident how malnutrition will affect (two) physiological mechanisms essential for normal brain function.

Myelin deposition represents another event which is very active after birth. The myelination of regions above the brainstem, necessary for the uniquely human brain expressions, to a large extent takes place only after environmental cues stimulate the brain into higher mental activity. Miller reviews in detail the extensive sequence of events which must follow a precise temporal program to assure that by the age of 2-3 years, myelination of designated axons has been completed. The high requirements for proteins (amino acids) and essential lipids during this period, with a temporal sequence which is different for various brain regions, makes myelination one of the most vulnerable processes during undernutrition and malnutrition. With a slowing in the speed of conduction, the communication and integration of physiological signals is less rapid and, therefore, learning and information assimilation become less efficient. Over the years, such regionally and functionally specific deficits become increasingly evident compared to the norm of the peer group(s). In turn, social prejudisms and expectations may then hinder rehabilitation, giving rise to greater intellectual slowing than the biological anomalies might have caused if the social environment were more enriched. The observation that myelination by mature oligodendrocytes may continue throughout life, although at a slower rate, seems to suggest that with more precise knowledge of the nutritional and sensory factors needed to maintain or accellerate myelination, recovery from a period of nutrient or social impoverishment will become increasingly successful.

Protein synthesis and the needed supply of essential amino acids are obviously indispensable during organ formation and maturation. Intuitively one accepts that anabolic processes have a preponderance over catabolic reactions under these circumstances. However, as the work by Lajtha and his collegues indicate, it seems that during brain development protein breakdown is as important as is amino acid assimilation into proteins. Contrary perhaps to expectation, malnutrition and undernutrition do not necessarily spare protein synthesis more than protein catabolism and may even shift the balance in favour of protein breakdown. Several reasons may account for this apparent anomaly.

More than any organ, the brain may escape the worst effects of essential amino acid deficiencies by reutilizing a large percentage of the amino acids liberated during protein turnover. Such protein turnover may be required to prevent that genetic or environmental factors modify the structure of an existing protein, thereby producing aberrant function; turnover therefore seems an efficient process to ensure that proteins maintain their conformation and amino acid sequence necessary for their designated function(s).

One problem associated with providing an adequate supply of amino acids to cells is the fact that amino acid transfer across membranes is not determined exclusively by the availability of a particular amino acid and the properties of its transport systems. Patterns of organ amino acid content or biological fluid concentrations are interdependently regulated: transport competition, incorporation in constant proportion into proteins, selective vulnerability of certain exposed or labile amino acids in peptide sequences, are some of the factors which determine the local free amino acid spectrum of organs. As Lajtha points out, each region or, even, cell may demonstrate a unique pattern of free amino acids available for use. Thus, during amino acid imbalances, where the level of one or more transport or metabolically related amino acids are either higher or lower than normal, the effect on functional development may vary in different brain regions or may affect especially one type of (maturing) brain cell.

Many proteins act as enzymes in the brain and these require vitamins as co-factors. During brain development, designated enzyme activities may wax and subsequently wane as particular formative periods of maturation are replaced by others. All vitamins are supplied to the infant by either the maternal circulation, milk, and later, the diet. In the early phases of infant brain development malnutrition or undernutrition may result mostly in a deficiency of the water soluble vitamins. These have to be continuously supplied by the diet, whereas fat soluble vitamins can be stored for long periods either by the mother or infant. Unless dietary insufficiencies are very severe and very prolonged, vitamin deficiencies in the foetus and nursing neonate pertain especially to the water soluble co-factors. Such deficiencies are discussed and reviewed by Butterworth. Since many of the vitamins are supplied by fresh and raw vegetables, avitaminosis is especially prevalent in world regions where drought conditions prevail and occur frequently. Nonetheless, it is becoming increasingly apparent that even in industrialized or wealthy nations, deficiencies of one or more water soluble vitamins may be quite widespread. The poor often subsist on staple foods lacking in vitamins, while among the rich a preference of children for processed foods and diets, high in carbohydrates but poor in fresh vegetables and fruits, may have similar results. The teen-age mother represents therefore a particularly vulnerable class in a population. Ironically, among the population which does follow nutritional advice, overdosage of certain vitamins is not uncommon because of facile access to mega-vitamin doses.

Paradoxically, although knowledge about the chemical structure and exact catalytic functions of practically all vitamins is quite precise, far less certainty exists as to the number and nature of the biological mechanisms in which they obligatorily participate; nor are the minimum or maximum permissible daily requirements all that well defined. One may cite as examples the controversy regarding the minimum requirement for vitamin C or the anti-oxidant action of vitamin E; the complexities of vitamin D metabolism are also as yet not totally worked out. Clearly then, much research is still needed in this area, as well as on the potential role of specific vitamins in preventing or attenuating certain disease entities.

Similarly to the vitamins, minerals are essential components of the diet. Many functional centers of proteins contain one or more metal atoms where they often serve in electron transfer (oxidation-reduction), in molecular group chelation, and in transport function. Unlike the vitamins, however, the dietary requirements for specific trace minerals and their exact biological roles, especially during brain development, remain in many cases very imprecise. It is therefore all the more valuable that Keen and his collegues consented to contribute a chapter to discuss some of these issues.

The wide-spread dietary need for specific trace minerals is indisputable. However, how do the various elements interact biologically, how does intestinal absorption regulate intake and maintain adequate but not excessive biological levels, which are the metabolic cues implicated in regulatory mechanisms? Does zinc in the Zn^{2+} finger domains of transcription factors serve the same function as this metal in carbonic anhydrase? Why are, particularly, the group 8 transitional metals- Fe, Co, Ni - such powerful epileptogenic agents? Investigations into the role of trace metals, and their exact role in health and disease, are clearly lacking and need increased attention.

Finally, throughout human (brain) development probably one event, more than any other, marks a critical period in the life of an individual. The abrupt transition from a docile, rather anaerobic foetus to a screaming and kicking infant, fighting to stay alive and to assimilate the meriad of stimuli bombarding its sensory systems, is one of the greatest marvels of nature. The need to transform in only 2-3 years an as yet primitive neural tissue into a sophisticated organ of integration and cognition requires enormous amounts of energy. That energy exists primarily in the form of ATP, which phosphate groups in precise configuration can incorporate increased electron bond vibration without breaking apart (high energy bonds). The metabolic process which car. meet the sudden 5-10 fold need for energy requires a food source which is always readily and abundantly available during life while its use does not add excessively to body waste. Since survival of the human depends primarily on brain function, the nervous system must have access under all life conditions to an assured supply of energy substrate. The complete metabolism of glucose, a substance transportable in blood at high concentrations, entirely meets the high energy requirements of the brain. However, complete metabolism of the sugar implies an absolute dependency on oxygen combined with an enzymic system which efficiently captures and transforms latent atomic bond energy into a useful form (ATP). Prevention of energy loss in the form of heat during the complex series of electron transfer steps is eminently accomplished by placing most of the oxidative enzymes and reactive surfaces together in units within special cell organs: the mitochondria.

Clark presents a comprehensive overview of the oxidative mitochondrial enzyme system and the developing transition in brain from an anaerobic, cytosolic (glycolytic) metabolism to the aerobic, mitochondrial (citric acid) enzyme system. The investigator discusses the development of the pyruvate dehydrogenase (PDH) complex as a key event in brain metabolic maturation, in that the complex represents the essential enzymic link between the glycolytic and oxidative uses of energy substrates. These substrates, in the neonate, include ketone bodies which supplement but only partially replace the need for glucose. With advancing CNS maturation, the brain becomes increasingly more dependent on glucose.

As already indicated by Butterworth and, in this chapter by Clark, interference with the PDH system can have devastating consequences for the intellectual development of the infant. Because of the complexity of this enzyme system and its localization in the mitochondrial membrane, the system appears highly vulnerable to biological interference. Many factors ranging from panthotenic-vitamin B deficiencies, to genetic influences, (ammonia) toxicities, and anoxia or hypoxia, will leave permanent sequelae in the brain, marked by mental and coordination underdevelopment. In what measure, how, and until which age such damage can be reversed remains undetermined but clinical observations to date would suggest that the time window for repair may be exceptionally small.

Nico M. van Gelder

(Mal)Nutrition and the Infant Brain, pages 161–174
© 1990 Wiley-Liss, Inc.

MATURATION OF NEURONAL-GLIAL INTEGRATION AND THE DEVELOPMENT OF BRAIN FUNCTION.

Nico M. van Gelder

Centre de recherche en sciences neurologiques, Dép. physiologie, Université de Montréal, C.P. 6128, succursale A, Montréal (Québec), H3C 3J7

The first 2-3 years after birth represent in the human a critical phase of brain maturation, when many of the higher expressions of intelligence become established. Speech, abstraction and conceptualisation, precise motor coordination, self awareness and socialization, among others, are all characteristic human attributes which emerge only with the final anatomical and functional integration of the CNS (Werker, 1989); myelination, essential for rapid signal transmission, also occurs for the most part within this time window (Agrawal and Davison, 1973). The vulnerability of the brain to damage during this developmental period stems directly from the fact that the infant has as yet no autonomy over its nutrition or environment. While the genome guides the primary patterns of brain development, these patterns are fine tuned into a sophisticated, unified communication network under the postnatal influence of the social and intellectual environment, in combination with an adequate nutrition. Much of the maturation process at this time represents an elaboration and strenghtening of anatomical interconnectivity and the integration of numerous neurochemical mechanisms of individual cells into interdependent metabolic linkages. It is this metabolic integration which to a large extent is responsible for establishing efficient communication between neurons, and between these and the various glial cell types.

Intercellular metabolic communication involves and requires the participation of many neurobiological components. The development of each of these depends in turn on anatomical configuration, characteristically sequenced electrophysiological stimuli, and the carefully timed appearance of serial neurochemical reactions (Dobbing, 1976; Le Douarin, 1986). With many possibilities for error and the need for each neurobiological function to develop within a particular time frame, it is not surprising that the neonatal stage of brain development is so susceptible to damage. The consequences of interference with, or a delay in the appearance of even only a few isolated neurobiological events may cause a chain reaction of amplifying functional errors, as misdirected, mistimed, or absent developmental cues increasingly perturb the normally ordered progression towards the highly complex expressions of human intelligence (Hickey, 1977).

Neurobiological Directives versus Environment

Since all humans belong to a single species it may be assumed that variations in the genomic developmental directives are slight. This may also be inferred from the observation that most noticeable genetic mutations affecting brain function, when they occur, have pathological consequences which are for the most part biologically incompatible with survival to a reproductive age (discounting modern medicin). Similarly, the minimum nutritional requirement for optimal brain development is biologically determined and should not differ much among individuals. Nevertheless, each human being soon after birth begins to express the same neurobiological properties of the brain in such widely divergent manner that even at two years of age, every individual is unique and can be distinguished from all others. Accepting that subtle genetic variability may determine the dominance of broad behavioral traits, one must nonetheless come to the conclusion that only one developmental influence demonstrates sufficient diversity to account, on interaction with these traits, for the emergence of the incredibly unique personality of each individual (Birch, 1972; Butzer, 1977). That influence is represented by the interaction of sensory (environmental) cues, with the ongoing process of neural functional integration (Hubel and Wiesel, 1970; Sutula et al, 1988).

Electrophysiological Signals into Neurochemical Events

The electrophysiological signals, their pattern of arrival and duration, their frequency, their repetition and their regional target in the brain, will produce neurochemical changes which, superimposed upon genetic directives, determine the final modifications in the maturing brain (Grenel et al, 1988). The more the environment is diversified, the more complex the combination of electrical signals will become and the more regions of the brain are affected simultaneously or in precise sequence. Herein probably lies the foundation for interregional associations, reinforcement of functional circuitry, and regional or intercellular metabolic integration. The transduction of electrophysiological signals into neurochemical cues can take many forms. To mention but a few: phosphorylation-dephosphorylation, calcium mobilization, patterns of hormone and transmitter release, activation of cytokines; those mechanisms can in turn influence such basic neurochemical processes as gene activation-repression, protein synthesis, and the balance between anabolic and catabolic reactions. Anatomically, anyone of these neurochemical changes, or in combination, will stimulate glial proliferation, direct and guide axonal growth cones to their destination, and selectively reinforce synaptic pathways (Ruoslahti and Pierschbacher, 1987; Abbott, 1988).

The manner in which electrophysiological and neurochemical events interact are innumerable (Svaetichin et al, 1965), and most important, not always predictable since local metabolic conditions are also determinant. Conceptually it is therefore not difficult to accept that almost identical types of neurobiological phenomena can nevertheless give rise to expressions of brain functions which are unique for each individual (Bennett et al, 1974). No environmental experience is likely to produce an identical electrophysiological response pattern and, thus, neurochemical transduction. However, it is predictable that , with increasing complexity of the environment to which the infant is exposed, the electrophysiological signal patterns and neurochemical responses also become more varied and pervasive. The resulting diversity and enrichment of neural interconnectivity and integration eventually becomes expressed as a greater ability of the brain to receive, assimilate, interpret and transform information. This ability is the essence of intelligence.

Appreciable evidence is beginning to suggest that this interplay between the environment and intellectual ability, to a considerable extent continues during the entire life span of an individual. Nevertheless the phenomenon is most essential and beneficial during the neonatal period when the process of neural integration is most active. This explains why malnutrition in the neonate can have such a devastating and possibly permanent deleterious effect on brain function (Hillman and Chen, 1981a,b). Without the trace metals, vitamins, protein precursors or adequate energy supplies, the transduction process fails or slows down. Much of the final complexities of brain development may never take place or are delayed so that information processing remains deficient. If the nutritional deficiencies are only temporary, most genetic directives are still operant and rehabilition appears quite successful. However, the longer the interval is between nutritional deficiencies and the restitution of nutritional quality and quantity, the more lasting the neurological consequences will be. This pessimistic outcome is also contributed to by a deteriorating social environment.

Poor nutrition usually occurs in the context of an impoverished social environment, increased disease susceptibility in combination with poor hygenic conditions, and scholastic underachievement. In malnourished societies child care standards are often inadequate which in turn can cause neural underdevelopment in the next generation as well. This creates a viscious circle as nutritional deficiencies, which were the initial cause of intellectual underachievement, become seemingly indigenous and begin to be confounded with genetic factors. It may cause grave social injustices by creating prejudices in terms of decreasing expectations for intellectual success, within the malnourished population itself, as well as among the more privileged societies. Neonatal brain growth thus represents a period which determines in many instances both the intellectual as well as social success of an individual. Since major events during this developmental phase concern the functional integration of the neuron and its support cells, the glia, it seems useful to discuss some of the more important aspects of this type of metabolic and anatomic interaction.

The Extracellular Guidance Matrix

The availability of cytochemical markers, models of development ranging from tissue cultures to brain implants, and molecular biology, in recent years have demonstrated the importance of glia in guiding axons to their final innervation (Kater and Letourneau, 1985, de Vellis et al, 1988;). In the human, much of the glial expansion process occurs during the neonatal period, well after most of the primary neuronal pathways are already in place (Dobbing, 1976; Hickey, 1977). However, at birth these pathways are as yet not very elaborate and it is the complexity of neuronal interconnectivity which determines the eventual functional intricacy of the brain. The elaboration process seems to be intimately associated with the proliferation of the glial systems.

Astrocytes and their extensions appear to provide the major adhesive pathways to guide neuronal arborization towards the proper target fields (Hammarback et al , 1985; Rutishauser, 1985). While anatomically these cells may appear to represent a homogeneous lineage, it is now becoming evident that populations of astrocytes in different brain regions do not elaborate identical chemical cues for neurite outgrowth and synaptogenesis (Herrup, 1987; Autillo-Touati et al, 1988). In addition, growth cones of different neurons are morphologically distinct. Their speed of progression to the target as well as neurite and growth cone number also vary considerably (Haydon et al, 1985; Roberts and Patton, 1985). Such cones in turn may confer, by secretion of cytokines, different biochemical specificity on a proliferating glial population in their viscinity (Espinosa de los Monteros and de Vellis, 1988; Giulian et al, 1988). Thus even if the chemical nature of the adhesive pathways may be restricted to only a small group of molecules, their combination with other guiding cues will provide sufficient complexity to assure that similarly destined axons reach their target as a bundle and form the proper synapses (Tessier-Lavigne et al, 1988). These determinant factors include variations in axon to axon cell adhesion molecules, the neuron-specificity of neurite elaboration and outgrowth, diffusible chemical factors originating from the glial cells in target fields, and secretion of synapse stimulating proteins on arrival of each growth cone at the destination (Trinkaus, 1985; Davies, 1988; Burry and Hayes, 1989). Once on site, stimulus frequency dependent release of peptidergic substances, co-localised with more transiently acting transsynaptic messenger substances, may strengthen and consolidate permanency of synaptic connections.

Regeneration versus Rehabilitation

One area of great interest for which at this time existing data still is insufficient to have practical application, is the anatomical role of glia after synaptogenesis has occurred. Neuron-specific and, even, neurite-specific rates of axonal elongation will account for the subsequent degeneration of redundant neuronal extensions which arrive too late at a target to participate in synaptogenesis (Mattson et al, 1988). However, not much is known about the subsequent biochemical specialization of the glia in this area. Some evidence indicates that a certain degree of biochemical specificity may remain (Schousboe et al, 1980). Whether such fully differentiated glia still retain the chemical potential to guide axons to their target is a crucial question to resolve. There appears to exist a fundamental difference in the requirements for successful regeneration, as opposed to those which may be needed to rehabilitate an underdeveloped brain.

Axonal sprouting and reactive gliosis following trauma to the CNS is often initiated by the increased appearance of macrophages and microglia (Perry and Gordon, 1988). These cells may secrete cytokines to promote astrocytosis

(Giulian, 1987). However, if the newly proliferating glial cells do not elaborate the regionally specific chemical cues needed for axonal guidance, because the event falls outside the developmental time frame when it usually occurs (Agrawal and Davison, 1973), the new astrocytic network may represent a barrier rather than promoting correct reinnervation.

In contrast to CNS damage, neural underdevelopment caused by adverse nutritional or environmental conditions may have persisted for some time. Underdevelopment of the glial guidance systems results in only a fraction of the growing axons population to reach their target. Moreover, those nerve terminals which do participate in forming functional contacts, afterwards may no longer incorporate the ability to secrete the same cytokines as were needed during the period of synaptogenesis. Nor would nutritional or environmental rehabilitation necessarily represent a trigger to reactivate the genetic program required to once more synthetise such cytokines. Hence, rehabilitation may be most successful during the developmental period when astrocytic and oligodendrocytic proliferation are still part of the normal sequence of gene expression. Outside this time window, it may be necessary to reinitiate this process by activating the production of special glial promoting growth factors which not only stimulate glial proliferation, but in addition confer regional metabolic specificity upon the network being elaborated. Some of that specificity requires that intact axons still secrete the appropriate cytokines (Parnavelas and Cavanagh, 1988). Thus, the later nutritional and/or environmental rehabilitation occurs during the developmental period, the less likely that this will entirely reactivate the complete neurochemical program required for the interactions between an elaborating glial guidance network and renewed arborization of axons.

Nonetheless, even late in development or after a prolonged period of insufficiencies, rehabilitation may still produce surprising improvements in brain function (Davenport et al, 1976). Existing synaptic surfaces can still expand, transynaptic messenger synthesis and release can become more efficient, and sequestration as well as transport mechanisms for messenger storage or inactivation in glia and nerve terminals may enhance their capacity. This inherent functional plasticity in neural tissue assures that whatever communication system survives a period of social or nutritional deprivation, it can be made to operate more efficiently and at greater speed by enrichment of the social environment, greater intellectual stimulation,and a balanced diet (Grenel et al, 1988).

The fact that the CNS seemingly demonstrates considerable anatomical and functional redundancy, makes the consequences of underdevelopment and the outcome of rehabilitation quite unpredictable for any one individual. In some cases the residual developmental imperfections remaining are only expressed as a diminished resistance to subsequent neurobiological or psychological trauma to the brain. On the other hand, in view of the now emerging understanding regarding the complex interactions between neurons and glia which are required for proper development, true rehabilitation may only become possible after (biochemical) methods are found to reactivate with appropriate cytokines the regionally specific guidance pathways and target selective innervation factors. Because a primitive neuronal network is already in place before the glial support structures make their appearance (Vitiello and Gombos, 1987), the most important initial chemical cues for development probably originate from the neurons (Banker, 1980). This is further corroborated by the observation that the oligodendrocytes, responsible for axonal myelination, also represent several subpopulations with different biochemical properties (Espinosa de los Monteros and de Vellis, 1988). At least two types of neuronal cytokines influence oligodendrocyte proliferation and differentiation (Giulian et al. 1988). Unlike recovery from trauma or damage, therefore, where glial specificity should be of primary importance, recovery from brain underdevelopment may require a different strategy since here the neurons may be the initial target for paliative intervention.

Chemical Interconnectivity: Metabolic Compartmentation

As the brain begins to mature anatomically, the biochemical properties and anatomical location of the glial support structure become increasingly essential to sustain neuronal activity. Some of the most important functions include the maintenance of water homeostasis, and the regulation of the inhibition-excitation balance in the CNS. In general, this requires that substances released from neuronal structures, on excitation, are taken up by glia. Here, they then can be transformed or they can be sequestered for later release or metabolism. The end result is the same, in that electrophysiological substances liberated during impulse generation are rapidly removed from the extracellular environment. This type of transsynaptic messenger inactivation was first suggested by Elliott, when it became evident that GABA, unlike acetylcholine, could not be easily destroyed by metabolic mechanisms situated on the external neuronal membrane (Elliott and van Gelder, 1958). The close apposition of the astrocytic structures around synaptic contacts (Sandri et al, 1977) is very compatible with this notion, even though no direct proof has yet been obtained to demonstrate that this is indeed the method by which the actions of transmitter substances are limited to milliseconds. Because the hypothesis is so attractive and indirect pharmacological interpretations are imminently compatible with the suggestion, the hypothesis now is so well accepted that most of the literature reports it as an established fact.

The movement of substances across semi-permeable membranes causes the transfer of water; the transfer or release of 300 mOsmole is accompanied by 1000 ml of water. Thus, the fact that a solute interchange occurs between closely adjacent structures indicates that this also causes water movement between neurons, and their glial envelope. A release of substances from neurons should tend to shrink the cells whereas the uptake process would tend to swell cells, as in the case for glia. The electrical conducting properties of the neuron are intimately dependent on intracellular to extracellular concentration gradients, the equilibrium potentials of various ions, as well as intermolecular distances of membrane constituents (Boggs, 1980; Di Perri et al, 1983; Fisher and Agranoff, 1987). It is evident therefore that neural volume changes will severely affect such physico-chemical parameters. Hence, it is to be anticipated that neurons maintain a constant volume, by continuous adjustment of their intracellular osmotic solute content. This can be accomplished, for example, if intracellularly a substance was available which can either be sequestered (osmotically inactive), exist free in solution, or be liberated from the cell (excesss water removal). One requisite property of a substance serving in osmotic regulation must be that varying concentrations of the free solute form do not directly affect ongoing cellular metabolism while, at the same time, that metabolism does influence the partition between inactive osmoles and the amount free in solution.

Osmotic Role of Taurine

Such a solute in the form of the amino acid taurine is in fact present in brain; very high levels are moreover found in cells still immature. Since cytoplasmic osmotic pressure is low before cellular differentiation, the cell would have need for high amounts of free taurine during the maturation stage. As cytoplasmic colloidal osmolarity increases with intracellular differentiation, the cell content of this solute would be expected to decrease. This too is observed for taurine. Finally, few biochemical actions of taurine are known and the amino acid can be liberated or captured by neural tissue in proportion to neuronal excitability and in response to changes in the transmembranal osmotic pressure (van Gelder and Barbeau, 1985; Wade et al, 1988). Also, taurine can form a sequestered complex in association with zinc (Wen et al, 1979).

Among various mammalian species taurine content in adult brain varies between   1-10 μmole/g tissue. In adult brain, the greatest threat to neuronal volume change comes from water which is continually produced from glucose metabolism. Taking into account that glucose metabolism increases with enhanced excitation and that certain brain structures have a higher metabolic rate than others, a simple calculation suggests that any substance used as an osmole to counter neuronal water production must be present at roughly 10% of glucose consumed. When taurine content is plotted against cerebral metabolic rate of various species, such a relationship seems to exist (Fig. 1; van Gelder, 1989)

One can envisage the osmotic function of taurine in the adult brain in the following manner: In proportion to intracellular glucose metabolism, taurine release from neurons maintains their constant volume and osmolarity. The taurine is taken up (+ water) into surrounding glial elements (swelling). These cells can synthetise glutamine, also proportional to excitation and glucose metabolism. The release of glutamine with water in effect represents CSF formation and leaves the astrocyte hyper-osmotic from an excess taurine, which is then released (Wade et al, 1988) and taken up in a sequestered form in the neuronal structures; sequestration renders taurine osmotically inactive (A summarizing scheme is presented in Fig. 2). In this manner, taurine can help in maintaining interstitial water homeostasis without a net loss of the amino acid from the CNS, compatible with the observed unusually low turnover of taurine in mammalian brain. This contrast with the rapid turnover of the glucose carbon through the glutamic acid-glutamine metabolic cycle.

Glutamate Compartmentation and Water Homeostasis

The synthesis of glutamic acid via the amination of 2-oxoglutarate by glutamic acid dehydrogenase represents one of the most important mechanisms of nitrogen fixation in the brain (Balazs and Haslam, 1965). The availability of 2-oxoglutarate from oxidative glucose metabolism, and that of ammonia,

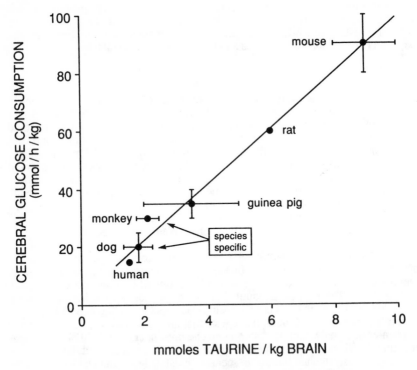

Fig. 1. A plot of brain taurine content against the cerebral metabolic rate (CRM) of several species. The neural tissue taurine content in a species may be determined by the amount of solute which is needed to osmotically balance the excess water produced during glucose consumption. Release of taurine from cells causes water efflux which can then be processed as CSF, while (re)uptake of taurine and intracellular sequestration renders the amino acid osmotically inert. (From data: McIlwain and Bachelard, 1971; van Gelder, 1989; Wetherell et al, 1989).

increases with increased excitability. Because of the very low solubility of the negatively charged ion and its extreme acidity, the high cellular glutamic acid content must be in a sequestered form (Cell pH>7; negative resting potential). One of the most effective stimuli for glutamic acid release is an increase in the intracellular ionic calcium content which occurs, among other circumstances, during neuronal excitation or a fall in cellular pH (Fig. 3). Extracellular glutamic acid has a strong excitatory-depolarizing action on neurons and this is probably the (evolutionary) reason why astrocytes posses a very efficient mechanism to capture extracellular glutamic acid and to transform this acidic amino acid to glutamine by transamidation; the latter demonstrates no electrophysiological actions. Thus, again, neuronal excitation tends to cause glial swelling during uptake of glutamic acid which can only be balanced by enhanced release of glutamine (Oligodendrocytes do not posses glutamine synthetase and this could explain why white matter is more sensitive to oedema; van Gelder, 1983a).

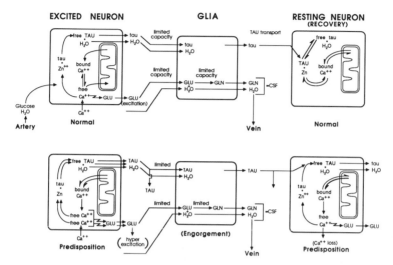

Fig. 2. Upon neuronal excitation, taurine is released in response to enhanced glucose derived water production, as is glutamic acid in response to increased ionic calcium levels. Both amino acids are captured by apposing glial elements; an additional water load is imposed upon the glia by bicarbonate-chloride exchange (van Gelder, 1983a). During and following excitation, enhanced glutamine production and its ostmotic release restores glial volume, but the extra taurine now tends to render the intracellular environment hyperosmotic in relation to the extracellular milieu. This triggers the release of taurine (Wade et al, 1988) which then is resequestered in the neuron.

In cells predisposed to hyperexcitation, an exaggerated release of glutamic acid promotes hypersynchrony or Spreading Depression, an enhanced loss of neural water, and increased swelling of surrounding astrocytes. Limits in glutamine production will tend to cause a net loss of these amino acids from the CNS (van Gelder et al., 1972; van Gelder 1990; with permission, Alan R Liss, Inc, 1990).

Whereas taurine may serve in intercellular water homeostasis (Fig. 1,2), the continuous export of glutamine to the blood while maintaining 0.3-0.5 mM CSF concentrations implies two phenomena. First, it indicates a continuous flow through of glutamine (and water) from glia to ventricles into the blood. Second, aside from having to replenish the glutamine precursors, i.e. glutamic acid and ammonia, the brain also needs to replenish its water content. Once more, some unambiguous calculations appear to balance the water efflux due to glutamine export with water influx due to glucose ouptake.

Without going into details (van Gelder, in press), the equation can be represented by the following events. At a brain glucose consumption of 15-20 mmoles/kg/hr, the amount of water entering the brain is around 60-70 ml. An osmotic pressure differential between blood and neural tissue proper adds another 20-25 ml (Hatashita et al, 1988). In all, the hourly volume of water entering neural tissue can be estimated at approximately 100 ml. Export of water has been reported at around 25 ml/hr/kg. Thus, overall, approximately 75 ml

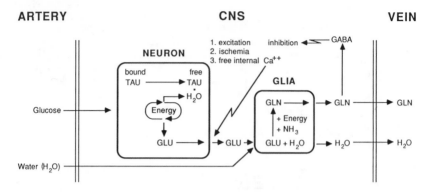

Fig. 3. Pictorial summary of glucose and glutamic acid metabolism in neural tissue, in combination with intracranial water movements. Since practically all glucose is immediately oxidized on intracellular entrance, the osmotic pressure changes little. The water accompanying glucose uptake by the CNS must thus be considered to remain outside the cells; calculated at about 100 ml/hr under basal glucose consumption, this volume approximates the ventricular CSF volume. Solute mediated CSF efflux from the CNS, estimated at 20-30 ml/hr, can be accounted for by transport of glutamine into the blood. With permission, Alan R Liss, Inc, 1990.

water in excess of tissue content must be present intracranially, which approaches in effect the reported volume of the CSF in the ventricular spaces. These seemingly simplistic calculations, without any assumptions and based on solid evidence, therefore provides a direct mechanism to explain how the brain maintains both its intracranial water balance as well as its constant intracellular water volume. More of the details have been discussed elsewhere (van Gelder, 1983a; van Gelder and Barbeau, 1985) and are schematically summarized in Figs 2 and 3 (with permission, Alan R Liss, Inc). The postulated relationship between calcium, taurine, and zinc has also been outlined previously (van Gelder, 1983b).

Compartmentation, Function and Development

The compartmentalised metabolism of glutamic acid-glutamine (Berl, 1975), in conjuction with the compartmentalised distribution of taurine, serves as a good example to underline the importance of the proper development of neuronal-glial metabolic integration. A malfunction in that process will have many ramification, including, to mention a few, disturbances in the excitation (glutamate)- inhibition (GABA) balance, intercellular anatomical integrity and calcium regulation (taurine, glutamic acid), and the innumerable synthetic metabolic pathways which need the glucose carbon, glutamic acid-transaminase reactions for amino acid metabolism, and intracellular pH regulation. Because many of these neurochemical cycles are very complex, even subtle deficiencies during development of the neuron-glia network may leave a number of metabolic weaknesses which however may only be expressed when the brain is subsequently stressed by disease or specific environmental conditions (van Gelder, 1987). In addition to the readily apparent sequelae of severe malnutrition or environmental isolation, the effects of moderate but chronic undernutrition and psychological trauma during infancy are far more difficult to assess or to use as predictors for the final outcome of brain development.

Fortunately, even more than the ability of the (neonatal) brain to be anatomically and physiologically rehabilitated, brain function appears to depend on more than the sum of fixed neurobiological circuities. Rather, the expressions of the human intellect are infinitely varied and, within certain anatomical limits, persist or recover despite seemingly very severe damage to the CNS. With a better understanding of the neurobiological integration which must occur during development, and the influence of life experiences on this process, one can be optimistic that the future will bring increasingly more efficient methods to prevent functional disabilities of the brain, or to provide more efficient methods to improve rehabilitation. This does not diminish the need, however, to provide the infant with every opportunity to develop optimum intelligence, by assuring a maximally nurturing social environment and a well balanced diet. That diet in the form of human milk can be best guaranteed by adequate health care, both mentally and physically, of the mother.

REFERENCES

Abbott NJ (1988). The milieu is the message. Nature 332:490-491.

Agrawal HC, Davison AN (1973). Myelination and amino acid imbalance in developing brain. In Himwich W (ed): "Biochemistry of the Developing Brain," New-York : Marcel Dekker, Inc., pp 146-183.

Autillo-Touati A, Chamak B, Araud D, Vuillet J, Seite R, Prochiantz A (1988). Regions-specific neuro-astroglial interactions: ultrastructural study of the in vitro expression of neuronal polarity. J Neurosci Res 19:326-342.

Balazs R, Haslam RJ (1965). Exchange transamination and the metabolism of glutamate in brain. Biochem J 94:131.

Banker GA (1980). Trophic interactions between astroglial cells and hippocampal neurons in culture. Science 209:809-810.

Bennett EL, Rosenzweig MR, Diamond MC, Morimoto H, Hebert M (1974). Effects of successive environments on brain measures. Physiol and Behavior 12:621-631.

Berl S (1973). Biochemical consequences of compartmentation of glutamate and associated metabolites. In Balazs R, Cremer JE (eds): "Metabolic Compartmentation in the Brain," London: Macmillan pp 3-17.

Birch HG (1972). Malnutrition, learning, and intelligence. Am J. Public Health 62:773-784.

Boggs JM (1980). Intermolecular hydrogen bonding between lipids: influence on organization and function of lipids in membranes. Can J Biochem 58:755-770.

Burry RW, Hayes DM (1989). Highly basic 30- and 32- kilodalton proteins associated with synapse formation on polylysine-coated beads in enriched neuronal cell cultures. J Neurochem 52:551-560.

Butzer KW (1977). Environment, culture and human evolution. Am Scientist 65:572-584.

Davenport JW, Gonzalez LM, Carey JC, Bishop SB, Hagquist WW (1976). Environmental stimulation reduces learning deficits in experimental cretinism. Science 191:578-579.

Davies AM (1988). The emerging generality of the neurotrophic hypothesis. Trends Neurosci 11:243-244.

de Vellis J, Ciment G, Lauder J (1988). Neuroembryology. Cellular and molecular approaches. J Neurosci Res 21: various chapters.

Di Perri B, Calderini G, Battistella A, Raciti R , Toffano G (1983). Phospholipid methylation increases [^{3}H] Diazepam and [^{3}H] GABA binding in membrane preparations of rat cerebellum. J Neurochem 41:302-308.

Dobbing J (1976). Malnutrition et développement du cerveau. La Recherche 7:139-145.

Elliott KAC, van Gelder NM (1958). Occlusion and metabolism of gamma-aminobutyric acid by brain tissue. J Neurochem 3:28-40.

Espinosa de los Monteros A, de Vellis J (1988). Myelin basic protein and transferrin characterize different subpopulations of olygodendrocytes in rat primary glial culture. J Neurosci Res 21:181-187.

Fisher SK, Agranoff BW (1987). Receptor activation and inositol lipid hydrolysis in neural tissues. J Neurochem 48:999-1017.

Grenel JM, Luhmann HJ, Singer W (1988). Pharmacological induction of use-dependent receptive field modifications in the visual cortex. Science 242:74-77.

Giulian D (1987). Ameboid microglia as effectors of inflammation in the central nervous system. J Neurosci Res 18:155-171.

Giulian D, Vaca K, Johnson B (1988). Secreted peptides as regulators of neuron-glia and glia-glia interactions in the developing nervous system. J Neurosci Res 21:487-500.

Hammarback JA, Palm SL, Furcht LT, Letourneau PC (1985). Guidance of neurite outgrowth by pathways of substratum-adsorbed laminin. J Neurosci Res 13:213-220.

Hatashita S, Hoff JT, Salamat SM (1988). Ischemic brain and osmotic gradient between blood and brain. J Cereb Blood Flow 8:552-559.

Haydon PG, Cohan CS, McCobb DP, Miller HR, Kater SB (1985). Neuron-specific growth cone properties as seen in identified neurons of Helisoma. J Neurosci Res 13:135-147.

Herrup K (1987). Glial cells and the formation of invisible boundaries in development (or, peanut barrels in the brain). Trends Neurosci 10:443-444.

Hickey TL (1977). Postnatal development of the human lateral geniculate nucleus: relationship to a critical period for the visual system. Science 198:836-838.

Hillman DE, Chen S (1981a). Vulnerability of cerebellar development in malnutrition-I. Quantitation of layer volume and neuron numbers. Neurosci 6:1246-1262.

Hillman DE, Chen S (1981b). Vulnerability of cerebellar development in malnutrition-II. Intrinsic determination of total synaptic area on Purkinje cell spines. Neurosci 6:1263-1275.

Hubel DH, Wiesel TN (1970). The period of susceptibility to the physiological effects of unilateral eye closure in kittens. J Physiol (London) 206:419-436.

Kater S, Letourneau P (1985). Biology of the nerve growth cone. J Neurosci Res 13: various chapters.

Le Douarin NM (1986). Cell line segregation during peripheral nervous system ontogeny. Science 231:1515-1522.

Mattson MP, Guthrie PB, Kater SB (1988). Intracellular messengers in the generation and degeneration of hippocampal neuroarchitecture. J Neurosci Res 21:447-464.

McIlwain H, Bachelard HS (1971). "Biochemistry and the Central Nervous System, London: Churchill Livingstone, pp 61-97.

Parnavelas JG, Cavanagh ME (1988). Transient expression of neurotransmitters in the developing cortex. Trends Neurosci 11:92-93.

Perry VH, Gordon S (1988). Macrophages and microglia in the nervous system. Trends Neurosci 11:273-277.

Roberts A, Patton DT (1985). Growth cones and the formation of central and peripheral neurites by sensory neurons in amphibian embryos. J Neurosci Res 13:23-38.

Ruoslahti E, Pierschbacher MD (1987). New perspectives in cell adhesion: RGD and Integrins. Science 238:491-497.

Rutishauser U (1985). Influence of the neural cell adhesion molecule on axon growth and guidance. J Neurosci Res 13:123-131.

Sandri C, Van Buren JM, Akert K (1977). Membrane morphology of the vertebrate nervous system. Prog Brain Res 46:106-140.

Schousboe A, Drejer J, Divac I (1980). Reginal heterogeneity in astroglial cells. Trends Neurosci 3:1-2.

Sutula T, Xiao-Xian H, Cavazos J, Scott G (1988). Synaptic reorganization in the hippocampus induced by abnormal functional activity. Science 239:1147-1150.

Svaetichin G, Negishi K, Fatehchand R, Drujan BD, Selvin de Testa A (1965). Nervous function based on interactions between neuronal and non-neuronal elements. Prog Brain Res 15:243-266.

Tessier-Lavigne M, Placzek M, Lumsden AGS, Dodd J, Jessell TM (1988). Chemotropic guidance of developing axons in the mammalian central nervous system. Nature 336:775-778.

Trinkaus JP (1985). Further thoughts on directional cell movement during morphogenesis. J Neurosci Res 13:1-19.

van Gelder NM (1989). Brain taurine content as a function of cerebral metabolic rate: osmotic regulation of glucose derived water production. Neurochem Res 14:495-497.

van Gelder NM (1987). Calcium mobility and glutamic acid release associated with EEG abnormalities, migraine and epilepsy. In Andermann F, Lugaresi E (eds): "Migraine and Epilepsy," Boston: Butterworths, pp 367-378

van Gelder NM, Barbeau A (1985). The osmoregulatory function of taurine and glutamic acid. In Oja SS, Ahtee L, Kontro P, Paasonen MK (eds): "Taurine: Biological Actions and Clinical Perspectives", New York: Alan R Liss, Inc, pp 149-163.

van Gelder NM (1983a). Metabolic interactions between neurons and astroglia: glutamine synthetase, carbonic anhydrase and water balance. In Jasper HH, van Gelder NM (eds): "Basic Mechanisms of Neuronal Excitability," New York:. Alan R. Liss, Inc, pp 5-29.

van Gelder NM (1983b). A central mechanism of action for taurine: osmoregulation, bivalent cations and excitation threshold. Neurochem Res 8:687-699.

Vitiello F, Gombos G (1987). Cerebellar development and nutrition. In Rassin DK, Haber B, Drujan B (eds): "Basic and Clinical Aspects of Nutrition and Brain Development," New-York : Alan R. Liss , Inc., pp 99-130.

Wade JV, Olson JP, Samson FE, Nelson SR, Pazdernik TL (1988). A possible role for taurine in osmoregulation within the brain. J Neurochem 51:740-745.

Wen GY, Sturman JA, Wisniewski HM, Lidsky AA, Cornwell AC, Hayes KC (1979). Tapetum disorganization in taurine-depleted cats. Invest Ophthalmol Visual Sci 18:1201-1206.

Werker JF (1989). Becoming a native listener. Am Scientist 77:54-59.

Wetherell JR, Fosbraey P, French MC (1989). A comparison of the distribution of neurotransmitters in brain regions of the rat and guinea-pig using a chemiluminescent method and HPLC with electrochemical detection. J Neurochem 53:1519-1526.

DISCUSSION

(Discussion tape inaudible)

(Mal)Nutrition and the Infant Brain, pages 175–190
© 1990 Wiley-Liss, Inc.

EFFECTS OF UNDERNUTRITION ON MYELIN DEPOSITION

Sheldon L. Miller

The Wistar Institute, Philadelphia, Pennsylvania 19104, USA

The chronological events leading to myelin deposition, can be divided into 3 parts: (1) the development of oligodendrocytes, central nervous system cells which make myelin; (2) myelin production by the oligodendrocyte and ensheathment of the axon (myelination); and (3) maintenance of the established myelin sheath.

Tissue culture experiments using developing rat optic nerve indicate that a precursor cell, designated O-2A, can develop into a cell which further differentiates into an oligodendrocyte. Proliferation of oligodendrocyte precursor cells and differentiation into mature oligodendrocytes occur during a discrete period of brain development. Developmental age during which this discrete period occurs in brain is species-dependent and varies for different brain regions within a given species. Regulatory factors appear to control whether an O-2A cell develops into an oligodendrocyte or another type of brain cell, the type 2 astrocyte (McMorris and Dubois-Dalcq, 1988; Raff, 1989). Since a significant decrease in the number of oligodendrocytes could prevent normal myelination of the brain, differentiation of O-2A cells into oligodendrocytes represents a period of vulnerability, i.e. a period during which insults, such as undernutrition, could have a lasting effect on normal development.

Cellular events leading to and including myelination of the axon by oligodendrocytes, like oligodendrocyte development, occur during a discrete period of brain development. They are not synchronous for various brain regions and consist of a temporally related complex series of phenomena including: synthesis of various myelin components (distinctly in advance of the appearance of myelin membrane); recognition by oligodendrocytes of axons to be myelinated; production of myelin membrane and axon ensheathment; and cessation of axon ensheathment when the myelin wrappings are of appropriate thickness.

The biochemical composition of myelin is approximately 2/3 lipid and 1/3 protein, whereas most membranes are approximately 1/3 lipid and 2/3 protein. Although none of the lipids found in myelin are unique to this membrane, some are highly enriched as compared to most other membranes of the body. Foremost are galactosylceramide (cerebroside) and the sulfated form of cerebroside, sulfatide. The concentration of these lipids in myelin is many times the concentration found in other tissues. Although cerebroside and sulfatide can be synthesized *de novo*, essential dietary factors, e.g. vitamin B_6, are necessary for the enzymes involved in this *de novo* synthesis.

Quantitatively, 3 of the myelin proteins (myelin basic protein,MBP, Folch-Lees proteolipid protein, PLP, and 2',3'-cyclic nucleotide-3'-phosphohydrolase, CNPase), constitute ~90% of the total protein in myelin membrane. MBP appears to be specific for central and peripheral nervous system myelin; PLP is found only in central nervous system myelin; and CNPase, although found in other tissues of the body, is highly enriched in oligodendrocytes and myelin as compared to other tissues. Although the remaining myelin proteins constitute a small percentage of the total myelin protein, many are believed to play an important role in either the myelination process, normal functioning of myelin, or the metabolic maintenance of myelin. Myelin protein synthesis may be vulnerable to undernutrition during the myelination period because of the large quantity of protein being synthesized during the period of rapid myelination .During the myelination process, large amounts of myelin membrane are produced by the oligodendrocyte by altering the composition in localized areas of its plasma membrane. The newly formed myelin membrane is extruded from the oligodendrocyte and ensheaths the axon. Although a particular oligodendrocyte will myelinate a single internode on a specific axon, one oligodendrocyte can myelinate between 10 and 40 internodes each on a different axon (Wood and Bunge,1984). Enormous amounts of metabolic energy are required to synthesize the proteins and lipids which are assembled into myelin membrane during the period of brain development. During the peak period of myelination in rat brain, it has been estimated that the oligodendrocyte may synthesize in one day an amount of myelin membrane equal to twice the weight of the oligodendrocyte cell body (Norton and Cammer,1984). Requirements of both essential and non-essential nutrients, as well as a caloric source for *de novo* synthesis of the complex molecules which constitute the components of the myelin membrane, are high during this developmental period. Because of this demand, the developmental period during which myelination is taking place should be considered a potential period of vulnerability for the attainment of normal deposition of brain myelin.

Once the initial period of rapid myelination is complete, myelination continues at a slower rate making fewer demands on the synthetic metabolism of the oligodendrocyte. Myelin continues to accumulate in rats at a slow rate throughout its life (Norton and Poduslo, 1973). It is uncertain if myelin accumulation continues slowly throughout the life of humans, but it probably continues at least through the third decade of life (Rorke and Riggs, 1969). Myelin is a typical membrane in that the proteins and lipids are continually removed and replaced by newly synthesized molecules (e.g. Miller et al., 1977). The capacity of the oligodendrocyte to continually synthesize myelin components at a slow rate after the period of rapid myelination in infancy raises the possibilty that myelin deficits, developed during undernutrition in the infant years, could be reversed at a later time during nutritional rehabilitation.

In the newborn, the majority of the brain mass is poorly myelinated (Rorke and Riggs,1969; Brody et al., 1987). Only the brain stem, and to a varying extent a few other selected areas, show significant myelination before birth as judged by galactolipid accumulation (Martinez, 1982) or detection of myelin by histological methods (Rorke and Riggs, 1969). By two years of age, the infant's brain is extensively but not entirely myelinated (Brody et al., 1987). Little is known about the temporal development of mature oligodendrocytes in the human brain. However, since mature oligodendrocytes must be present before myelination can take place, the period of rapid oligodendrocyte precursor cell proliferation and oligodendrocyte maturation probably begins during the third trimester *in utero* and continues until sometime between the first and second year of life. Since much of the animal modeling of the undernourished infant brain and its effects on myelin deposition have been done in rat, it is important to compare rat brain oligodendrocyte development to myelination in the human. In rat, rapid oligodendrocyte precursor cell proliferation and oligodendrocyte maturation, begins during late gestation and continues to about 20 days post partum, but mostly overlaps the period of rapid myelination which occurs from approximately 16 to 30 days of neonatal age (Norton and Poduslo, 1973). Unlike the human where a substantial portion of oligodendrocyte maturation is believed to take place *in utero*, the same process in the rat is primarily a postnatal event.

UNDERNUTRITION: RELIABILITY AND INTERPRETATION OF DATA

The Human Infant.

Data concerning anatomical and biochemical development of the normal human infant brain and the effects of undernutrition have been collected by various methods: retrospective studies (autopsy); via non-invasive techniques (e.g., evoked potentials and imaging); or, indirectly, from analysis of body fluids such as blood. Knowledge of the age-related sequence of myelinaton in various brain regions of the "normal" infant central nervous system is based on autopsy of infants (e.g. Rorke and Riggs, 1969; Brody et al., 1987) and these findings serve as "normal controls" for determining myelin deficits in the brain of undernourished infants. Although some variations have been reported in the the temporally related quantity of myelin in several discrete brain areas, there is in general good agreement on the sequence of myelination in different brain areas of the human infant as related to age. Nevertheless, defining the nutritional history in studies of undernutrition in the human infant is particularly difficult.

Conditions designated as protein-calorie undernutrition usually involve other nutritional deficiencies (Holman et al., 1981), e.g. vitamins and trace metals. It may be difficult or impossible to determine the time period at which undernutrition began, its severity, and the commencement of nutritional rehabilitation. Although a long term follow up during the nutritional rehabilitation period is essential to determine whether the observed deficits can be reversed or are permanent, this type of study is usually not possible.In addition to the practical limitations of the research protocol, the criteria used to define the effects of undernourishment can vary between studies. The differing methods of evaluation may not be equivalent or may not even measure the same parameters. When equivalent methods of evaluation are used it is often difficult to interpret the findings in terms of primary and secondary deficits particularly in studies of surviving infants. For instance, if undernutrition begins early in development and continues throughout the vulnerable growth periods (during which myelin is normally deposited), it may be impossible to distinguish between a primary myelin deficit and a myelin deficit secondary to incomplete development of neurons and their associated axons and dendrites. However, despite such limitations, an overview of comparable studies of human undernutrition can reveal generally consistent and useful findings. Certain deficiencies resulting from human infant undernutrition, such as alteration in complex behavior patterns cannot be determined using animal models. Animal models are also poor predictors of the length of time required for nutritional rehabilitation to correct reversible deficits. This latter point is of practical importance if undernourishment affects higher brain functions since a protracted time period of rehabilitation could affect a child's normal educational development which is generally based on age.

Animal Models of Undernutrition.

Effects of undernutrition on myelin deposition in the neonatal brain have been studied extensively in animal models, principally in the rat. These studies have the advantage of being able to define the specific nutritional factor(s) which are limited. Decreases in overall myelin deposition, changes in the number of myelin membrane layers ensheathing the axon, and dysmyelination (accumulation of myelin which is altered in composition) can be studied quantitatively at the light and electron microscope level, and biochemically. Since more details are known about the temporal and anatomical correlates involved in the development of oligodendrocytes and myelination in the rat than in the human, the vulnerability of different developmental periods in rat brain development can be ascertained and the reversibility of myelin deficits determined. Composition of myelin and the developmental events leading to myelin accumulation appear, at the present time, to be similar in rat and human. Therefore, much of the knowledge gained from this animal model should be useful in understanding the effects of undernutrition in the human infant. However, specific aspects of the rat model may not be directly applicable to the human. For instance, the severity of undernutrition used in the rat model may not be quantitatively applicable in human terms. Also, the development of most rat brain oligodendrocytes from non-differentiated precursor cells occurs after birth and before weaning, where undernourishment can be directly manipulated by limiting the time pups have access to the nursing mother, or by addition of pups from a second litter to produce an overcrowded litter which the mother cannot adequately nurse. In the human a greater proportion of oligodendrocyte development takes place *in utero* (based on the relative amount of myelin present and the myelination which follows post partum; Rorke and Riggs, 1969; Brody et al., 1987). Undernourishment of the human fetus can be attenuated by the mother at the expense of her own nutritional needs.

Tissue Culture Methodology

Through tissue cultures it is possible to elucidate the "signal(s)" which initiates various steps in the sequence of glioblast development into an oligodendrocyte, oligodendroglial maturation, and the process of myelination. If undernutrition can prevent the initiation of myelination as has been suggested (Wiggins, 1986), then identification of the signal(s) could lead to devising a strategy that might be used during the period of nutritional rehabilitation to initiate myelination in stunted oligodendrocytes. A second important application of tissue culture research is to follow the sequence of events by which glioblasts evolve into oligodendrocytes.Since glioblasts have the potential to develop into type 2 astrocytes as well as oligodendrocytes, it has been proposed that chemical signals influence the type of cell which differentiates from the glioblast; recent findings support this hypothesis (McMorris and Dubois-Dalcq, 1988). Severe undernutrition in the rat has been found to result in a decrease of mature oligodendrocytes in the corpus callosum (Lai et al., 1980; Sikes et al., 1981) suggesting that glioblast development into an oligodendrocyte was adversely affected by the undernutrition. If experiments in tissue culture could delineate the factors that initiate glioblast differentiation and guide development towards a mature oligodendrocytes, more precise methods of nutritional rehabilitation, to stimulate and increase the rate of oligodendrocyte maturation, can be delineated.

EFFECT OF PROTEIN UNDERNUTRITION ON MYELIN DEPOSITION

A number of studies have focused on the effects on the developing brain of severe protein-calorie undernutrition. Also referred to as malnutrition or undernutrition, these studies refer to restriction of both protein and calorie intake. In human studies, protein-calorie undernutrition is also accompanied by other deficiencies (e.g. vitamins) and is better termed undernutrition, since the effects produced by different dietary components cannot be separated.

Human Studies

The effects on the brain of undernutrition in perinatal and early postnatal development (less than 2 years after birth) have been described by Winick and Rosso (1969) among others. The condition results in a lower body and brain weight and decreases in DNA, RNA, and protein per brain, when compared to well-nourished children of matched age and sex. The protein/DNA ratio appears however relatively unchanged, suggesting that these changes can be explained in terms of decreased number of brain cells. Early biochemical studies (Fox et al., 1972; Fishman et al., 1969) indicated that the concentration of lipids with which myelin is enriched may be preferentially decreased as a result of undernutrition while other brain lipids, not enriched in myelin, show little or no change in brain content.In a more recent study (Martinez, 1982), biochemical parameters from cerebrum, cerebellum, and brainstem were examined in 3 brains of undernourished small-for-date fetuses and 7 brains from undernourished infants whose body weight ranged from 30 to 44% of normal. Brain from well-nourished fetuses and infants who died of non-neurological causes were used for comparison.

In control brains at birth, galactolipid, which is enriched in oligodendrocytes and myelin, is 2.8 times greater (μmoles/g wet tissue) in the brain stem than in cerebellum and 25 times more concentrated when compared to the cerebrum. These differences in structure contents correspond to the temporal sequence in which myelination occurs during development. The content (μmoles/g wet tissue) of cholesterol and total phospholipids which are not more enriched in myelin than in other brain membranes, are not very different in the three brain regions. In brain stem and cerebellum, which are extensively myelinated *in utero*, undernutrition did not result in decreased levels of galactolipid with respect to controls either pre- or postnatally. In cerebrum, which is sparsely myelinated at birth but rapidly accumulates myelin postnatally, the low galactolipid concentration at birth also did not differ between the undernourished and control brains. Postnatally, however, the cerebral galactolipid concentration in undernourished brains was consistently lower than in controls. Also, total plasmalogens in the cerebrum before 32 weeks gestation did not differ from controls; after 32 weeks gestation and postnatally, total plasmalogen was however consistantly lower in undernourished brains than in controls.

Although these data indicate that postnatal myelination in the cerebrum is particularly vulnerable to undernutrition whereas the cerebellum and brainstem appear to be more refractory, the small number of brains used in the study and other problems inherent in human studies make it difficult to draw any firm conclusions. A more definitive understanding of the effects of undernourishment on the normal myelination process can be obtained from animal models.

Rat Studies

Protein-calorie undernutrition has been produced in rats before the age of 21 days (approximate time of weaning) using several different experimental protocols, including: (1) undernourishment of the dam during gestation and weaning periods; (2) combining the pups of two litters and using only one mother to nurse (overcrowding); and (3) providing, in lieu of free access, a limited time when the mother may nurse the young. Each protocol can be varied and the severity of undernourishment is reflected in the percent decrease in body weight and brain weight of the undernourished rats, as compared to well-nourished controls.

The developmental period during which the undernourishment takes place and the severity of undernourishment appear to be more important in affecting myelin deposition than the nutritional paradigm used to achieve these ends (Wiggins, 1982; Fuller et al., 1984). A graded increase in severity of undernourishment, as judged by decreasing body weight of the undernourished rat pups relative to controls, produces a greater decrease in myelin deposition (Fuller et al., 1984).When rat pups are undernourished from birth to approximately 21 days of age, resulting in a body weight of about 50% of well-nourished, age-matched controls, changes in the myelination process as well as in myelin deposition are observed. These reported changes are qualitatively as well as quantitatively consistent in the literature (Winick and Noble, 1966; Chase et al, 1969; Wiggins et al., 1974; Wiggins et al., 1976; Krigman and Hogan, 1976; Hamberger and Sourander, 1978; Wiggins and Fuller, 1979; Reddy et al., 1979; Lai and Lewis, 1980; Wiggins et al., 1985; Yeh, 1988).

The changes include: decreased brain weight (~20%); decreased amounts of myelin isoated per brain (~30%); deceased brain DNA; decreased rates of protein and lipid synthesis; and decreased levels of myelin enriched lipids and myelin specific proteins. On microscopic examination, the myelin of undernourished brain appears to have a normal multilamellar structure. However, both the number of myelinated axons as well as the ratio of the number of myelin lamellae to axon diameter are decreased (Krigman and Hogan, 1976; Wiggins, 1979; Lai and Lewis, 1980;Wiggins et al., 1985). In general, the nuber of oligodendrocytes is decreased in whole brain if developing rats are subjected to undernutrition beginning either *in utero* or at birth, and continuing through the second or third week of life (Robain and Ponsot, 1978; Lai et al., 1980; Giuffrida et al., 1980; Sikes et al., 1981; Patel, 1983). In one study (Sikes et al., 1981), little or no effect of undernourishment on oligodendrocytes was observed in several specific brain regions, but this refractoriness may have been related to the period of development during which the undernourishment was initiated.

The maturation of oligodendrocytes appears to be retarded during severe undernutrition especially in the corpus callosum where most of myelin deposition occurs during the later phase of brain myelination (Robain and Ponsot,1978; Lai et al.,1980).While the number of oligodendrocytes appears diminished in the undernourished corpus callosum, astrocytes are reported to increase (Lai et al.,1980). It is not known if these are type 2 astrocytes. Although a glioblast has the potential to develop into either oligodendrocytes or type 2 astrocytes, any conclusion as to whether this precursor cell has a greater propensity to develop into type 2 astrocytes during undernutrition is tenuous. Despite the increase in the number of astrocytes, these cells may also be developmentally delayed since undernutrition results in decreased levels of S-100 protein. This protein is normally enriched in astrocytes of mature brain and is found in only very low levels early in development.

Neuronal development is also affected by undernutrition (Bass et al., 1970; Noback and Eisenman, 1981).When only dietary protein is restricted (~5% of diet) from birth, at 21 days of age body weight and brain weight are reduced to approximately 65% and 80%, respectively, of that of well-nourished rat pups, and deficits in myelin deposition are present (Nakhasi et al., 1975; Reddy et al., 1979; Reddy and Horrocks, 1982). CNPase activity and myelin lipid galactose per brain, which reflect the amount of myelin deposition, are decreased in brain by 25 - 50%, and by ~20%, respectively. During protein undernutrition, a significant decrease in myelin proteolipid protein has also been reported (Reddy et al., 1979). As with protein-calorie undernourishment other cell types are also affected (West and Kemper, 1976; Deo et al., 1978). Thus, protein undernourishment results in myelin deficits similar to those found in protein-calorie undernourishment.

ESSENTIAL FATTY ACID (EFA) DEFICIENCY

Unsaturated fatty acids in the body can be classified into 3 groups, n-3, n-6, n-9, depending on the number of carbons from the methyl end of the molecule to the first carbon-carbon double bond. The n-9 series can be synthetized *de novo* whereas the n-3 and n-6 series must be obtained through the diet. Under conditions of normal nutrition, the shorter essential fatty acids, linoleic (n-6) and linolenic (n-3), as compared to the n-9 fatty acids, are better able to compete for the enzymes involved in chain lengthening and desaturation. These, therefore, are preferentially converted to long chain polyunsaturated fatty acids, used in the synthesis of phospholipids and other fatty acid-containing lipids. Myelin lipids tend to be more enriched in long chain polyunsaturated fatty acids than other membranes. In EFA deficiency, because of a higher relative concentration, the n-9 series fatty acids can compete more successfully for metabolic conversion to long chain polyunsaturated fatty acids. Thus, during undernutrition, the n-9 series represent a significant portion of the fatty acids incorporated into myelin.

Human studies

The importance of dietary EFA was first reported in nutrition experiments with rats (Burr and Burr, 1929). Thirty-four years later, the importance of EFA in human nutrition was demonstrated in over 400 newborn infants, who developed clinical symptoms when maintained on fat-free diet but who recovered when the diet was supplemented with EFA (Hansen et al., 1963). Although essential fatty acid deficiency can be found in older patients on long term total parenteral nutrition (e.g. as can occur post-surgically and in Crohn's disease, or in cases of cystic fibrosis), the most rapid development of EFA deficiency symptoms is classically found in infants (especially premature infants) where EFA may be missing from total parenteral nutrition (Friedman et al., 1976; Farrell et al., 1988). In infants suffering from undernutrition, EFA deficiency contributes to the abnormalities of general protein-calorie undernourishment (Schendel and Hansen, 959; Holman et al., 1981). Little is yet known about the biochemical consequences of EFA deficiency in humans.

Rat and Mouse Studies

Most experiments concerned with the effects of EFA deficiency on myelination and net myelin accumulation have been carried out in rats and mice. There appear to be no striking differences in the response of rats and mice to EFA deficiency, so no distinction will be made between these species in discussing the experimental findings.When EFA deficiency is initiated *in utero* and continues for at least several weeks past the weaning period, several differences are seen in EFA deficient animals relative to controls, including: decreased body and brain weight; decreased total brain DNA, protein, and myelin isolated; alteration in levels of cerebroside and myelin specific proteins (markers for myelin); and changes in the fatty acid composition of phospholipids (Galli, 1973; Alling et al., 1973; Sun et al., 1974; Miller et al., 1981; Berkow and Campagnoni, 1981; Menon and Dhopeshwarkar, 1982; Bourre et al., 1984; Miller et al., 1984). The phospholipid changes reflect an increase in the proportion of n-9 derived polyunsaturated, long chain fatty acids and a decrease in the n-3 and n-6 polyunsaturated, long chain fatty acids (the relative composition of the different phospholipid classes remain unchanged). The degree of EFA deficiency, as measured by the decrease in n-3 and n-6 fatty acids and the increase in long chain polyunsaturated n-9 fatty acids, is proportional to the deficiency of n-3 and n-6 fatty acids in the diet (Alling et al., 1973). Relative protein composition in myelin was not found to be significantly changed (McKenna and Campagnoni, 1979; Berkow and Campagnoni, 1981; Miller et al., 1984). Reports differ as to whether myelin proteolipid protein decreases (McKenna and Campagnoni, 1979; Berkow and Campagnoni, 1981) or remains unchanged (Miller et al., 1984)). Changes in the metabolism of myelin proteins and phospholipids include an increased reutilization of myelin fatty acids (Miller et al., 1981) and a decreased uptake of isoleucine into myelin proteins (Menon and Dhopeshwarkar, 1984). As in protein-calorie undernutrition, the effects of EFA deficiency are not restricted to oligodendrocytes and myelin. The changes in fatty acid composition of phospholipids found in myelin are altered in a parallel fashion in astrocytes, neurons, whole brain microsomes, and a synaptosomal fraction isolated from essential fatty acid deficient animals (Sun et al., 1974 ; Bourre et al., 1984). The observed composition changes have been shown to be related to the severity of essential fatty acid deprivation (Sun et al., 1974).

REHABILITATION FROM UNDERNUTRITION DEFICITS

In a practical sense, the major concerns with the effects of undernutrition on myelin deposition are whether the biochemical deficit(s) produced leads to functional deficit(s), and the reversibility of the deficit(s) by refeeding with a nourishing diet (rehabilitation). The rehabilitation can be viewed at two levels: first, are any biochemical and structural deficits, produced by undernourishment, returned to the expected norm by feeding a therapeutic diet. This problem is best approached in the animal model where direct biochemical measurements and observations at the light and electron microscopic levels can be obtained. The second aspect of rehabilitation deals with recovery of functional deficits, since it is possible that either the biochemical and/or structural alterations do not result in a detectable functional deficit, or that only partial recovery of structural and biochemical abnormalities can lead to total functional recovery, so that no deficits are measurable. Assessment of the amount of functional recovery cannot be completely determined in the animal model for reasons discussed above.

Rehabilitation of Protein-Calorie Undernutrition Deficits

When several litters of rat pups are placed on a protein-calorie undernutrition regimen of various degrees of severity, from 1 through 20 days of age, the decrease of whole brain myelin accumulation varies relative to the severity of undernutrition. The success of rehabilitation from 20 to 60 days of age was related to the severity of protein-calorie undernutrition (Fuller et al., 1984). At 60 days of age, body weight, brain weight and the rate of accumulation of myelin per gram of brain did not differ significantly between the control and all the undernourished groups. However, the total amount of myelin/g of brain after rehabilitation was the same for the control and only the least severely undernourished litter. Although the ratio of myelin/g of brain did not significantly differ among the more severly undernourished litters, it was significantly below that of the control litter. Thus, the deficit in the more severely undernourished litters appears to be permanent. It is unclear from this study whether the relationship between the severity of undernutrition and rehabilitation of the myelin deficit is a graded phenomenon or exhibits a threshold effect. Since all the undernourished litters had the same brain weight at the end of the rehabilitation period even though the more severely undernourished pups had a deficit in total myelin deposition, this study also demonstrated that brain weight is not a useful measure of recovery from decreased myelin deposition (see also Yeh, 1988).

When pups were protein-calorie undernourished for various periods during postnatal development, attempts at rehabilitation up to 60 days of age were not successful if the undernutrition occurred from birth to 14 days of age, or from birth to 20 days of age. If, on the other hand, the undernutrition occurred from birth to 8 days, or started at 14 days and continued to 20 or even 30 days, followed by rehabilitation to 60 days of age, no significant myelin deficit was found in different brain regions (Wiggins and Fuller, 1978). This indicates that between birth and 14 days of age the brain is vulnerable to a protein-calorie undernutrition regimen which produces a myelin deficit not completely reversible by rehabilitation, although partial rehabilitation is possible even for undernutrition occurring during this period of vulnerability (Yeh, 1988; Fuller et al., 1984). During this period, DNA, RNA, and protein in brain are significantly reduced and rehabilitation up to 133 days of age does not restore the reduced levels of these brain components to those of the control (Winick and Noble, 1966). Decreases of protein and lipid synthesis which occur in undernutrition during this period do not appear to be reversed (Wiggins et al., 1976). On the cellular level, undernutrition for the first 3 weeks of life, decreased the number of myelinated fibers and the ratio of the number of myelin lamellae to axon diameter in the corpus callosum. When this undernutrition was followed by two weeks of rehabilitation, a partial restoration of these deficits was achieved although the ratio of the number of myelin lamellae to axon diameter was increased principally in the smaller diameter fibers.

Rehabilitation of EFA deficits

Although rehabilitation in EFA deficiency has not been studied as extensively as protein-calorie undernutrition, it has been firmly established that the altered long chain, polyunsaturated EFA deficiency pattern in lipids is readily reversed by rehabilitation, as are some of the overt clinical symptoms such as scaly skin (e.g., Hansen et al., 1963). In a case study of a 6 year old child who was inadvertently put on a linolenic acid deficient diet, blurring of vision and impairment of lower limbs resulted, but when linolenic acid was included in the diet the clinical symptoms were reversed (Holman et al., 1982).Mice, born to an EFA deficient dam and cross fostered at birth to a well-nourished dam, had decreased brain DNA and protein levels for up to 9 weeks of rehabilitation (duration of experiment; Berkow and Campagnoni, 1981). In the same study, although brain levels of myelin proteolipid protein were unaffected by the essential fatty acid deficiency regimen, brain levels of cerebrosides were decreased and 9 weeks of postnatal rehabilitation did not restore the cerebrosides to control levels. Some motor and behavioral deficits in EFA deficient animals have also been found and appear to be irreversible (Menon and Dhopeshwarkar, 1982). Additional research is needed to identify vulnerable period(s) and the nature of the deficit resulting from EFA deficiency.

MYELIN DEFICITS IN UNDERNUTRITION: GENERAL CONSIDERATIONS

Vulnerability to an Undernutrition Insult

Enhanced vulnerability of an organism to an insult can occur during well defined critical period(s) of development, when there is a greatly increased probability that damage will produce a lasting deficit (Dobbing and Smart, 1973). For myelin deposition in brain, this period was originally defined as the entire period of the developmental growth-spurt. In the human, this begins *in utero* during the latter part of the third trimester and ends in the latter part of the second year of life. For rat, it is primarily a postnatal event beginning around the time of birth and ending around the third week of life. Subsequently, it was proposed that the rapid growth period be viewed as consisting of 2 phases, cell division and cell growth, and the that vulnerable period was the phase involving cell division (see Dobbing and Smart, 1973, for summary). More recently, a third proposal (Wiggins, 1986) has been advanced, focussing more specifically on which of the developmental event(s) culminating in myelin deposition are most susceptible to a metabolic insult and will result in a lasting myelin deficit, i.e. a deficit which cannot be reversed by rehabilitation. The reasons cited as the basis of the latter definition of vulnerability are: (1) the lack of distinct separate periods of cell growth and division; (2) the vulnerability of myelin deposition to permanent deficits is from birth to 14 days of age in rats, before the bulk of brain myelination has begun (Wiggins and Fuller, 1978); and (3) the lack of a significant a diminution of oligodendrocytes under a regimen which produces a lasting myelin deficit (Wiggins,1986). The latter proposal suggests that the event that correlates best with a permanent myelin deficit is the period of myelinogenesis and probably involves the signal which initiates myelination.

A proposed outline of the developmental steps leading to myelin formation is shown in Fig 1. Although a metabolic insult to one or more of these steps might potentially result in a permanent myelin deficit, designating an age of vulnerability is problematic. Since process of myelination does not occur simultaneously in all brain regions (Rorke and Riggs, 1969; Brody et al., (1987), then an event, such as oligodendroglial maturation, will be occurring in brain stem *in utero*, whereas oligodendroglial maturation in the globus pallidus probably occurs in the second year of life.

The problem of temporal heterogeneity of brain development culminating in myelin deposition remains whether the focus is restricted to a particular brain region, or to a functional system of the brain (Brody et al., 1987). Thus, rather than specifying for each particular event, implicated in myelin deposition, a period of maximum vulnerability, it may be more meaningful to designate for each brain region and/or brain function(s) the developmental age when undernutrition no longer affects these parameters of maturation. A second problem in dealing with vulnerability of processes leading to the deposition of myelin is that susceptibility of a given developmental event is almost certainly related to the severity of undernutrition. However, at a given age, a particularly severe undernutritional paradigm may affect only a single developmental event and because

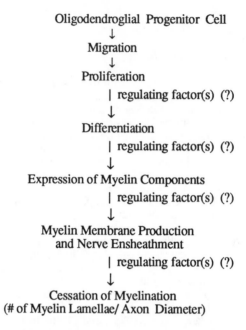

Fig. 1. Developmental steps,culminating in myelin deposition, which may be susceptible to an undernutritional insult.

of the temporal heterogeneity of brain maturation, may implicate just a limited number of anatomical sites, resulting in little or no measurable dysfunction. On the other hand, at the same age a less severe undernutritional paradigm may affect several developmental events simultaneously, resulting in myelin deficits at an increased number of anatomical sites and therefore causing more extensive dysfunction. A third problem, involving the concept of vulnerability and the production of deficits, is how to define a deficit. For example, even if a biochemical deficit can be detected and measured, but does not produce a measurable dysfunction, it may be of little practical importance. This is especially true in human terms where the concern is about rehabilitation and how to minimize the impact of a permanent dysfunction. Thus, it may be more practical in the undernutrition of the human infant to speak of different types and severity of undernutrition, the types of developmental events which are susceptible, the brain regions or nerve tracts which may be affected at a particular developmental age, and the resulting dysfunction.

Rehabilitation

Rehabilitation of insufficient myelin deposition caused by undernutrition, inherently depends on stimulation of the myelination process. Since there are a number of critical steps in development (see Fig. 1) which culminate in myelin deposition, the question becomes whether these vulnerable step(s) arrested by undernutrition, and the subsequent metabolic events leading to myelin deposition, can be reinstituted or extended beyond the developmental period during which most myelination normally occurs.At least two developmental steps leading to myelin deposition appear vulnerable to undernutritional insult-oligodendroglial maturation (Robain and Ponsot, 1978; Lai et al., 1980) and the initiation of myelination (Krigman and Hogan, 1976; Wiggins and Fuller, 1978). The arrested developmental step may not be reinitiated solely by nutritional re-habilitation, but this does not necessarily infer that a rehabilitation paradigm cannot be devised. For instance, a protein factor may be needed to promote the transformation of glioblasts into oligodendrocytes (McMorris and Dubois-Dalcq, 1988). If a period of sufficiently severe undernutrition coincides with the transient appearance of this factor during development, the metabolic precursors for normal development may be insufficient for glioblast proliferation and differentiation, and this window of opportunity may be lost. Rehabilitation of a myelin deficit in this case may require that some activator factors must sup-plement nutritional rehabilitation to renew the development of glioblasts into oligodendrocytes. That approach is based on the assumption that the arrested development is reversible, which may not be true for all developmental steps.

Acknowledgements: I gratefully acknowledge the useful suggestions offered by Dr. David Klurfeld and Ms. Shirley Peterson in preparation of this manuscript. Supported in part by U.S. Public Health Service Grant HD 19661-03.

REFERENCES

Alling C, Bruce A, Karlsson I, Svennerholm L(1973). The effect of dietary lipids on the central nervous system. In Galli,C.,Facini,G., Pecile,A. (eds): "Dietary lipids and postnatal development", New York: Raven Press pp 203-215.

Bass NH, Netsky MG, Young E (1970). Effect of neonatal malnutrition on developing cerebrum. I. Microchemical and histologic study of cellular differentation in the rat. Arch Neurol 23: 289-302.

Berkow SE, Campagnoni AT (1981). Essential fatty acid deficiency: effects of cross-fostering mice at birth on brain growth and myelination. J Nutr 111:886-894.

Bourre JM, Pascal G, Durand G, Masson M, Dumont O, Piciotti M (1984). Alterations in the fatty acid composition of rat brain cells (neurons, astrocytes, and oligodendrocytes) and of subcellular fractions (myelin and synaptosomes) induced by a diet devoid of n-3 fatty acids. J Neurochem 43:342-348.

Brody BA, Kinney HC, Kloman AS, Gilles FH (1987). Sequence of central nervous system myelination in human infancy. I. An autopsy study of myelination. J Neuropath Exper Neurol 46::283-301.

Burr GO, Burr MM (1929). A new deficiency disease produced by the rigid exclusion of fat from the diet. J Biol Chem 82:345-367.

Chase HP, Lindsley Jr WFB, O'Brien, D (1969). Undernutrition and cerebellar development. Nature 221:554-555.

Deo K, Bijlani V, Deo MG (1978). Effects of malnutrition on cell genesis and migration in developing brain in rats. Exper Neurol 62:80-92.

DobbingJ, Smart JL (1973). Early undernutrition,brain development and behavior.In Barnett, SA (eds.): "Ethology and Development", Philadelphia: J.B. Lippincott and Company, pp 16-36.

Farrell PM, Gutcher,GR, Palta M, DeMets D. (1988). Essential fatty acid deficiency in premature infants. Am J Clin Nutr 48:220-229.

Fishman MA, Prensky AL, Dodge PR (1969). Low content of cerebral lipids in infants suffering from malnutrition. Nature 221:552-553.

Fox JH, Fishman MA, Dodge PR, Prensky AL (1972). The effect of malnutrition on human central nervous system myelin. Neurol 22:1213-1216.

Friedman Z, Danon A, Stahlman MT, Oates JA (1976). Rapid onset of essential fatty acid deficiency in the newborn. Pediatr 58:640-649.

Fuller GN, Johnston DA, Wiggins RC (1984). The relationship between nutritional adequacy and brain myelin accumulation: a comparison of varying degrees of well fed and undernourished rats. Brain Res 290:195-198.

Galli C (1973). Dietary lipids and brain development. In Galli C, Facini G, Pecile A (eds): "Dietary lipids and postnatal development", New York: Raven Press pp 191-202.

Giuffrida AM, Hamberger A, Serra I, Geremia E (1980). Effects of undernutrition on nucleic acid synthesis in neuronal and glial cells from different region of developing rat brain. Nutr Metab 24:189-198.

Hamberger A, Sourander P (1978). The influence of early protein-calorie malnutrition on neuronal and glial protein synthesis. Neurochem Res 3:535-547.

Hansen AE, Wiese HF, Boelsche AN, Haggard ME, Adam DJD, Davis H (1963). Role of linoleic acid in infant nutrition. Pediatr 31:171-192.

Holman RT, Johnson SB, Mercuri O, Itarte HJ, Rodrigo MA, DeTomas ME (1981) Essential fatty acid deficiency in malnourished children. Am J Clin Nutr 34:1534-1539.

Holman RT, Johnson SB, Hatch TF (1982). A case of human linolenic acid deficiency involving neurological abnormalities. Am J Clin Nutr 35:617-623.

Krigman MR, Hogan EL (1976). Undernutrition in the developing rat: effect upon myelination. Brain Res 107:239-255.

Lai M, Lewis PD (1980). Effects of undernutrition on myelination in rat corpus callosum. J Comp Neurol 193:973-982.

Lai M, Lewis PD, Patel AJ (1980). Effects of undernutrition on gliogenesis and glial maturation in rat corpus callosum. J Comp Neurol 193:965-972.

McKenna MC, Campagnoni AT (1979). Effect of Pre- and Postnatal essential fatty acid deficiency on brain development and myelination. J Nutr 109:1195-1204.

Martinez M (1982). Myelin lipids in the developing cerebrum, cerebellum, and brainstem of normal and undernourished children. J Neurochem 39:1684-1692.

McMorris FA, Dubois-Dalcq M (1988). Insulin-like growth factor I promotes cell proliferation and oligodendroglial commitment in rat glial progenitor cells developing in vitro. J Neurosci Res 21:199-209.

Menon NK, Dhopeshwarkar GA (1982). Essential fatty acid deficiency and brain development. Prog Lipid Res 21:309-326.

Menon NK, Dhopeshwarkar, GA (1984). Incorporation of [U-^{14}C] isoleucine into myelin in essential fatty acid (EFA) deficiency in the rat. Nutr Rep Intern 29:783-789.

Miller SL, Benjamins JA, Morell P (1977). Metabolism of glycerophospholipids of myelin and microsomes in rat brain. J Biol Chem 252:4025-4037.

Miller SL, Klurfeld DM, Weinsweig D, Kritchevsky D (1981). Effect of essential fatty acid deficiency on the synthesis and turnover of myelin lipid. J

Neurosci Res 6:203-210.

Miller SL, Klurfeld DM, Loftus B, Kritchevsky D (1984). Effect of essential fatty acid deficiency on myelin proteins. Lipids 19:478-480.

Nakhasi HL,Toews AD, Horrocks LA (1975). Effect of postnatal protein deficiency on the content and composition of myelin from brains of weanling rats. Brain Res 83:176-179.

Noback CR, Eisenman LM (1981). Some effects of protein-calorie undernutrition on the developing central nervous system of the rat. Anat Rec 201:67-73.

Norton WT, Poduslo SE (1973). Myelination in rat brain: Changes in myelin composition during brain maturation. J Neurochem 21:759-773.

Norton WT,Cammer W (1984). Isolation and Characterization of myelin. In Morell,P(ed): "Myelin", NewYork: Plenum Press, pp 147-195.

Patel AJ (1983). Undernutrition and brain development. Trends Neurosci 6:151-154.

Raff MC (1989). Glial cell diversification in rat optic nerve. Science 243:1450-1455.

Reddy PV, Das A, Sastry PS (1979). Quantitative and compositional changes in myelin of undernourished and protein malnourished rat brains. Brain Res 161:227-235.

Reddy TS, Horrocks LA (1982). Effects of neonatal undernutrition on the lipid composition of gray matter and white matter in rat brain. J Neurochem 38:601-605.

Robain O, Ponsot G (1978). Effects of undernutrition on glial maturation. Brain Res 149:379-397.

Rorke LB, Riggs HE (1969). Myelination of the brain in the newborn. Philadelphia: J.B.Lippincott Company, pp 1-91.

Schendel HE, Hansen JDL (1959). Studies of serum polyenoic fatty acids in infants with kwashiorkor. S African Med J 33:1005.

Sikes RW, Fuller GN, Colbert C, Chronister RB, DeFrance J, Wiggins RC (1981). The relative numbers of oligodendroglia in different brain regions of normal and postnatally undernourished rats. Brain Res Bull 6:385-391.

Sun GY, Go J, Sun AY (1974). Induction of essential fatty acid deficiency in mouse brain: Effects of fat deficient diet upon acyl group composition of myelin and synaptosome-rich fractions during development and maturation. Lipids 9:450-454.

West CD, Kemper TL (1976). The effect of a low protein diet on the anatomical development of the rat brain. Brain Res 107:221-237.

Wiggins RC (1979). A comparison of starvation models in studies of brain myelination. Neurochem Res 4:827-830.

Wiggins RC (1982). Myelin development and nutritional insufficiency. Brain Res Rev 4:151-175.

Wiggins RC (1986). Myelination: A critical Stage in development.Neurotoxicol 7:103-120.

Wiggins RC, Benjamins JA, Krigman MR, Morell P (1974). Synthesis of myelin proteins during starvation. Brain Res 80:345-349.

Wiggins RC, Miller SL, Benjamins JA, Krigman MR, Morell P (1976). Myelin synthesis during postnatal nutritional deprivation and subsequent rehabilitation. Br Res 107:257-273.

Wiggins RC, Bissell AC, Durham L, Samorajski T (1985). The corpus callosum during postnatal undernourishment and recovery: a morphometric analysis of myelin and axon relationships. Brain Res 328:51-57.

Wiggins RC, Fuller GN (1978). Early postnatal starvation causes lasting brain hypomyelination. J Neurochem 30:1231-1237.

Wiggins RC, Fuller GN (1979). Relative synthesis of myelin in different brain regions of postnatally undernourished rats. Brain Res 162:103-112.

Winick M, Noble A (1966). Cellular response in rats during malnutrition at various ages. J Nutr 89:300-306.

Winick M, Rosso P (1969). The effect of severe early malnutrition on cellular growth of human brain. Pediat Res 3:181-184.

Wood P, Bunge RP (1984). The biology of the oligodendrocyte. In:Norton,WT (ed): "Oligodendroglia", New York: Plenum Press, pp 1-46.

Yeh Y-Y (1988). Maternal dietary restriction causes myelin and lipid deficits in the brain of offspring. J Neurosci Res 19:357-363.

DISCUSSION

(Discussion tape inaudible)

(Mal)Nutrition and the Infant Brain, pages 191–206
© 1990 Wiley-Liss, Inc.

NUTRITIONAL ALTERATIONS OF AMINO ACIDS AND PROTEINS DURING CEREBRAL DEVELOPMENT

Abel Lajtha, Miriam Banay-Schwartz, David Dunlop

Center for Neurochemistry, The Nathan S. Kline Institute for Psychiatric Research, Orangeburg, New York 10962, USA

In principle the supply of amino acids might be expected to have an important influence on protein metabolism and protein composition in the brain, since precursor availability is often the rate-limiting factor in metabolic reactions. And changes in amino acid levels should influence protein metabolism of the immature brain, in which metabolic controls are not fully developed, to a greater degree than that of the mature brain. The amino acid supply should be more important, and greater sensitivity can be expected, in the immature brain.

Although these are reasonable expectations, they are far from being well established. The relationship of amino acids to protein metabolism is made more complex by changes in the control mechanisms during development. At birth many processes are already operational, some even at higher activity than in the adult brain. That regulation of amino acids involves the processes of transport, activation, incorporation into proteins, release from proteins, reincorporation, and compartmentation indicates the multiplicity and diversity of the controlling factors. Additional complexity is evident in the multiple mechanisms of protein breakdown. Perhaps because of these many complex processes, information about metabolic influences on cerebral proteins, and about metabolic controls in general in young and adult, is still rather scant.

This chapter is an attempt to briefly survey various aspects of the problem, to discuss some areas studied in detail where consensus has been reached, and to indicate what further work is needed. With the rapid expansion in technology and the recognition of the importance of nutritional influences on macromolecular composition of the brain, great advances can be expected.

Heterogeneity of Amino Acid Pools

The distribution of amino acids is not homogeneous throughout the brain. The regional heterogeneity is different for the various amino acids, and changes during development and aging.

Recently in a series of papers (Banay-Schwartz et al., 1989a,b,c,d) we analyzed the amino acid content in tissue from 53 discrete brain areas microdissected with the punch technique (Palkovits, 1973). These samples, though only a small portion of the whole brain, represented many functionally different nuclei. We found very large regional variations in concentrations, as illustrated in Table 1. For each amino acid, the highest concentration was 6 to 30-fold the level in the area of lowest concentration. These differences were not restricted to only a few areas; even if the average of the 5 highest areas was compared to the average of the 5 lowest, the concentration difference was 3-5 fold. Although the areas investigated were small (a few mg of fresh tissue) each may be a heterogeneous sample containing multiple functional areas, cells, and fine subcellular structures in which amino acid levels differ from the average. Thus the differences shown in Table 1 represent minimum values, with the actual heterogeneity in the various structures likely to be considerably greater.

Examination of the distribution of amino acids revealed that there were a number of areas in which most amino acids, or at least a group of amino acids transported by the same system, had either high or low levels. There were also many areas where some amino acids were high, and others low. For the various amino acids the area with the highest level was different. This heterogeneity in composition is illustrated in Table 2, where the rank order of the five most concentrated amino acids is given for a few areas. In each of the areas selected, a different amino acid is highest; glutamate, which is highest in the sensory cortex, is not among the top 5 in the ventromedial nucleus, and similarly, taurine is the amino acid at highest level in the caudate nucleus but is not among the five highest in the superior colliculus or in the posterior hypothalamic nucleus. Such heterogeneity in distribution is not specific for the neurotransmitter amino acids but is seen with most amino acids, although as mentioned above, in a number of areas the levels of related amino acids are all similarly high or low. Our recent studies of regional heterogeneity in cerebral amino acid distribution were not the first on this subject - a number of previous studies established such heterogeneity (Battistin and Lajtha, 1970; Perry, 1982). Because the previous studies examined larger tissue samples, the heterogeneity did not appear to be as great as it did in our recent work examining small areas. Glutamate and aspartate showed significant regional heterogeneity when small regions were microdissected and compared (Palkovits et al., 1986).

Because the regional heterogeneity of protein turnover in these brain areas has not been measured, there is little information on whether amino acid levels are related to rates of incorporation (such studies are in progress in our laboratory). The available data on regional heterogeneity of protein synthesis would indicate considerably less regional variation in protein synthesis than in amino acid levels.

Further important aspects of heterogeneous distribution of cerebral amino acids include the metabolic compartmentation of glutamic acid (Patel and Balazs, 1975; van den Berg et al., 1975; Hamberger et al., 1982) and the synaptic transport of neurotransmitter amino acids (Kvamme et al., 1988).

TABLE 1. Ratio of the Highest to the Lowest Concentration of Amino Acid in Brain Areas

Amino Acid	Concn. ratio	Amino Acid	Concn. ratio
Aspartic acid	9	Valine	10
Glutamic acid	5	Leucine	12
Glutamine	6	Isoleucine	11
GABA	21	Phenylalanine	9
Taurine	34	Tyrosine	9
Threonine	9	Methionine	13
Glycine	8	Histidine	12
Serine	8	Lysine	15
Alanine	7	Arginine	23

Amino acids were assayed in 53 microdissected areas from rat brain (Banay-Schwartz et al., 1989a,b,c,d).

TABLE 2. Concentration Order of the Levels of Amino Acids

Brain Area	1	2	3	4	5
Sensory cortex	Glu	Gln	Tau	Asp	GABA
Superior colliculus	GABA	Gln	Asp	Glu	Gly
Caudate nucleus	Tau	Glu	Gln	GABA	Asp
Ventromedial nucleus	GABA	Asp	Gln	Gly	Tau
Posterior hypo-thalamic nucleus	Gln	GABA	Glu	Asp	Gly

Amino acids are shown in the order of their levels (1 the highest) in some areas in adult rat brain (Banay-Schwartz et al., 1989b).

These important and extensive studies of heterogeneous amino acid pools deal with neurotransmitter function of specific amino acids rather than with aspects of relevance to protein metabolism and nutrition, and are outside the scope of this chapter. A recent example of such studies is the report (Kish et al., 1989) that the uptake of GABA, glycine, and glutamate into synaptic vesicles occurs through three separate transport systems, with heterogeneous regional distribution of the uptake systems. Having a significant portion of these amino acids stored in specific vesicles containing only one amino acid at high levels, and heterogeneous distribution of these vesicles possibly according to amino acidergic pathways, would constitute further compartments, and extension of the regionally heterogeneous distribution of amino acids.

A further aspect of regional heterogeneity of amino acids is the difference in their levels in various cells, with neuronal/glial ratios varying in different areas. We note that recent advances in amino acid analysis (Cheng and Dovichi, 1988) have pushed the limit of detection to the subattomole (amol = 10^{-18} mol) level. Thus it may be technically feasible to measure at least glutamate in a single large neuron. The distribution of amino acids is likely to be heterogeneous even within the cell, with concentrations occurring at sites of protein synthesis and amino acid activation, in synaptic vesicles, and at sites of protein breakdown.

Developmental Changes in Amino Acid Levels

Since in this chapter possible changes in proteins in response to nutritional factors and the differences in these changes in different developmental stages are examined, it is important to emphasize how metabolite levels and metabolic rates are altered during development in the brain. As with the heterogeneity of regional distribution, where the distribution of each amino acid is different, developmental changes also vary with each amino acid.

Developmental changes in cerebral amino acid levels, which were found early and are now well established, are discussed in several review chapters (Perry, 1982; Himwich and Agrawal, 1969; Lajtha et al., 1988). Developmental changes are illustrated in Table 3, from one of our early papers. As seen in this table, and as found in numerous other studies, the levels of glutamate, aspartate, and GABA increase and those of valine, leucine, phenylalanine, and lysine decrease in development. This led to the oft-repeated statement that amino acids primarily utilized for protein synthesis decline with the decline in protein metabolism during development and amino acids with neurotransmitter function increase with increasing functional activity. Probably this is an oversimplification, as shown by the decrease in glycine levels and the major decrease in taurine levels. In contrast to the other amino acids, cerebral taurine levels are highly species dependent, being rather high in mice, lower in rats, and much lower in other species including monkey and man (Perry, 1982).

The variations in the patterns of change are illustrated in Table 3. Some amino acids such as glutamate and aspartate change gradually (even go through several periods of increase and decrease) (Piccoli et al., 1971), others such as alanine change rapidly around birth, and some such as lysine and threonine change rapidly perinatally and continue to change till adult values are reached. The developmental alterations in amino acid levels were somewhat different in the various brain areas, although only gross brain areas were analyzed for these studies. We found further changes in aging in our studies (Banay-Schwartz et al., 1989a,b,c,d) comparing the levels of amino acids in 53 brain areas of 3-month-old and 29-month-old Fischer male rats. Most amino acids showed changes in the old rat brain in the majority of the areas. Though there were some increases in concentration the changes were primarily decreases, in complex patterns differing among the various amino acids.

TABLE 3. Changes in Brain Amino Acids During Development

Amino Acid	Fetus		Newborn		Adult
	15 days	19 days	1h	24 h	
Tau	14	12	15	16	8.0
Asp	2.4	2.0	2.0	2.3	3.8
Glu	7.5	5.7	4.4	5.0	12
Gln	3.7	6.0	6.0	6.6	5.6
Thr	4.3	0.90	1.2	0.90	0.56
GABA	0.50	1.8	2.0	1.6	2.4
Gly	2.3	1.6	2.2	2.3	1.3
Ala	5.1	3.0	5.0	0.80	0.56
Val	0.56	0.30	0.46	0.28	0.10
Leu	0.53	0.26	0.30	0.18	0.06
Phe	0.24	0.22	0.19	0.13	0.07
Lys	0.86	0.88	1.1	0.41	0.29

Content in whole brain of Swiss mice was analyzed. Values are expressed as μmol of free amino acid per g of fresh tissue (Lajtha and Toth, 1973).

In summary, regional amino acid levels and amino acid distribution in the brain are markedly heterogeneous and undergo large changes during development and aging. Concentration ratios vary from 5 to 30-fold between areas, and there are undoubtedly larger differences in finer structures such as synaptic vesicles, glia, and neurons. The distribution pattern is specific for each amino acid, as are the developmental and aging changes.

Changes in Amino Acid Transport in Development

Since most nutrients probably are taken up by the brain via mediated transport processes, most nutritional influences on brain content may be influenced by, and dependent upon, transport activity. It has been shown with drugs and other marker compounds that the immature brain is more permeable than the adult organ. Especially with the poorly penetrating amino acids, it was also shown that a comparable increase in plasma levels results in a greater increase in the immature brain (Seta et al., 1972). On the other hand blood-brain barrier transport activity for amino acids was shown to be higher in the immature brain (Sershen and Lajtha, 1976a; Cremer et al., 1976). The developmental change of transport is different for the different transport classes (Nagashima et al., 1987). Such an increase in amino acid transport may reflect increased needs during net protein deposition and this increased need for metabolites may imply a greater sensitivity to transport inhibition in the immature organism. The difference in transport activity was significant, 30-100% higher in growing brain; the portion of uptake that was not inhibitable by analogs, i.e., the diffusion component, was, as might be expected from the studies discussed above, also much greater in the immature brain. These developmental aspects of the blood-brain barrier were the subject of a recent review (Johanson, 1989).

The transport systems for amino acids in the brain are heterogeneously distributed. Some specific systems are present only in synaptic regions or structures (Kish et al., 1989), and a number of systems active in brain cells are absent or are present only at low activity in the blood-brain barrier capillaries. The cellular and synaptic transport systems may play a role as important in the determination of tissue amino acid distribution as do the capillary endothelial transport systems. The transport system for glutamate is of low activity in the capillaries and high in the cells, while phenylalanine transport is of high activity in the capillaries and low in the cells, reflecting the differing transport requirements for a neurotransmitter and an essential amino acid used largely for protein synthesis. Such findings indicate that if transport is one of the determinants of tissue levels, cellular transport may be of greater importance than capillary transport.

Cellular transport systems are heterogeneous, and not all transport systems are present in all cells. For example, the synaptic vesicle transport systems seem to be specific for transmitter amino acids and are present only in these structures. Thus there are many amino acid transport systems present in the brain - we identified in cells at least ten such systems (Sershen and Lajtha, 1979a), and probably more are present. Some systems transport a number of structurally related amino acids, and a change in the level of any one, altering the concentration ratios, may alter transport rates of the other members of the group; for example, an increase in the blood concentration of one amino acid may competitively inhibit the transport of the others in the group. A well- studied example is the L transport system for the large neutral amino acids, which includes neurotransmitter precursors such as tyrosine and tryptophan (Wurtman et al., 1976; Acworth et al., 1988). Changes in plasma ratios do indeed lead to corresponding though lesser changes in the brain (Smith, 1988). For some amino acids such as glutamate, multiple transport systems were found, some specific for glutamate alone, others for glutamate and aspartate, hence a change in aspartate levels would influence glutamate transport in only those structures in which the system shared by both is the dominant entrance route for glutamate. Synaptosomal systems show significant differences in such properties as substrate specificity, ion dependence, and source of energy (Kvamme et al., 1988; Naito and Ueda, 1985). Both cell-specific and non-cell-specific systems have also been described for GABA and taurine transport (Seiler and Lajtha, 1987).

Thus we have multiple transport systems, some specific for cells or synaptosomes, some present in capillaries, all of which must play a part in regulating the levels of amino acids throughout the brain. One would expect the heterogeneous pattern of developmental change in amino acid distribution to be reflected in a diversity of developmental alterations in transport. We found a complex pattern of developmental changes in amino acid uptake in brain slices which was different from capillary transport. Cellular amino acid transport as measured by uptake in brain slices increased, especially for the essential amino acids, with development (Sershen and Lajtha, 1976b) while capillary transport decreased. The greatest developmental changes seem to be quantitative changes rather than alterations in the properties of the transport systems. However, developmental changes in properties do occur: both the maximal rate (V_{max}) and the affinity (K_m) of GABA transport in neurons increased during development as did the effect of neuronal transport inhibitors (Balcar et al., 1989).

Changes in Protein Synthesis in Development

Several laboratories found some time ago that the rate of incorporation of amino acids into brain proteins is higher in the developing brain than in the adult brain (Dunlop et al., 1977a,b; Oja, 1967). The overall rate of incorporation in adult mice or rats was 0.6-0.8 percent/hour and in the young brain (1-3 days old) 1.8-2.2 percent/hour. These figures are clearly the averages of multiple pools, some proteins with much higher, others lower, metabolic rates than the average, but they are a true measure of the amount of amino acid incorporated, i.e., a measure of ribosomal activity. We examined in some detail whether the higher incoporation rate in the young brain is due to a very active small fraction of proteins. We compared rates of incorporation into young and adult brain proteins of different brain areas and in neuronal and glial fractions (Shahbazian et al., 1986a), incorporation into various subcellular particulate fractions (Shahbazian et al., 1986b), and into protein fractions separated according to molecular weight (Shahbazian et al., 1986c). Although we found some regional, cellular, particulate, and molecular weight differences in turnover, in each fraction the ratio of metabolic rates of young versus adult was rather similar. We concluded that the developmental difference in metabolic rate reflects a general change in metabolic rate that is generally similar in extent for most brain proteins. Since the average metabolic rate in the newborn is about 3 times that in the adult, this is not unexpected - a small fraction could not account for the 3-fold change in rates in development. When metabolic rates were broken down into fractions of protein, estimated from the changes in incorporation rates of amino acids with time, there were indications of a small active pool in the adult brain with a rate higher than the average rate in young brain (Lajtha et al., 1976; Lajtha et al., 1979). This small fraction of protein with a more active metabolism in the adult brain is probably composed largely of regulatory proteins.

Although protein metabolism as expressed as half-life, or percent replaced per hour, is more active in the immature brain, if amino acid incorporation is expressed per unit of RNA in brain, the rates do not change during development (Dunlop et al., 1984), suggesting that RNA may be rate-determining in protein synthesis. That is, the number of ribosomes rather than ribosomal efficiency (Dunlop, 1983) appears to be the variable.

Differences in protein turnover between species have also been noted. In a recent study (Sayegh and Lajtha, 1989) we compared protein synthesis rates of brain (and muscle and liver) in the chicken, lizard, fish, frog, and mouse. As found before (Lajtha and Sershen, 1975), protein metabolism rates are strongly dependent on body temperature, but even if extrapolated to similar temperatures, protein turnover in lizard brain was lower than in the other

TABLE 4. Rates of Brain Protein Synthesis

Species	Age	Body Temperature	Incorporation % per hour
Rat	Adult	38	0.6
Rat	Newborn	37	2.0
Mouse	Adult	38	0.7
Chicken	30 days	39	0.7
Goldfish	Adult	10	0.03
Goldfish	Adult	34	0.5
Lizard	Adult	26	0.13
Lizard	Adult	38	0.27

(Lajtha and Sershen, 1975; Sayegh and Lajtha, 1989; Dunlop et al., 1977a).

species. Thus in addition to the temperature effect, brain protein turnover is inherently lower in some species. In fish, where body temperature can show a 15-20°C seasonal variation, turnover rates of brain proteins can change as much as 10-15 fold (Lajtha and Sershen, 1975) (Table 4). Turnover is a property of most proteins in the brain (Lajtha and Toth, 1966), with only a small fraction being permanent or having a very long half-life (Shapira et al., 1981).

That proteins in the brain are in a dynamic state, continuously broken down and resynthesized, and that most proteins undergo large changes in metabolic rates during development, suggests that external factors may influence protein composition by altering synthetic or degradative steps, and mechanisms of distribution and posttranslational modification.

It should also be considered that a particular protein may be metabolized differently in different cells, such as glia and neurons, and in different structures, such as cytoplasm and membranes. It is well known that the metabolic rates of proteins in various myelin regions (Lajtha et al., 1977) and synaptic regions (Sedman et al., 1986) vary. A recent example of regional heterogeneity is the report that the turnover rate of microtubule-associated protein (MAP2) in the axons differs from that in the dendrites (Okabe and Hirokawa, 1989). The consequences of this metabolic heterogeneity are that nutritional or pathological influences such as hyperphenylalaninemia may influence the metabolism of only some proteins, in some brain structures, in some developmental stages (Hughes and Johnson, 1978).

Although there have been many studies on brain protein metabolism in *in vitro* systems, such studies have to be interpreted with caution. We found that protein synthesis rates are much higher (over ten-fold) in the living brain than in most isolated systems (Dunlop et al., 1977a). It is of interest that the differences between protein synthesis rates *in vivo* and *in vitro* (slices) are much greater in the adult brain (Dunlop et al., 1981). Similarly, though rates of degradation in brain slice preparations appeared fairly close to *in vivo* rates at one hour, they vary in time and magnitude in a manner quite different from those observed *in vitro.*

Changes in Protein Breakdown in Development

Like protein synthesis rates, the rates of protein degradation are high in the immature brain and decrease during development (Dunlop et al., 1978; 1982). The changes are less than those of synthesis but are highly significant; in the cerebral hemisphere in rats from 2 to 30 days protein breakdown decreases from 1.3 to 0.8 percent per hour, in the cerebellum from 1.9 to 0.8 percent per hour. The rate of breakdown during the active growth of brain is in excess of net protein deposition so that growth involves restructuring as much as the simple addition of new material.

We know less about the mechanism of protein breakdown than of synthesis, and it is not clear what regulatory factors account for this developmental decrease of catabolism. Assays of brain proteases showed an increase in cathepsin D during development (Banay-Schwartz et al., 1983a) but in calpains, the Ca-dependent neutral proteinases, a decrease in activity during development (Simonson et al., 1985). Neither activity is parallel with *in vivo* protein breakdown changes - the decrease in calpain activity is much greater than *in vivo* breakdown decrease and cathepsin D content increases during this period. Of course it is difficult to make conclusions from changes in enzyme activity *in vitro* about the activity of the enzymes under *in vivo* conditions. In general, estimates are that the content of proteolytic enzymes is in great excess of that needed for physiological protein turnover (Banay-Schwartz et al., 1983b).

There are a number of proteinases in the brain, many with sufficiently broad substrate specificity to enable them to play a quantitatively significant role in protein turnover - but it has not yet been established which proteins are in fact substrates of these enzymes *in vivo.* We found that though cathepsin D has a strongly acidic pH optimum, this is not the case with all substrates (Banay-Schwartz et al., 1985); thus this enzyme could also participate in turnover. The important role of proteolytic enzymes is underscored by the finding that the life span of many species is in inverse proportion to their cerebral calpain content (Baudry et al., 1986). The activity of these enzymes may change under various conditions, for example, with some pathological degenerative changes (Smith et al., 1981), and inhibition of proteases under these conditions may have therapeutic significance (Smith and Amaducci, 1982). It is of interest in this respect that tissue damage may activate not only latent proteolytic activity but also latent amino acid transport activity (Bracco et al., 1982a).

The proteinases themselves may contribute to the heterogeneity of protein degradation by exercising some unexpected specificities, as indicated by the finding of rapid degradation of cytoplasmic tubulin by cathepsin D while membrane-bound tubulin was resistant to the enzyme (Bracco et al., 1982b).

Alterations of Cerebral Protein Metabolism

The effects of amino acids on protein turnover were studied in some detail in liver and muscle. These are organs that rapidly break down under low protein diet and therefore are known to be organs that can supply needed amino acids during malnutrition. Thus, lowered amino acid levels in the organism should stimulate protein degradation in these organs, and when amino acids are supplied in plenty, degradation should decrease (Mortimore and Neely, 1975). Such processes are also evident for protein synthesis and degradation in muscle in response to fasting (Morgan et al., 1971; Li et al., 1979; Li and Goldberg, 1976). Refeeding decreases proteolysis in muscle (Goodman and Del Pilar Gomez, 1987). In liver, amino acids seem to regulate the lysosomal pathway of proteolysis (Mortimore and Poso, 1984; Mortimore et al., 1977). This occurs through alterations in autophagy, the internalization and degradation of proteins in lysosomes. The regulation is rapid: in perfused liver within minutes autophagy is increased if amino acids are absent in the perfusion medium, and is restored to normal (close to *in vivo* rates) just as quickly if amino acids are added to the perfusate. This rapid response is interesting since the amino acids that are derived from intralysosomal protein degradation form a pool in the lysosomes that does not equilibrate rapidly with the cytosolic amino acid pool in the liver (Ward and Mortimore, 1978). The regulation is rather complex, and all amino acids do not have a similar effect; leucine is the most active in inhibiting proteolysis (Mortimore and Poso, 1984; Mortimore et al., 1984). Such effects on protein turnover are not specific for amino acids, since a number of other factors, such as ischemia (Williams et al., 1981) and ethanol (Morland and Sjetnan, 1976; Poso et al., 1987) exhibit similar interactions.

The incorporation rate at a high flooding dose of a labeled amino acid was not different from the rate when a tracer dose was administered (Dunlop et al., 1977b), indicating that increasing one amino acid has little effect on overall metabolic rates.

Diets deficient in protein affect cerebral protein metabolism, but the effects are different from those observed with muscle and liver, since brain proteins do not serve as an auxiliary amino acid supply. Amino acid transport *in vivo* after protein deficiency is altered in a complex way, with the uptake of some amino acids increased, especially of histidine, and others decreased or unchanged (Toth and Lajtha, 1980; Ója and Korpi, 1972). Although free histidine in the brain increases under these conditions, the levels of a number of essential amino acids, such as valine, decrease. Thus the changes in transport processes into the brain do not sustain the pre-diet balance.

A mildly protein-deficient diet does not affect protein metabolism in the adult brain, but in the developing brain both synthesis and breakdown are decreased, with no change in protein content (Banay-Schwartz et al., 1979). If the deficiency is prolonged and is extensive, synthesis and breakdown are decreased at all ages, with the changes in growing brain greater. Under these conditions the decrease of synthesis is greater than that of breakdown, resulting in some decrease in brain protein content in the malnourished young as compared to control. If the period of protein deficiency is limited some recovery can be found, but with a longer period of deficiency cerebral protein content remains diminished (Banay-Schwartz et al., 1979; Zamenhof et al., 1971); the effects are complicated in that various proteins are affected to a different degree (Wiggins et al., 1974; Moore et al., 1977). Clearly the effects of malnutrition are far-reaching, since they include many metabolic pathways in addition to protein metabolism and result in structural alterations. Synaptosomal membrane fluidity is altered in protein-free diet, without significant changes in protein composition (Felipo et al., 1989), and cell formation is specifically affected in young (Patel et al., 1973).

Protein metabolism in brain, although fairly stable, can be altered, in addition to malnutrition, by drugs such as nicotine (Sershen and Lajtha, 1979b). Now that technical developments make it possible to study changes in individual brain proteins, these changes can be reinvestigated to find which protein components are affected and how such effects change during development of the brain.

REFERENCES

Acworth IN, During MJ, Wurtman RJ (1988). Processes that couple amino acid availability to neurotransmitter synthesis and release. In Huether G (ed): "Amino Acid Availability and Brain Function in Health and Disease", Berlin-Heidelberg: Springer-Verlag, pp 118-136.

Balcar VJ, Hauser KL, Demieville H (1989). Developmental changes in high-affinity uptake of GABA by cultured neurons. Neurochem Res 14:229-233.

Banay-Schwartz M, Bracco F, Dahl D, DeGuzman T, Turk V, Lajtha A (1985). The pH dependence of breakdown of various purified brain proteins by cathepsin D preparations. Neurochem Int 7:607-614.

Banay-Schwartz M, Bracco F, DeGuzman T, Lajtha A (1983a). Developmental changes in the breakdown of tubulin by cerebral cathepsin D. Neurochem Res 8:51-61.

Banay-Schwartz M, Bracco F, Dunlop DS, Lajtha A (1983b). Alterations and heterogeneity of protein breakdown in the nervous system. In Austin L, Jeffrey PL (eds): "Molecular Aspects of Neurological Disorders," Sidney: Academic Press, pp 159-171.

Banay-Schwartz M, Giuffrida AM, DeGuzman T, Sershen H, Lajtha A (1979). Effect of undernutrition on cerebral protein metabolism. Exp Neurol 65:157-168.

Banay-Schwartz M, Lajtha A, Palkovits M (1989a). Changes with aging in the levels of amino acids in rat CNS structural Elements I. Glutamate and related amino acids. Neurochem Res 14:555-562.

Banay-Schwartz M, Lajtha A, Palkovits M (1989b). Changes with aging in the levels of amino acids in rat CNS structural elements II. Taurine and small neutral amino acids. Neurochem Res 14:563-570.

Banay-Schwartz M, Lajtha A, Palkovits M (1989c). Changes with aging in the levels of amino acids in rat CNS structural elements III. Large neutral amino acids. J Neurosci Res (in press).

Banay-Schwartz M, Lajtha A, Palkovits M (1989d). Changes with aging in the levels of amino acids in rat CNS structural elements IV. Methionine and basic amino acids. J Neurosci Res (in press).

Battistin L, Lajtha A (1970). Regional distribution and movement of amino acids in the brain. J Neurol Sci 10:313-322.

Baudry M, DuBrin R, Beasley L, Leon M, Lynch G (1986). Low levels of calpain activity in Chiroptera brain: Implications for mechanisms of aging. Neurobiol Aging 7:255-258.

Bracco F, Gennaro J Jr, Lajtha A (1982a). Relationship of morphologic damage and amino acid uptake in incubated slices of brain. Exp Neurol 76:606-622.

Bracco F, Banay-Schwartz M, DeGuzman T, Lajtha A (1982b). Membrane-bound tubulin: Resistance to cathepsin D and susceptibility to thrombin. Neurochem Int 5:501-511.

Cheng YF, Dovichi NJ (1988). Subattomole amino acid analysis by capillary zone electrophoresis and laser-induced fluorescence. Science 242:562-564.

Cremer JE, Braun LD, Oldendorf WH (1976). Changes during development in transport processes of blood-brain barrier. Biochim Biophys Acta 448:633-637.

Dunlop DS (1983). Protein turnover in brain: Synthesis and degradation. In Lajtha A (ed): "Handbook of Neurochemistry," New York: Plenum Press, Vol 5, pp 25-63.

Dunlop DS, Bodony R, Lajtha A (1984). RNA concentration and protein synthesis in rat brain during development. Brain Res 294:148-151.

Dunlop DS, van Elden W, Lajtha A (1977a). Developmental effects on protein synthesis rates in regions of the CNS in vivo and in vitro. J Neurochem 29:939-945.

Dunlop DS, Lajtha A, Toth J (1977b). Measuring brain protein metabolism in young and adult rats. In Roberts S, Lajtha A, Gispen WH (eds): "Mechanisms, Regulation and Special Functions of Protein Synthesis in the Brain," Amsterdam: Elsevier, pp 79-96.

Dunlop DS, McHale DM, Lajtha A (1982). The rate of protein degradation in developing brain. Biochem J 208:659-666.

Dunlop DS, van Elden W, Lajtha A (1978). Protein degradation rates in regions of the central nervous system in vivo during development. Biochem J 170:637-642.

Dunlop DS, van Elden W, Plucinska I, Lajtha A (1981). Brain slice protein degradation and development. J Neurochem 36:258-265.

Felipo V, Minana MD, Grisolia S (1989). A protein-free diet changes synaptosomal membrane fluidity and tyrosine and glutamate transport. Neurochem Res 14:531-535.

Goodman MN, Del Pilar Gomez M (1987). Decreased myofibrillar proteolysis after refeeding requires dietary protein or amino acids. Amer J Physiol 253:E52-E58.

Hamberger A, Jacobsson I, Molin SO, Nystrom B, Sandberg M, Ungerstedt U (1982). Metabolic and transmitter compartments for glutamate. In Bradford HF (ed): "Neurotransmitter Interaction and Compartmentation," New York: Plenum Press, pp 359-378.

Himwich WA, Agrawal HC (1969). Amino acids. In Lajtha A (ed): "Handbook of Neurochemistry", New York: Plenum Press, Vol 1, pp 33-52.

Hughes JV, Johnson TC (1978). Experimentally induced and natural recovery from the effects of phenylalanine on brain protein synthesis. Biochim Biophys Acta 517:473-485.

Johanson CE (1989). Ontogeny and phylogeny of the blood-brain barrier. In Neuwelt EA (ed): "Implications of the Blood-Brain Barrier and its Manipulation," New York: Plenum Press, Vol 1, pp 157-198.

Kish PE, Fischer-Bovenkerk C, Ueda T (1989). Active transport of γ-aminobutyric acid and glycine into synaptic vesicles. Proc Natl Acad Sci USA 86:3877-3881.

Kvamme E, Roberg B, Johnansen L (1988). Uptake and release of amino acids from synaptosomes. In Huether G (ed): "Amino Acid Availability and Brain Function in Health and Disease," Berlin-Heidelberg: Springer-Verlag, pp 57-68.

Lajtha A, Dunlop DS, Patlak C, Toth J (1979). Compartments of protein metabolism in the developing brain. Biochim Biophys Acta 561:491-501.

Lajtha A, Latzkovits L, Toth J (1976). Comparison of turnover rates of proteins of the brain, liver and kidney in mouse in vivo following long-term labeling. Biochim Biophys Acta 425:511-520.

Lajtha A, Sershen H (1975). Changes in the rates of protein synthesis in the brain of goldfish at various temperatures. Life Sci 17:1861-1868.

Lajtha A, Sershen H, Dunlop DS (1988). Developmental changes in cerebral amino acids and protein metabolism. In Huether G (ed): "Amino Acid Availability and Brain Function in Health and Disease", Berlin-Heidelberg: Springer-Verlag, pp 393-402.

Lajtha A, Toth J (1966). Instability of cerebral proteins. Biochem Biophys Res Commun 23:294-298.

Lajtha A, Toth J (1973). Perinatal changes in the free amino acid pool of the brain in mice. Brain Res 55:238-241.

Lajtha A, Toth J, Fujimoto K, Agrawal HC (1977). Turnover of myelin proteins in mouse brain in vivo. Biochem J 164:323-329.

Li, JB, Goldberg AL (1976). Effects of food deprivation on protein synthesis and degradation in rat skeletal muscles. Amer J Physiol 231:441-448.

Li, JB, Higgins JE, Jefferson LS (1979). Changes in protein turnover in skeletal muscle in response to fasting. Amer J Physiol 236:H222-H228.

Moore BW, Menke R, Prensky AL, Fishman MA, Agrawal HC (1977). Selective decreases of S-100 in discrete anatomical areas of undernourished rat brain. Neurochem Res 2:549-553.

Morgan HE, Earl DCN, Broadus A, Wolpert EB, Giger E, Jefferson LS (1971). Regulation of protein synthesis in heart muscle. I. Effect of amino acid levels on protein synthesis. J Biol Chem 246:2152-2162.

Morland J, Sjetnan AE (1976). Reduced incorporation of [^{3}H]leucine into cerebral proteins after long-term ethanol treatment. Biochem Pharmacol 25:220-221.

Mortimore GE, Neely AN (1975). Regulatory effects of insulin, glucagon and amino acids on hepatic protein turnover in association with alterations of the lysosomal system. In Schimke RT, Katunuma N (eds): "Intracellular Protein Turnover," New York: Academic Press, pp 265-279.

Mortimore GE, Poso AR (1984). Lysosomal pathways in hepatic protein degradation: regulatory role of amino acids. Fed Proc 43:1289-1294.

Mortimore GE, Schworer CM (1977). Induction of autophagy by amino acid deprivation in perfused rat liver. Nature 270:174-176.

Mortimore GE, Surmacz CA (1984). Liver perfusion: an in vitro technique for the study of intracellular protein turnover and its regulation in vivo. Proc Nutr Soc 43:161-177.

Nagashima T, Lefauconnier JM, Smith QR (1987). Developmental changes in neutral amino acid transport across the blood-brain barrier. J Cerebr Blood Flow Metab S1:524.

Naito S, Ueda T (1985). Characterization of glutamate uptake into synaptic vesicles. J Neurochem 44:99-109.

Oja SS (1967). Studies on protein metabolism in developing rat brain. Ann Acad Sci Fenn (Med) 131:7-81.

Oja SS, Korpi ER (1972). Amino acid transport. In Lajtha A (ed): "Handbook of Neurochemistry," New York: Plenum Press, Vol 7, pp 311-333.

Okabe S, Hirokawa N (1989). Rapid turnover of microtubule-associated protein MAP2 in the axon revealed by microinjection of biotinylated MAP2 into cultured neurons. Proc Nat Acad Sci USA 86:4127-4131.

Palkovits M (1973). Isolated removal of hypothalamic or other brain nuclei of the rat. Brain Res 59:449-450.

Palkovits M, Lang T, Patthy A, Elekes I (1986). Distribution and stress-induced increase of glutamate and aspartate levels in discrete brain nuclei of rats. Brain Res 373:252-257.

Patel AJ, Balazs R (1975). Factors affecting the development of metabolic compartmentation in the brain. In Berl S, Clarke DD, Schneider D (eds): "Metabolic Compartmentation and Neurotransmission," New York: Plenum Press, pp 363-383.

Patel AJ, Balazs R, Johnson AL (1973). Effect of undernutrition on cell formation in the rat brain. J Neurochem 20:1151-1165.

Perry TL (1982). Cerebral amino acid pools. In Lajtha A (ed): "Handbook of Neurochemistry," New York: Plenum Press, Vol 1, pp 151-180.

Piccoli F, Grynbaum A, Lajtha A (1971). Developmental changes in Na^+, K^+ and ATP and in the levels and transport of amino acids in incubated slices of rat brain. J Neurochem 18:1135-1148.

Poso AR, Surmacz CA, Mortimore GE (1987). Inhibition of intracellular protein degradation by ethanol in perfused rat liver. Biochem J 242:459-464.

Sayegh JF, Lajtha A (1989). In vivo rates of protein synthesis in brain, muscle, and liver of five vertebrate species. Neurochem Res 14:1165-1168

Sedman GL, Jeffrey PL, Austin L, Rostas JAP (1986). The metabolic turnover of the major proteins of the postsynaptic density. Mol Brain Res 1:221-230.

Seiler N, Lajtha A (1987). Functions of GABA in the vertebrate organism. In Redburn DA, Schousboe A (eds): "Neurotophic Activity of GABA During Development," New York: Alan R. Liss, pp 1-56.

Sershen H, Lajtha A (1976a). Capillary transport of amino acids in the developing brain. Exp Neurol 53:465-474.

Sershen H, Lajtha A (1976b). Perinatal changes of transport systems for amino acids in slices of mouse brain. Neurochem Res 1:417-428.

Sershen H, Lajtha A (1979a). Inhibition pattern by analogs indicates the presence of ten or more transport systems for amino acids in brain cells. J Neurochem 32:719-726.

Sershen H, Lajtha A (1979b). The effect of nicotine on the metabolism of brain proteins. Neuropharmacology 18:763-766.

Seta K, Sershen H, Lajtha A (1972). Cerebral amino acid uptake in vivo in newborn mice. Brain Res 47:415-425.

Shahbazian FM, Jacobs M, Lajtha A (1986a). Regional and cellular differences in rat brain protein synthesis in vivo and in slices during development. Int J Dev Neurosci 4:209-215.

Shahbazian FM, Jacobs M, Lajtha A (1986b). Rates of amino acid incorporation into particulate proteins in vivo and in slices of young and adult brain. J Neurosci Res 15:359-366.

Shahbazian FM, Jacobs M, Lajtha A (1986c). Amino acid incorporation in relation to molecular weight of proteins in young and adult brain. Neurochem Res 11:647-660.

Shapira R, Wilhelmi MR, Kibler RF (1981). Turnover of myelin proteins of rat brain, determined in fractions separated by sedimentation in a continuous sucrose gradient. J Neurochem 36:1427-1432.

Simonson L, Baudry M, Siman R, Lynch G (1985). Regional distribution of soluble calcium activated proteinase activity in neonatal and adult rat brain. Brain Res 327:153-159.

Smith QR (1988). Regulation of amino acid transport at the blood-brain barrier. In Huether G (ed): "Amino Acid Availability and Brain Function in Health and Disease," Berlin-Heidelberg: Springer-Verlag, pp 57-68.

Smith ME, Amaducci LA (1982). Observations on the effects of protease inhibitors on the suppression of experimental allergic encephalomyelitis. Neurochem Res 7:541-554.

Smith ME, Chow SH, Rolph RH (1981). Partial purification and characterization of neutral proteases in lymph nodes of rats with experimental allergic encephalomyelitis. Neurochem Res 6:901-912.

Toth J, Lajtha A (1980). Effect of protein-free diet on the uptake of amino acids by the brain in vivo. Exp Neurol 68:443-452.

van den Berg CJ, Matheson DF, Ronda G, Reijnierse GLA, Blokhuis GGD, Kroon MC, Clarke DD, Garfinkel D (1975). A model of glutamate metabolism in brain: A biochemical analysis of a heterogeneous structure. In Berl S, Clarke DD, Schneider D (eds): "Metabolic Compartmentation and Neurotransmission," New York: Plenum Press, pp 515-543.

Ward WF, Mortimore GE (1978). Compartmentation of intracellular amino acids in rat liver. J Biol Chem 253:3581-3587.

Wiggins RC, Benjamins JA, Krigman MR, Morrell P (1974). Synthesis of myelin proteins during starvation. Brain Res 80:345-349.

Williams EH, Kao RL, Morgan HE (1981). Protein degradation and synthesis during recovery from myocardial ischemia. Amer J Physiol 240:268-273.

Wurtman RJ, Fernstrom JD (1976). Control of brain neurotransmitter synthesis by precursor availability and nutritional state. Biochem Pharmacol 25:1691-1696.

Zamenhof S, van Marthens E, Grauel L (1971). DNA (cell number) and protein in neonatal rat brain: Alteration by timing of maternal dietary protein restriction. J Nutr 101:1265-1270.

DISCUSSION

Q (Haber): It is interesting that particularly larger proteins have a certain turnover rate. Is that true irrespective of the amino acid tracer which you use?

A: Yes this is true. Developmental changes are fairly uniform for all proteins; this 4-5 fold change from young to adult. We tried to fractionate for molecular weight, and so on, but the heterogeneity for the larger proteins seems to be true, as a rule.

Q (Diamond): In housing your animals for your protein metabolism, how did you house your old animals and measure decrease (in protein synthesis) with aging.

A: We adopted two measures with old animals. These are Fisher rats from NIH, housed 2-3 per cage in a non-enriched environment i.e. no toys! The protein metabolism *in vivo* as you measure it in the old brain does decline rather slightly from the adult values. But interestingly, the brain protein content doubles; although the enzyme (protein) doubles, the enzyme activity *in vivo* as far as we can tell is not. I am not sure what that means, we don't know what the function of the enzyme is. My feeling is that this doubling of the enzyme indicates that, perhaps, utilization of the enzymes becomes less efficient (or) represent a stress response at normal protein utilization. I have a number of theories but no proofs.

Q (Huether): The amino acids which enter protein synthesis: Are they preferentially derived from proteolysis or do they come from uptake. What is the ratio?

A: Not an easy question to answer. If you look at what is the real incorporation of the locally liberated protein under physiological conditions, the best guess, and this is difficult to test, is about 50%. It does differ for each amino acid. There is a significant proteolysis in the lysozomes although we usually don't think that this occurs to an appreciable extend under physiological conditions *in vivo*. Again, the guess is (and no more) that this may amount to 50%. These amino acids equilibrate less rapidly than in other pools, so that there are several such pools which need to be considered.

Q (Huether): Yes, what I mean is, as long as you have a release of amino acids by protein breakdown you will never be able to affect protein synthesis by supply; also, efficacy may change and protein breakdown will be depending (more) on supply.

A: Yes, but of course under extreme malnutrition there may be a loss of free amino acids.

Q (Huether): You lose the capacity to release amino acids and then you get a greater dependency on supply?

A: Yes.

Q (S. Hashim): There may be a role of insulin in protein synthesis in brain, and I don't mean pancreatic insulin. It is now known that the brain contains even more insulin than the pancreas, I wonder what it is doing there.

A: Is there a function of insulin? I think if you increase insulin, it does somewhat increase incorporation. I have not seen dependency on insulin. I think that, in general, the insulin effects in brain are more indirect with respect to protein metabolism.

(Mal)Nutrition and the Infant Brain, pages 207–224
© 1990 Wiley-Liss, Inc.

VITAMIN DEFICIENCIES AND BRAIN DEVELOPMENT

Roger F. Butterworth

Laboratory of Neurochemistry, André-Viallet Clinical Research Centre, (Hôpital St-Luc) H2X 3J4 and Dept. of Medicine, Université de Montréal, Montréal, Québec, Canada

In pregnancy, maternal nutrients are ingested, processed by the placenta and provided to the fetus. As the fetus develops and biochemical maturation takes place, nutritional requirements change to respond to changing fetal demands. Vitamins are essential to fetal and infant brain development. The vitamins most likely to be deficient during pregnancy are the water-soluble vitamins, vitamin B_6 (pyridoxine), vitamin B_1 (thiamine) and folic acid (Rassin, 1984).

Vitamin deficiencies in pregnancy and lactation may result from:

1. Poor diet
2. Malabsorption due to gastrointestinal disease
3. Increased requirements
4. Alcohol abuse
5. Interference by drugs
6. Genetic factors

There is evidence to suggest that several developmental neurological conditions may result from maternal vitamin deficiencies of vitamin B_1, B_6 and folate (summarized in Table 1).

In this review, the prevalence of hypovitaminemia in pregnant and lactating women from various world communities will be summarized. In addition, evidence for an etiologic role for vitamin deficiencies in certain developmental brain disorders in humans will be evaluated and possible neurochemical mechanisms by which vitamin deficiencies may lead to such disorders will be discussed.

TABLE 1. Developmental Neurological Disorders Associated with Vitamin
Deficiencies in Humans

Vitamin Deficiency	Neurological Disorder
Folate	Neural Tube Defects Fetal Alcohol Syndrome
Thiamine (B_1)	Infantile Beri Beri Fetal Alcohol Syndrome Sudden Infant Death Leigh Disease
Pyridoxine (B_6)	Convulsions

Folate Deficiency in Humans

Megaloblastic anemia caused by folate deficiency has been reported by numerous workers throughout the world, suggesting that this disease constitutes a major world health care problem (Herbert, 1968). A majority of cases are associated with pregnancy, malabsorption of the vitamin, or alcoholism. Nutritional megaloblastic anemia of pregnancy is the major form of megaloblastic anemia in tropical areas. Vegetarian communities, particularly Hindu Indians are particularly at risk (Chanarin, 1979).

The recommended daily allowance for total folate intake ranges from 50 µg for infants under 1 year old to 600 µg for lactating women and 800 µg for pregnant women (Colman, 1977). Foods rich in folates include legumes, spinach and whole grains. Meats and dairy products are generally poorer sources of folate (Perloff and Butrum, 1977). There are many reports demonstrating that pregnant women from various world populations (both developed and underdeveloped) have dietary folate intakes far lower than those recommended. In the USA, Baker et al., (1975) found folate deficiency in 53% of 174 mothers from low-income groups at the time of admission to obstetrics services. In another study, folate deficiency was observed in 44% of pregnant black South African women (Colman et al., 1975). A Nutrition Canada report published in 1977 showed that the daily dietary intake of folates in pregnant Canadian women was less than 20% of recommended values (Table 2). Women from low-income groups and from the native population were found to have the lowest dietary intake of folates. In the same survey, the prevalence of folate deficiency, as defined by serum folate levels of less than 5 ng/ml in Canadian women of childbearing age was found to be greater than 60%. Eskimo women were again found to have particularly low serum folates with 96% being below normal values (Nutrition Canada Survey, 1977). Folate deficiency in pregnancy is probably attribuable to poor diet and to increased requirements for the vitamin (Colman, 1977).

A report by Gross et al. (1974) demonstrated that 8 of 14 African children aged six weeks to four years, whose mothers had been severely folate deficient during pregnancy, showed abnormal or delayed development as revealed by The Denver Developmental Screening Test.

The importance of lactation in preventing the restoration of normal folate status following pregnancy has been emphasized (Metz, 1970); in a report of the effect of previous pregnancy and lactation on the incidence of folate deficiency in non-pregnant women of childbearing age, folate deficiency was found to last up to 2 years following the former pregnancy (Colman, 1977).

Folate deficiency in pregnancy is aggravated by alcoholism. Chronic alcoholism leads to impairment of folate coenzymes, accelerates the appearance of hematolytic indices of megaloblastic anemia and causes malabsorption of folates (Blocker and Thenen, 1987). Within hours of even moderate alcohol ingestion by humans, serum folate levels are found to be decreased (Eichner and Hillman, 1973).

The effects of folate deficiency on brain development have been receiving increased attention in recent years. This is due to reports of the possible relationship of folate deficiency to the incidence of pregnancies complicated by neural-tube defects such as anencephaly, spina bifida and myelomeningocele (Smithells et al., 1976). In a report by Laurence et al., (1980), 174 women in South Wales who had previously had a child with a neural-tube defect (NTD) were studied prospectively during the first trimester of 186 subsequent pregnancies; 103 women were given dietary counselling before the pregnancy (78 complied), and 71 women were not counselled (9 improved their diet). There were 8 recurrences of NTD's, all of which occured in the 45 pregnancies in women taking poor diets. In another related study, UK women who had previously given birth to one or more infants with NTD were recruited into a trial of periconceptional multivitamin supplementation; 1 of 178 (0.6%) of infants/fetuses of vitamin-supplemented mothers had a NTD compared to 13 among 260 (5.0%) of infants/fetuses of unsupplemented mothers (Smithells el al., 1980). Some available evidence suggests that these beneficial effects of vitamin supplementation result from folate. A double-blind randomized

TABLE 2. Mean Dietary Intake of Folate in Pregnant Women in Canada (Nutrition Canada Report, 1977)

Population studied	Mean daily intake of folate (μg)
All	184
Low income	159
Lowest income	141
Eskimo	72

Average daily folate intake in Canada and USA (men and women): 200-300 μg.
Recommended daily folate intake in Canada and USA (pregnant women): 800 μg.

controlled trial before conception to prevent recurrence of NTD's revealed a significant protective effect of folate (Table 3, Laurence et al, 1981).

However, folate deficiency may not be the only cause of recurrence of NTD's. In a study by Molloy et al., (1985), serum folate levels were measured in 32 mothers with pregnancies affected by NTD's and in 395 non-affected pregnant women. No significant differences in the median values and frequency distributions of folate levels between the two groups was observed. Of 16 blood samples from mothers whose infants had NTD's, 11 were found to have folate levels within the normal range. Similar negative findings were reported in a group of 24 pregnant women who had previously given birth to a child with an NTD in Norway (Magnus et al., 1986). A subsequent study of vitamins in amniotic fluid from pregnancies complicated by NTD's revealed abnormalites of vitamin B_{12} metabolism (Gardiki-Kouidou and Seller, 1988). Further studies to better delineate the metabolic abnormality of folate or vitamin B_{12} in relation to the recurrence of NTD's is clearly required.

TABLE 3. Results of a Double-Blind Controlled Trial of Folate Treatment before Conception to Prevent Recurrence of Neural-Tube Defects

Outcome of pregnancy	Folate group		Placebo group
	Compliers	Non-compliers	
Normal fetus	44	14	47
Neural-Tube Defect	0	2	4

(from Laurence et al., (1981), Brit Med J 282: 1509-1511

There may also be an association between folate deficiency, NTD's and the fetal alcohol syndrome. NTD's were found in a case of fetal alcohol syndrome by two independent groups (Goldstein and Arulanantham, 1978; Fuster et al., 1979). Brain malformations were observed in four infants born to alcoholic women. All four brains showed similar malformations resulting from errors in the migration of neuronal and glial elements; two of the infants had hydrocephalus (Clarren et al., 1979).

Experimental Folate Deficiency and Brain Development

Several studies have clearly demonstrated the deleterious effects of folate deficiency on the differentiation of the embryonic nervous system. CNS malformations have been consistently produced by the use of folate antagonists in mammalian species (Nelson et al., 1952). Folate deprivation in pregnant rats resulted in up to 95% having litters with congenital abnormalities of various organs including the nervous system; hydrocephalus was noted in significant numbers of offspring (Nelson et al., 1952). Whitley et al., (1951) reported that rats born to mothers fed a folate-deficient diet showed inferior maze-learning ability as compared to controls.

Folic acid is important in neurogenesis and in subsequent cell growth and myelination. Folate is required for cell multiplication in the central nervous system probably due to its role in the synthesis of thymidine and purine. Reductions of DNA in brain tissue of rats born to folate deficient mothers have been reported (Tagbo and Hill, 1977). Haltia et al., (1970) showed evidence of impaired RNA synthesis in cerebellar Purkinje cells in developing chicks caused by folate deprivation. Similar effects were observed by Shaw et al., (1973) in mice exposed to folate deficiency prenatally and continued through lactation. Johnson et al., (1963) studied the effects of maternal folate deficiency on cytologic phenomena in rat embryos and found decreased mitotic rates and reduced amounts of ribosomes as well as RNA in the cytoplasm of the cells of the neural tube.

Arakawa et al. (1969) showed that there was a significant decrease in both cholesterol and phospholipid content of the myelin fraction isolated from 6 week old folate-deficient rats. In a subsequent study by Hirono and Wada (1978), rats were fed a folate-deficient diet from day 12 of gestation throughout lactation. Offspring were fed the same diet after weaning. Myelin yield in brain was found to be significantly decreased in folate-deficient animals. Furthermore, the developmental increase in percentages of 22:6, 22:4 and 20:1 in non-hydroxy fatty acids of myelin lipids from folate deficient rats was significantly lower than controls. It was suggested that folate may play an important role in the desaturation of chain elongation of polyunsaturated fatty acids in the brain of developing rats.

Prevention of Folate Deficiency

There is now a general consensus that folate supplements should be administered to pregnant women. If the findings of the protective effect of folate in the recurrence of NTD's are confirmed in larger controlled trials, folate supplementation should be started at the time of conception. The problem remains, however, that antenatal care is not available to (or not taken advantage of by) large numbers of pregnant women (Colman, 1977). To illustrate this latter point, one report showed that, of 110 consecutive women seeking prenatal care in the South Bronx, 61 were in the second trimester and 26 in the third trimester of pregnancy (Herbert et al., 1975).

As an alternative approach, feasibility studies of folate fortification of maize and cornmeal, the staple food in some world communities, have been done (Colman, 1977). Folate in fortified maize meal was stable for up to 18 months under normal storage conditions and resisted prolonged cooking for 1-2 hours.

Vitamin B_1 Deficiency in Humans

Thiamine is a water-soluble vitamin found in high concentrations in brewer's yeast, wheatgerm and whole grains. Milling of grain as well as prolonged cooking results in substantial losses of the vitamin. Normal daily thiamine requirements in humans are of the order of 1 mg. Human milk contains 21 mg thiamine per 100 Kcal. Formulas prepared for preterm infants, on the other hand, contain thiamine in concentrations of up to 250 mg per 100 Kcal

(Rassin, 1984). Large discrepancies are observed between content of other vitamins in preterm formulas. A systematic re-evaluation of recommended daily allowances for both preterm and term infants is long overdue.

Thiamine malnutrition is still a problem in some parts of Asia where it has been repeatedly shown that babies suckling from thiamine-deficient mothers develop signs of beri beri (Kywe-Thein et al., 1968; Pongparich et al., 1974). Beri beri usually presents itself in the first few months postnatally. It is generally sudden in onset and runs a fulminating course with acute cardiovascular symptoms and subsequent death, often within hours. The central nervous system is frequently involved as evidenced by nystagmus and convulsions (Nicholls, 1951; Sturman and Rivlin, 1975). According to one estimate, up to two-thirds of the infant mortality in The Phillipines in the 1950's was due to beri beri (Nicholls, 1951). Beri beri frequently occurs in infants breast-fed by mothers who themselves have no clinical symptoms of beri beri but who secrete milk with a low thiamine content (Davidson et al., 1975). A joint WHO-FAO report published in 1967 suggested that thiamine deficiency was still an important problem in The Philippines, Vietnam, Burma and Thailand (WHO Technical Report #302, Rome, 1967). Although a more recent report suggested a reduction in the incidence of beri beri, thiamine deficiency as evaluated by biochemical means may still be a problem of considerable magnitude in certain world populations (Butterworth, 1987). For example, a study carried out on Ghanaian children revealed evidence of severe thiamine deficiency in 34% of those studied (Neumann et al., 1979). Thiamine deficiency was also reported in 36% of malnourished children in Jamaica (Hailemariam et al., 1985) as well as in children from Northeastern Thailand (Sornmani et al., 1981). Thiamine requirements increase during pregnancy and lactation. Significant numbers of pregnant women were found to be thiamine deficient in studies in Malaysia (Chong Ho et al., 1970) and in India (Bamji, 1976). Furthermore, thiamine deficiency in *developed countries* is more common than is generally presumed. In a study published in 1974, 30% of a group of pregnant women in Europe were found to be thiamine deficient (Heller et al., 1974); 16% of a group of 37 parturient women in Holland were reportedly thiamine deficient (Van den Berg et al., 1978) and studies of vitamin profiles of 174 mothers and their newborns in the U.S. revealed thiamine deficiency in a significant number of cases (Baker et al., 1975).

Chronic alcoholism results in thiamine deficiency and, even when a normal diet is ingested, chronic alcohol consumption may lead to thiamine deficiency due to alcohol-induced reduction of thiamine absorption or decreased synthesis of the active (cofactor) form of thiamine in brain (Butterworth, 1987; 1989). In 1968, Lemoine and associates reported a high incidence of intrauterine growth retardation (IUGR), psychomotor abnormalities and congenital defects in children born to alcoholic mothers. Since then, numerous studies have confirmed these findings and the syndrome is now generally referred to as "the fetal alcohol syndrome". Thiamine deficiency in the pregnant rat results in IUGR in the offspring and it has been proposed that thiamine deficiency may play a role in the pathogenesis of the fetal alcohol syndrome (Roecklin et al., 1985).

It has also been suggested that a disorder of thiamine neurochemistry may play a role in the etiology of the "Sudden Infant Death Syndrome" (SIDS). Unexpected deaths have been described in apparently thriving infants of thiamine-deficient mothers (Read, 1978) and sleep apnea, a symptom frequently described in "near miss" SIDS infants, has been described in children with Leigh Disease, a genetic disorder of thiamine metabolism (Butterworth, 1985). However, direct studies of thiamine status in SIDS cases did not reveal any evidence of thiamine deficiency (Peterson et al., 1981).

Neurochemistry of Thiamine Deficiency

Thiamine deprivation results in decreased tissue thiamine stores. Studies of thiamine deficiency in experimental animals show that animals become symptomatic when thiamine levels in brain fall below 20% of normal values (Dreyfus, 1961). Thiamine, in the form of its diphosphate ester, thiamine

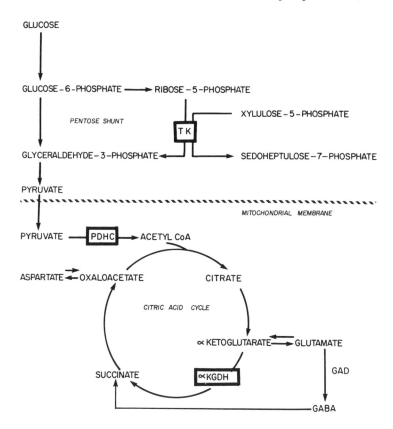

Fig. 1. Thiamine-dependent enzymes

pyrophosphate (TPP) is a cofactor for three enzymatic reactions involved in cerebral glucose utilization. These enzymes are the Pyruvate Dehydrogenase Complex (PDHC), α-ketoglutarate dehydrogenase (αKGDH) and transketolase (TK). The position of these enzymes in relation to glucose metabolism is shown schematically in Figure 1 (from Butterworth, 1989).

Studies in rat pups suckling from dams receiving a thiamine deficient diet revealed evidence of deficits of memory and learning (Bell and Stewart, 1979) as well as significant growth retardation (Trostler and Sklan, 1977). Analysis of milk composition from thiamine-deficient rats showed that the percentage transfer of thiamine was significantly reduced. Lactose content of the milk was decreased whereas fatty acid levels were increased and it was suggested that such changes in milk composition resulting from thiamine deficiency could have clinical significance (Trostler and Sklan, 1977). As part of a series of studies of the effect of thiamine deficiency on brain development, Butterworth and coworkers fed a thiamine-deficient diet to pregnant rats from the 14th day of gestation. Brain weights of the offspring were found to be decreased and reductions in the specific activities of thiamine-dependent enzymes in the brains of rats 13 days posnatally were observed (Fournier and Butterworth, 1989). PDHC and αKGDH activities were significantly reduced in cerebral cortex; TK activities on the other hand were reduced in cerebral cortex, cerebellum and brainstem of 13 day-old rat pups born to thiamine-deficient mothers (Table 4).

Table 4. Effects of Maternal Thiamine Deficiency onThiamine-Dependent Enzymes in Brain Regions of 13 Day Old Rat Pups.

Enzyme	Treatment Group	Enzyme Activity $(nmole.min^{-1}.mg^1.prot)$		
		Cerebral cortex	Cerebellum	Brainstem
PDHC	Control	22.17 ± 1.68	7.98 ± 1.15	35.82 ± 2.22
	B_1 deficient	$17.36 \pm 0.38*$	8.52 ± 1.62	37.48 ± 1.87
αKGDH	Control	10.06 ± 0.41	8.77 ± 0.80	12.99 ± 0.88
	B_1 deficient	$7.63 \pm 0.45**$	8.51 ± 0.15	12.82 ± 0.66
TK	Control	5.81 ± 0.17	7.95 ± 0.08	5.76 ± 0.62
	B_1 deficient	$4.10 \pm 0.13**$	$4.05 \pm 0.34**$	$4.01 \pm 0.35*$

$*p < 0.05$, $** p < 0.01$ compared to control (from Fournier and Butterworth, 1989)

In contrast to the developing young, thiamine-deficient mothers remained asymptomatic and brain enzyme activities remained within normal limits. These findings again suggest that developing brain is more susceptable to a dietary lack of thiamine than is that of the adult. It has been suggested that the pattern of PDHC development in brain may be of key importance in the establishment of adult patterns of brain energy metabolism (Butterworth, 1985; see Clarke, this volume). Furthermore, there may be very little surplus activity of either PDHC or αKGDH over that required to maintain metabolic fluxes in brain (Butterworth et al., 1986), suggesting that even modest decreases of enzyme activity could have serious metabolic consequences. Indeed, significant accumulation of brain pyruvate, consistent with decreased activities of PDHC or αKGDH, have been reported in the brains of rat pups born to thiamine-deficient mothers (Trostler et al., 1977).

The period of myelination in rat brain is most rapid between 10 and 20 days postnatally and this period is considered to be a particularly vulnerable one in brain development (Davison and Dobbing, 1966). Decreases in the incorporation of ^{14}C-glucose into myelin lipids has been described in the brains of the offspring of thiamine-deficient rats (Table 5; Trostler et al., 1977; Trostler and Sklan, 1978). Such reductions in lipid synthesis could result from decreased availability of acetyl CoA resulting from diminished activities of PDHC in the brains of these animals (Trostler and Sklan, 1978; Fournier and Butterworth, 1989).

Table 5. Incorporation of U-^{14}C-Glucose into Brain Lipids in 21-Days Old Pups of Thiamine-Deficient Rats.

Brain region	U-^{14}C-glucose incorporated (% dose per 100g.tissue)	
	Pair-fed control	Thiamine-deficient
Cerebrum	0.63 ± 0.05	0.25 ± 0.06*
Cerebellum	0.70 ± 0.07	0.21 ± 0.04 *

*$p< 0.01$ compared to controls (Data from Trostler and Sklan, 1978)

Vitamin B_6 Deficiency in Humans

Vitamin B_6 deficiency in humans is rare. One major outbreak resulted from over-heating of infant formula milk during manufacturing leading to almost complete loss of pyridoxine. Babies fed this formula milk suffered convulsions (Coursin, 1954); administration of pyridoxine resulted in relief of these symptoms.

The RDA for pyridoxine during pregnancy is 5.5 µg per day (Schuster et al., 1981). Studies of vitamin status of pregnant women from various world populations reveals significant evidence of B_6 deficiencies. For example, 50% of a series of pregnant women in Europe were found to be B_6 deficient (Heller et al., 1973). Vitamin B_6 deficiency has also been reported in pregnant women in the USA (Baker et al., 1975). Lower socio-economic groups are particularly vulnerable to development of B_6 deficiency. Shuster et al., (1981) measured vitamin B_6 status of low income pregnant women in Florida and found 68% to be deficient. In a study by Smithells et al., (1977), daily intake of vitamin B_6 in pregnant women from lower social classes in Northen England was found to be less than one third of the RDA. There is evidence to suggest that preterm infants may be succeptible to the development of B_6 deficiency; vitamin B_6 levels in milk from mothers of preterm infants was found to be lower than normal throughout the first month postpartum (Udipi et al., 1985). Human milk contains 13 µg of pyridoxine per 100 Kcal. Preterm infant formulas, on the other hand contain between 60 and 240 µg pyridoxine per 100 Kcal (Rassin, 1984).

Diabetic patients as well as patients with renal disease may be at increased risk for the development of vitamin B_6 deficiency (Dakshinamurthi, 1982). Chronic alcohol abuse results in alterations of B_6 metabolism resulting in deficiency of the coenzyme from pyridoxal phosphate (Hines, 1973).

Two siblings with seizures unresponsive to anticonvulsants were described by Hunt et al., (1954). Large doses of pyridoxine were found to control the seizures. Since that time, many reports of pyridoxine-dependent or pyridoxine-responsive infantile convulsions have appeared (Dakshinamurthi, 1982).

Experimental Vitamin B_6 Deficiency and Brain Development

Feeding of a vitamin B_6 deficient diet to pregnant rats during the last two weeks of gestation results in a 50% reduction of pyridoxal phosphate levels in brain at birth (Dakshinamurthi and Stephens, 1969). The progeny of rats fed a low vitamin B_6 diet during pregnancy and lactation show symptoms of pyridoxine deficiency (ataxia, convulsions) between 10 and 18 days postnatally. Cerebellum is more seriously affected by vitamin B_6 deficiency than is neocortex. This is in contrast to the effects of protein restriction. The effects of different levels of dietary B_6 fed to dams from lactation to weaning resulted in reductions of granular and molecular layers of cerebellum. Under normal conditions, during the first week of postnatal life in the rat, Purkinje cells move to form a single row. It is suggested that this phenomenon of alignment of Purkinje cells results from movement of granule cells. In support of this view, inhibition of early granule cell formation by X-rays or viruses results in Purkinje cells remaining in multicellular arrangements (Altman and Anderson, 1972). Similar effects on Purkinje cell alignment are observed in cerebella of rat pups born to vitamin B_6 deficient mothers (Morré et al., 1978a). In a study of the effects of vitamin B_6 deficiency on cerebellar development, Chang et al., (1981) found serious reductions in dendritic growth of Purkinje cells of the progeny following maternal vitamin B_6 deficiency. Total length of Purkinje cell dendrites per cell was significantly reduced in the deficient animals (Figure 2).

The effects of reduced maternal intake of vitamin B_6 on myelination in the brains of the progeny have been studied. Electron micrographs showed markedly less myelination in deficient animals (Morré et al., 1978b). Biochemical studies similarly revealed adverse effects of vitamin B_6 deficiency during the critical period of brain development; incorporation of ^{14}C-acetate into all major lipid classes in brain was found to be significantly decreased (Dakshinamurthi, 1982). Specific radioactivities of purified cerebrosides and sulfatides from vitamin B_6-deficient rat brain were found to be < 20% of normal. Specific activities of the myelin marker-enzyme, 2'3'-cyclic nucleotide 3'-phosphohydrolase were found to be significantly reduced in vitamin B_6-deficient neonatal rat brain (Morré and Kirksey, 1978).

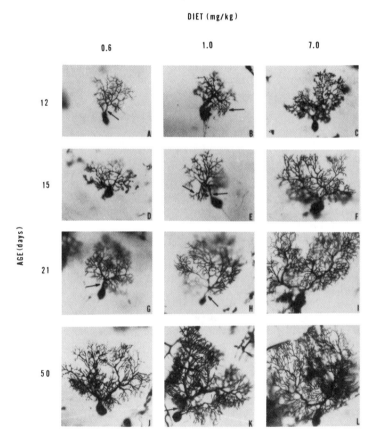

Fig. 2. Photomicrographs of Purkinje cells at 12, 15, 21 and 50 days of age in rat pups fed 0.6, 1.0 and 7.0 mg pyridoxine/Kg diet. Arrows indicate aberrations (From Chang et al., J. Nutr 111, 848 (1981), with permission).

Neurochemical studies of the brains of rat pups born to vitamin B_6-deficient mothers reveal decreases in the activities of glutamic acid decarboxylase (GAD) the enzyme responsible for GABA synthesis (Figure 1) in nerve terminals. GABA is an important inhibitory neurotransmitter in mammalian brain; GAD is a B_6-dependent enzyme. The convulsive disorders associated with vitamin B_6 deficiencies most likely result from decreased synthesis of GABA in brain.

Some Other Vitamin Deficiencies

Pellagra, although uncommon today, is still encountered in chronic alcoholism or in patients with cancer. The disease is characterized by dementia, diarrhea and dermatitis. Pellagra is caused by *niacin* deficiency. Treatment of newborn mice with the niacin antagonist 6-amino nicotinamide results in hydrocephalus and cytoplasmic vacuolation of aqueductal ependymal and glial cells in midbrain, as well as changes in glial cells of brainstem, cerebellum and spinal cord (Aikawa and Suzuki, 1986).

Deficiencies of *vitamin A* during the period of myelination in the rat result in decreases in the deposits of sulfatide in brain (Clausen, 1969). Myelin fractions isolated from the brains of deficient animals show a significantly lower sulfatide content.

CONCLUSIONS

There is substantial evidence showing that pregnant and lactating women from both underdeveloped and developed countries of the world are vitamin deficient. Vitamin deficiencies most frequently encountered in pregnancy are the water soluble vitamins folate, B_1 and B_6. Women from lower socio-economic groups are particularly vulnerable to develop vitamin deficiencies during pregnancy. Alcoholism as well as gastrointestinal disease and diabetes may exacerbate these vitamin deficiencies.

Folate supplementation during pregnancy appears to protect against the recurrence of neural-tube defects in susceptible pregnancies. Results of studies in experimental animals suggest that folate deficiency results in decreased brain DNA synthesis and in hypomyelination.

Vitamin B_1 deficiency remains a potentially important health care problem particularly during pregnancy and lactation. Alcoholic mothers are at particular high risk for development of B_1 deficiency. Maternal B_1 deficiency results in infantile beri beri and may also be associated with the fetal alcohol syndrome. Studies in rats show that maternal B_1 deficiency leads to alterations of glucose-metabolizing enzymes and in decreased synthesis of myelin in the brains of offspring.

Vitamin B_6 deficiency is common in pregnancy. In infants, B_6 deficiency results in convulsions, most probably resulting from decreased synthesis of the inhibitory neurotransmitter GABA.

Appropriate antenatal dietary counselling as well as vitamin-fortification of foods may be effective in the prevention of many developmental neurological disorders resulting from maternal deficiencies of these vitamins.

ACKNOWLEDGMENTS

Work described from the authors laboratory was funded by The Medical Research Council of Canada and Fonds de la recherche en santé du Québec. The author is grateful to Dominique D. Roy for assistance in the preparation of the manuscript.

REFERENCES

Aikawa H, Suzuki K (1986). Lesions in the skin, intestin and central nervous system induced by an antimetabolite of niacin. Am J Pathol 122:335-342.

Altman J, Anderson WJ (1972). Experimental reorganization of the cerebellar cortex. I Morphological effects of elimination of all microneurons with prolonged X-irradiation started at birth. J Comp Neuro 146:335-406.

Arakawa T, Mizuno T, Chida N, Narisawa K (1969). Electroencephalogram and myelin lipids of six-week old rats with aminopterin-treatment during suckling period. Tohoky J Exp Med 99:59-64.

Baker H, Frank O, Thomson AD, Langer A, Munves ED, De Angelis B, Kaminetzky HA (1975). Vitamin profile of 174 mothers and newborns at parturition. Am J Clin Nutr 28:59-65.

Bamji MS (1976). Enzymic evaluation of thiamin, riboflavin and pyridoxine status of parturient women and their newborn infants. Br J Nutr 35:259-265.

Bell JM, Stewart CN (1979). Effects of fetal and early postnatal thiamin deficiency on avoidance learning in rats. J Nutr 109:1577-1583.

Blocker DE, Thenen SW (1987). Intestinal absorption, liver uptake and excretion of ^{3}H-folic acid in folic acid-deficient alcohol consuming non-human primates. Am J Clin Nutr 46:503-510.

Butterworth RF (1985). Pyruvate Dehydrogeanse Deficiency Disorders. In McCandless DW (ed): "Cerebral Energy Metabolism and Metabolic Encephalopathy", New York: Plenum Press, pp 121-141.

Butterworth RF (1986). Cerebral thiamine-dependent enzymes in experimental Wernicke's Encephalopathy. Metab Brain Dis 1:165-175.

Butterworth RF (1987). Thiamin malnutrition and brain development. In Rassin D, Haber B, Drujan B (eds): "Basic and Clinical Aspects of Nutrition and Brain Development", New York: Alan R Liss Inc, pp 287-304.

Butterworth RF (1989). Effects of thiamine deficiency on brain metabolism: implications for the pathogenesis of the Wernicke-Korsakoff Syndrome. Alcohol and Alcoholism 24:273-279.

Chanarin I (1979). Distribution of Folate Deficiency. In Botez MI, Reynolds EH (eds): "Folic Acid in Neurology, Psychiatry and Internal Medicine", New York: Raven Press, pp 7-10.

Chang SJ, Kirksey A, Morre DM (1981). Effects of vitamin B_6 deficiency on morphological changes in dendritic trees of Purkinje cells in developing cerebellum of rats. J Nutr 111:848-857.

Chong YH, Ho GS (1970). Erythrocyte transketolase activity. Am J Clin Nutr 23:261-266.

Clarren SK (1979). Neural tube defects and fetal alcohol syndrome. J Pediatr 95:328.

Clausen J (1969). The effect of vitamin A deficiency on myelination in the central nervous system of the rat. Eur J Biochem 7:575-582.

Colman N, Barker EA, Barker M, Green R, Metz J (1975). Prevention of folate deficiency by food fortification. IV. Identification of target groups in addition to pregnant women in an adul rural population. Am J Clin Nutr 28:471-476.

Colman N (1977). Folate Deficiency in Humans. In Draper HH (ed): "Advances in Nutritional Research", New York: Plenum Press, pp 77-124.

Coursin DB (1954). Convulsive seizures in infants with pyridoxine-deficient diet. J Am Med Assoc 154:406-416.

Dakshinamurti K, Stephens MC (1969). Pyridoxine deficiency in the neonatal rat. J Neurochem 16:1515.

Dakshinamurti K (1982). Neurobiology of pyridoxine. Adv Nutr Res 4:143-180.

Davidson S, Passmore R, Brock JP, Truswell AS (1975). Human Nutrition and Dietetics, 6th ed, Edinburgh: Churchill Livingstone, pp 338-339.

Davison AN, Dobbing J (1966). Myelination as a vulnerable period in brain development. Brit Med Bull 22, 40-44.

Dreyfus PM (1961). The quantitative biochemical distribution of thiamine in deficient rat brain. J Neurochem 8:139-146.

Eichner ER and Hillman RS (1973). Effect of alcohol on serum folate level. J Clin Invest 52: S84-S87.

Fournier H, Butterworth RF (1989). Effects of maternal thiamine deficiency on the development of thiamine-dependent enzymes in regions of the rat brain. Neurochem Int (in press).

Fuster JS, Guell S, Tauli P, Cahuana AB, Garcia-Tornel S (1979). Neural tube defects and fetal alcohol syndrome. J Pediat 95:328-329.

Gardiki-Kouidou P, Seller MJ (1988). Aminiotic fluid folate, vitamine B_{12} and transcobalamius in neural tube defects. Clin Genet 33:441-448.

Goldstein G, Arulanantham K (1978). Neural tube defect and renal anomalies in a child with fetal alcohol syndrome. J Pediatr 93:636-637.

Gross RL, Newberne PM, Reid JVO (1974). Adverse effects on infant development associated with maternal folic acid deficiency. Nutr Rep Internat 10:241-248.

Hailemariam B, Landman JP, Jaulson AA (1985). Thiamin status in normal and malnourished children in Jamaica. Br J Nutr 53:477-483.

Haltia M (1970). The effect of folate deficiency on neuronal RNA content. A quantitative cytochemical study. Brit J Exp Pathol 51:191-196.

Heller S, Balkeld RM, Korner WF (1974). Vitamin B_1 status in pregnancy. Am J Clin Nutr 27:1221-1224.

Herbert V (1968). Megaloblastic anemia as a problem in world health. Am J Clin Nutr 21:1115-1125.

Herbert V, Colman N, Spivack M, Ocasio E, Ghanta V, Kimmel K, Brenner L, Freundlich J, Scott J (1975). Folic acid deficiency in the United States: Folate assays in a prenatal clinic. Am J Obstet Gynecol 123:175-185.

Hines JD (1975). Hematologic abnormalities involving vitamin B_6 and folate metabolism in alcoholic subjects. Ann NY Acad Sci 252:316-327.

Hirono H, Wada Y (1978). Effects of dietary folate deficiency on developmental increase of myelin lipids in rat brain. J Nutr 108:766-772.

Hunt AD jnr, Stokes J jnr, McCrory WW, Stroud HH (1954). Pyridoxine dependency: report of a case of intractable convulsions in an infant controlled by pyridoxine. Pediatrics 13:140-142.

Johnson EM, Nelson MM, Monie IW (1963). Effects of transitory pteroylglutamic acid (PGA) deficiency on embryonic and placental development in the rat. Anat Rec 146: 215-224. See also Johnson EM, Anat Rec 149:49-57 (1964).

Kywe-Thein, Thane-Toe, Tin-Tin-Oo, Khn-Khn Tway (1968). A study of infantile beri beri in Rangoon, Union of Burma. J Life Sci 1:62-72.

Laurence KM, James N, Miller M, Campbell H (1980). Increased risk of recurrence of pregnancies complicated by fetal neural tube defects in mothers receiving poor diets, and possible benefit of dietary counselling. Brit Med J 281:1592-1594.

Laurence KM, James N, Miller MH, Tennant GB, Campbell H (1981). Double-blind randomised controlled trial of folate treatment before conception to prevent recurrence of neural-tube defects. Brit Med J 282:1509-1511.

Lemoine P, Harrousseau M, Borteyru JP, Menuet JC (1968). Les enfants de parents alcooliques. Anomalies observées. A propos de 127 cas. Quart Med 21:476-482.

Magnus P, Magnus EM, Berg K (1986). Increased levels of apo-transcobalamins I and II in amniotic fluid from pregnant women with previous neural tube defect offspring. Clin Genet 30:167-172.

Metz J (1970). Folate deficiency conditioned by lactation. Am J Clin Nutr 23:843-853.

Molloy AM, Kirke P, Hillary I, Weir DG, Scott JM (1985). Maternal serum folate and vitamin B_{12} concentrations in pregnancies associated with neural tube defects. Arch Dis Childh 60:660-665.

Morre DM, Kirksey A (1978). The effect of a dietary deficiency of vitamin B_6 on the specific activity of 2'-3'-cyclic nucleotide 3'-phosphohydrolase of neonatal rat brain. Brain Res 146:200-204.

Morre DM, Kirksey A, Das GD (1978a). Effects of vitamin B_6 deficiency on the developing central nervous system of the rat. Gross measurements and cytoarchitectural alterations. J Nutr 108:1250-1259.

Morre DM, Kirksey A, Das GD (1978b). Effects of vitamin B_6 deficiency on the developing central nervous system of the rat. Myelination. J Nutr 108:1260-1265.

Nelson M.M., Asling C.W., Evans H.M. (1952). Production of multiple congenital abnormalties in young by maternal pteroylglutamic acid deficiency during gestation. J Nutr 48:61-79.

Neumann CG, Swendseid ME, Jacob M, Steihm ER, Dirige OV (1979). Biochemical evidence of thiamine deficiency in young Ghanaian children. Am J Clin Nutr 32:99-104.

Nicholls L (1951). Tropical Nutrition and Dietetics, London: Balliere, pp 140-141.

Perloff BP, Butrum RR (1977). Folacin in selected foods. J Amer Dietet Ass 70:161-172.

Peterson DR, Labbe RF, Vanbelle G, Chinn NM (1981). Erythrocyte transketolase and sudden infant death. Am J Clin Nutr 34:65-57.

Pongparich B, Spikrikkrich N, Dhanamitta S, Valyasevi A (1974). Biochemical detection of thiamine deficiency in infants and children in Thailand. Am J Clin Nutr 27:1399-1408.

Rassin DK (1984). Nutritional Requirements for the Fetus and the Neonate. In Ogra PL (ed): "Neonatal Infectious: Nutritional and Immunologic Interactions", Grune and Stratton, pp 205-227.

Read DJC (1978). The aetiology of the sudden infant death syndrome: Current ideas on breathing and sleep and possible links to deranged thiamine neurochemistry. Aust NZ Med J. 8:322-336.

Roecklein B, Levin SW, Comly M, Mukherjee AB (1985). Intrauterine growth retardation induced by thiamine deficiency and pyrithiamine during pregnancy in the rat. Am J Obstet Gynecol 151:455-460.

Schuster K, Bailey LB, Mahan CS (1981). Vitamin B_6 status of low-income adolescent and adult pregnant women and their condition of their infants at birth. Am J Clin Nutr 34:1731-1735.

Shaw W, Schreiber RA, Zemp JW (1973). Perintal folate deficiency: effects on developing brain in C57BL/6J mice. Nutr Rep Internat 8:219-228.

Smithells RW, Sheppard S, Schorah CJ (1976). Vitamin deficiencies and neural tube defects. Arch Dis Childh 51:944-950.

Smithells RW, Sheppard S, Schorah CJ, Seller MJ, Nevin NC, Harris R, Read AP, Fielding DW (1980). Possible prevention of neural-tube defects by periconceptional vitamin supplementation. Lancet: 339-340.

Summani S, Schelp FP, Vivatanasesth P, Pongpaew P, Sritabutra P, Supawan V, Vudhivai N, Egormaphol S, Harinasuta C (1981). An investigation of the health and nutritional status of the population in the NamPong Water Resource Development Project, Northeast Thailand. Ann Trop Med and Parasitol 75:335-346.

Sturman JA, Rivlin RS (1975). Pathogenesis of Brain Dysfunction in Deficiency of Thiamine, Riboflavin, Pantothenic Acid or Vitamin B_6. In Gaull GE (ed): "Biology of Brain Dysfunction", New York: Plenum Press, Vol 3, pp 425-475.

Tagbo IF, Hill DC (1977). Effect of folic acid deficiency on pregnant rats and their offspring. Can J Physiol Pharmacol 55:427-433.

Trostler N, Guguenheim K, Havivi E, Sklan D (1977). Effect of thiamine deficiency in pregnant and lactating rats on the brain of their offspring. Nutr Metab 21:294-304.

Trostler N, Sklan D (1978). Lipogenesis in the brain of thiamine-deficient rat pups. J Nutr Sci Vitaminol 24:105-111.

Udipi SA, Kirksey A, West K, Giacoia G (1985). Vitamin B_6, vitamin C and folacin levels in milk from mothers of term and preterm infants during the neonatal period. Am J Clin Nutr 42:522-530.

Van den Berg H, Schreyrs WHP, Joosten GPA (1978). Evaluation of the vitamin status in pregnancy. Int J Vit Nutr Res 43:12-21.

Whitley JR, O'Dell BL, Hogan AG (1951). Effect of diet on maze learning in second generation rats. Folic acid deficiency. J Nutr 45:153-160.

DISCUSSION

Q (Jhaveri): Could you indicate how deficiency was defined.

A: It was defined by dietary intake figures, I believe (not my work) by using dietary questionaires. In some cases this was backed up by actual vitamin levels being measured, and in some cases by an even more specific definition, by measuring enzymes which are vitamin dependent.

Q (Jhaveri): I wonder whether we may not be overestimating the magnitude of the problem if we only consider the dietary survey.

A: We may well be. But I think in all these cases we had low serum levels. I was careful not to look at just the dietary history. I believe that, in almost all cases, we had low serum or red cell levels of vitamins or their enzymes. You are absolutely right, one has to be careful with that kind of information.

Comment (Harper): I think it is very important to emphasize this difference between estimates of inadequate intake by dietary surveys and estimates which are made on biochemical or clinical measurements. I looked at some of the information from the U.S., from our U.S. DA surveys, and the estimates of dietary intake range up to 15% of the population having an inadequate intake. If you look at the clinical measurements, at least at the iron inadequacies which is one of the major ones, and look at the feritin stores which are a direct measure of iron status, the figures come down to below 5%. But, one has a proportion of people which have an inadequate income even in a rich country, and a proportion of people who suffer from some sort of local dislocation, and some people, especially young persons, which suffer from neglect. And in this population these figures (15%) are not out of line at all.

Q (Rassin): Another consideration, rather than looking at undernutrition, one area of increasing concerns paticularly in the U.S and other rich countries, is over-vitamin intake rather then under-intake. Certainly, there are neuropathies associated with excess B_6 and there are probably also similar problems with folate and other vitamins. There is a real concern about what the recommended daily dietary intake should be and what people are doing in taking too many vitamins.

A: I could not agree more. I was talking yesterday with Harvey Anderson, and I think that the situation may be worse than that. We don't even know what the levels should be. I mean, it is fine recommending things, but I am not even sure that we have the numbers yet.

Comment (Harper): Well that was one reason why the Food and Nutrition Board included recommendations for some of the minor (trace) mineral elements; even though they could not set a recommended allowance, they gave a range. This was primarily for this reason, because they were concerned about some of these minor elements being put into vitamin capsules. And this was a guideline primarily for the Food and Drug Administration (U.S.). Not in terms of the appropriate intake for the population but rather to set an appropriate upper level of intake which the FDA needed for their enforcement policy.

(Mal)Nutrition and the Infant Brain, pages 225–236
© 1990 Wiley-Liss, Inc.

ZINC AND MANGANESE DEFICIENCIES IN PRENATAL AND
NEONATAL DEVELOPMENT, WITH SPECIAL REFERENCE TO THE
CENTRAL NERVOUS SYSTEM

John M. Rogers, Patricia Oteiza, Carl L. Keen

Developmental Toxicology Division (MD-67), HERL, US
Environmental Protection Agency, Research Triangle Park, North
Carolina 27711 and Department of Nutrition, University of
California Davis, CA 95616

Central nervous system development in mammals is a long and complex process. The brain is one of the first organs to become recognizable during embryonic development, and continued development, including increases in the number of cells, kinds of cells, and intercellular connections, proceeds until long after birth in many species. A consequence of this long period of development is that it renders the brain susceptible to developmental insults over a protracted period. A number of trace elements including zinc (Zn), manganese (Mn), copper, iron, iodine, and selenium have been shown to be essential for normal development in a wide variety of mammalian species with the central nervous system defects being prominent among the developmental anomalies produced by a deficiency of one or more of these elements. In this paper we will review the effects of Zn and Mn deficiencies during prenatal or neonatal development, with emphasis on the sensitivity of the developing brain to deficiencies of these trace elements. The reader is directed to other recent reviews for information concerning the effects of copper, iron, selenium and iodine deficiencies on the developing brain (Prohaska, 1987; Hetzel and Mano, 1989; Rogers et al., 1985a; Yehuda and Youdim, 1989).

Zinc

Prenatal effects of maternal Zn deficiency. Hurley and Swenerton (1966) first reported the production of congenital malformations in a mammal by maternal Zn deficiency, in the Sprague-Dawley rat. Fetuses of Zn-deficient rats are characterized by multiple skeletal abnormalities including misshapen heads, clubbed feet, fused or missing digits, micrognathia, fusions of the ribs, spinal curvature, missing caudal vertebrae, and incomplete ossification of ribs, vertebrae, cranial bones, and digits. Brain, cardiac, and urogenital malformations were also common (Rogers et al., 1985b; Keen and Hurley,

1989; DaCunha Ferreira et al., 1989). The frequency and severity of congenital malformations resulting from Zn deficiency can be correlated both with the concentration of Zn in the maternal diet and with the timing of the deficiency. For example, when rats were fed a Zn-deficient diet for the first 10 days of pregnancy, 22% of the fetuses were malformed at term; when the Zn-deficient diet was fed until day 12, 56% were malformed. When the deficient period was days 6-14, almost 50% of fetuses were malformed at term (Hurley, 1981). The rapid effect of dietary Zn deficiency suggests that the pregnant rat cannot mobilize adequate Zn from body stores to supply the developing embryo. Consistent with this idea is the observation that plasma Zn concentration is significantly decreased in rats within 6 hours of the introduction of a Zn-deficient diet (Hurley et al., 1982). A rapid effect of Zn deficiency on preimplantation embryos has also been shown (Hurley and Shrader, 1975). In eggs flushed from the oviducts of control rats on day 3 of pregnancy, all of the eggs appeared normal and were at the 8- or 16-cell stages; in contrast, only 20% of the eggs collected from dams fed a Zn-deficient diet during the first 3 days of pregnancy were found to be normal, and all of these were at the 8-cell stage.

Postnatal effects of prenatal Zn deficiency. Even when gross malformations are not evident at birth, prenatal Zn deficiency can markedly affect postnatal development. For example, administration of a Zn-deficient diet during mid-pregnancy results in low birth weight and a high incidence of early postnatal death (Keen and Hurley, 1989). Less severe (marginal) maternal Zn deficiency during the perinatal period also results in poor survival of offspring; Rogers et al., 1984) have demonstrated a positive correlation between increasing maternal dietary Zn and survival of offspring. Zn deficiency during fetal or early postnatal development can also adversely affect growth and later function of lymphoid organs. In developing mice, Zn deficiency results in small thymuses, depressed response to mitogens, and severe reduction of serum IgM, IgG2A and IgA (Keen and Gershwin, 1990). Strikingly, Zn-deficiency-induced deficits in circulating immunoglobulins have been reported to persist for up to three generations, even when only the first generation was exposed to Zn deficiency, and that only during prenatal development (Beach et al., 1982).

Effects of Zn deficiency on brain development. Severe Zn deprivation during embryonic and fetal development in the rat results in profound effects on virtually all derivatives of the neural tube and associated structures including the brain, spinal cord, eyes, and olfactory tract (Warkany and Petering, 1973; Adeloye and Warkany, 1976; Rogers et al., 1985b). Typical brain malformations observed with early severe Zn deficiency, include hydrocephaly, anencephaly, hydranencephaly, and exencephaly (Rogers et al., 1985b). Hurley and Shrader (1972) and Warkany and Petering (1972, 1973) have also demonstrated that microscopic lesions in the brain tissue are often present in fetuses whose heads seem to be normal externally. Defects revealed by microscopic examination included tissue disorganization, missing commissures, and rosette and ductule formation.

Pathological closure of the aqueduct of Sylvius has been indicated as a cause of hydrocephaly and exencephaly in Zn-deficient fetuses (Hurley and Shrader, 1972), although it has been noted that occlusion of the aqueduct could be a secondary effect of hydrocephaly rather than the primary cause (Adeloye and Warkany, 1976).

One of the mechanisms underlying the induction of brain malformations with Zn deficiency is a reduction in cellular proliferation. Eckert and Hurley (1977) were able to show using autoradiograph that, compared to controls, there is a lower uptake of tritiated thymidine by Zn-deficient embryos with the primary difference being in the developing central nervous system. Consistent with the above, during this same stage of development, Zn-deficient rat embryos show a decrease cellularity of the neural tube, which is extremely thin-walled compared to conrols (Rogers et al., 1985a). With Zn deficiency the neural tube often contains more mitotic figures than are seen in controls, suggesting that the cells are unable to divide normally. Incorporation of tritiated thymidine into DNA is also depressed in brains of Zn-deficient rat fetuses in the third trimester of gestation (Dreosti et al., 1980). McKenzie and coworkers (1975) found lower brain weight and DNA and higher brain protein/DNA ratios (indicating larger cell size) in fetuses of dams fed a Zn-deficient diet during the last third of pregnancy than in controls, further demonstrating that Zn deficiency can impair cell division in the developing brain. Dvergsten (1984) has also reported retarded synaptogenesis and differentiation of cerebellar neurons in rat pups subjected to Zn deficiency during the suckling period.

The morphogenesis of the eye is particularly sensitive to maternal Zn deficiency in the rat. Anophthalmia or microphthalmia of varying severity was noted in 38% of the fetuses of rats fed a Zn-deficient diet throughout pregnancy (Rogers et al., 1985b). Colobomata of the retina have been described in Zn-deficient fetuses by several investigators (Warkany and Petering, 1972; Rogers and Hurley, 1987). This defect is due to failure of the choroid fissure to close. A persistent choroid fissure prevents development of vitreous pressure within the eye which is essential for normal expansion of the eye during later development. Microphthalmia can thus be the result of a persistent choroid fissure. Microphthalmic eyes from Zn-deficient fetuses also often contain large retinal folds. However, histogenesis of the retina has not been severely affected, with the cell layers of retinas of Zn-deficient fetuses at term being reported to be similar to those of controls in terms of thickness and degree of differentiation, even when retinal folding occurred (Rogers and Hurley, 1987).

Mechanisms of Zn deficiency. It is evident from the above that severe maternal Zn deficiency can result in embryonic and fetal abnormalities; however, the mechanisms underlying these defects are not well understood. A fundamental question is whether the effects of Zn deficiency on the embryo/fetus are due directly to a deficiency of Zn in embryonic cells, or do they occur in part through an indirect effect of Zn deficiency on the metabolism of the mother. The observation that feeding a Zn-deficient diet results in lower than normal embryonic and fetal Zn concentrations, is suggestive of a direct effect of Zn deficiency on the embryo/fetus, but does not prove a causative relationship between low fetal Zn and malformations.

For example, since one effect of Zn deficiency can be a marked reduction in food intake (Clegg et al., 1989), it has been argued that some of the teratogenic effects of Zn deficiency are secondary to maternal food restriction. This idea has been tested using restricted-fed controls. Although restricted-fed females gained almost no weight during pregnancy (in contrast to ad libitum-fed controls), and their fetuses were smaller than those of ad libitum-fed conrols, gross terata were not observed (Hurley, 1981). Thus, the gross teratogenic effects of Zn deficiency are not related to the depressed food intake produced by this condition. However, it is important to point out that while the gross structural defects associated with prenatal Zn deficiency are not due to maternal food restriction, more subtle biochemical lesions may be, in part, due to this effect of Zn deficiency. Thus, it is important that restricted-fed controls be used in investigations of the biochemical lesions underlying the teratogenicity of Zn deficiency.

One approach to the investigation of the direct effects of Zn deficiency on the embryo has been the use of embryo culture systems. In these systems the potential teratogenic effects of Zn-induced changes in maternal metabolism can be eliminated. Using the embryo culture system, embryos are removed from control dams during early development (typically from day 8 to day 9.5 in the rat). The embryos are then placed in culture tubes containing rat serum and distilled water, cultured up to 48 h and examined. The strength of this system is that an investigator can use serum collected from either control or Zn-deficient rats. Mieden et al. (1986) reported that rat embryos grown on serum collected from Zn-deficient dams developed abnormally. Abnormal embryos exhibited a single malformation complex; the heads were small, the optic sulci narrow and the optic placode ill-defined. In contrast to the above, when embryos were grown on Zn-deficient sera that were supplemented with Zn to a concentration similar to that of control sera, they developed normally, suggesting that the teratogenicity of the initial Zn-deficient sera was the direct result of the low Zn concentrations. Defects in neural tube closure have also been observed in early chick embryo explants cultivated in a Zn-deficient medium (Iniguez et al., 1978).

In contrast to the findings of Mieden et al. (1986) and Iniguez et al. (1978), Record et al. (1985a) were unable to produce the teratogenic effects of Zn deficiency in the rat embryo culture system using methodologies similar to those used by Mieden et al. (1986). These investigators reported that in their experiments, embryos collected from control dams developed normally for 48 h when grown on sera collected from deficient dams. Although the yolk-sac protein content was lower in the embryos grown on the deficient sera than in controls. The explanation for the difference in results between the two rat embryo culture studies has yet to be determined.

In a separate study Record et al. (1985a) did observe abnormal development in 9.5-day-old embryos collected from Zn-deficient dams which were then cultured on Zn-deficient sera for 48 h. An interesting observation in this study was that the embryos from the Zn-deficient dams fell into two morphological classes; the first being morphologically normal at day 9.5, the second class were smaller and the embryonic pole of the egg cylinder was developmentally abnormal and/or retarded. Culture of the first group of embryos in either Zn-deficient or Zn-supplemented serum produced morphologically normal embryos; while those that appeared abnormal at day 9.5 were grossly malformed after 48 h incubation in either serum. Future studies directed at investigation the biochemical differences between these two subgroups of embryos collected from Zn-deficient dams should provide valuable new information on the biochemical lesions underlying Zn deficiency teratogenicity.

With regard to biochemical lesions which may underlie the negative effects of Zn deficiency on embryonic and fetal development, several ideas have been advanced.

Considerable attention has been given to the idea that one of the basic defects underlying the abnormalities observed in Zn deficiency is abnormal nucleic acid metabolism. DNA synthesis is significantly depressed in Zn-deficient embryos and fetuses compared with controls, and this lower rate of synthesis has been linked to depressed activities of DNA polymerase and thymidine kinase (Keen and Hurley, 1989; Dreosti et al., 1986). If the impairment in nucleic acid synthesis or expression is sufficient, then this could result in alterations in the differential rates of cellular growth necessary for normal morphogenesis. Evidence that the rate of cellular growth is altered in Zn-deficient embryos is provided by the finding that the mitotic index in the brains of Zn-deficient embryos is higher than in control brain.

In addition to abnormalities in nucleic acid metabolism, there is evidence that cellular membranes and cytoskeletal integrity can be affected by Zn deficiency. Tubulin assembly has been shown to be impaired in brains of Zn-deficient fetal rats (Oteiza et al., 1990). The mechanism by which Zn deficiency affects tubulin polymerization has yet to be established; however, since the concentration of tubulin is similar in brain supernatants of Zn-deficient and control rats (Oteiza et al., 1990), it can be postulated that Zn plays a direct role in the regulation of tubulin polymerization *in vivo*, possibly through the formation of Zn mercaptide bridges between the tubulin dimer subunits. Abnormal tubulin polymerization resulting from cellular Zn deficiency could result in significant defects in cellular endo- and exocytosis. Defects in tubulin polymerization have also been postulated as a potential biochemical lesion underlying chromosomal aberrations, including gaps, fragments and terminal deletions, that are found in the tissues of Zn-deficient fetuses (Keen and Hurley, 1989).

Finally, it has been reported that in both maternal and fetal liver of Zn-deficient rats, there are significantly elevated levels of malondialdehyde, an indicator of lipid peroxidation (Dreosti, 1987). The increase in levels of lipid peroxidation products in the Zn-deficient fetus may reflect a role of Zn in membrane stabilization, an elevation in the pool of unsaturated fatty acids available for peroxidation, or a role for Zn in the antioxidant defense system. Evidence that the increased malondialdehyde products observed in Zn-deficient fetuses reflect cellular membrane lipid peroxidation has been suggested by Harding et al. (1987), who using electron microscopy observed that in the 11 days Zn-deficient fetus there is severe deterioration of cell membranes, especially those of the mitochondrion, in the period just preceding the appearance of cell death in the neural tube. This group has also shown that in the Zn- deficient fetus there is extensive cell necrosis in those areas of the embryos undergoing rapid cell division, prior to the development of identifiable malformations (Record et al., 1985b). Similar observations of large numbers of pyknotic cells and cellular debris in the wall and lumen of cells in all regions of the developing brain in Zn-deficient embryos examined on days 12-14 of gestation have been reported by Rogers et al. (1985b). Taken together, these results support the idea that an increased rate of cellular lipid peroxidation in the Zn-deficient fetus results in membrane damage with resultant cellular necrosis and cell death which leads to asynchrony in the development of the affected tissue primordia.

Zn deficiency in humans. While a direct link between maternal Zn deficiency and teratogenesis has not been established in humans, considerable data suggest that maternal Zn deficiency is correlated with abnormal fetal development. In several studies it has been found that mothers who gave birth to anencephalic infants, or infants with spina bifida, tended to have lower plasma Zn levels at term than mothers who gave birth to normal infants (Keen and Hurley, 1989; Hinks et al., 1989). In an extensive study by Jameson in 1976, low maternal Zn levels during the first and second trimesters of pregnancy were correlated with an increased risk of fetal abnormalities and overall poor pregnancy outcome. Strong evidence that Zn deficiency is teratogenic in humans also can be taken from studies on the outcome of pregnancies in women with untreated acrodermatitis enteropathica. Seven pregnancies have been registered to date: two gave birth to babies with malformations, one an anencephalic fetus and the other an achrondroplastic dwarf; two of the other pregnancies resulted in low birthweight infants (Hambidge et al., 1975). In contrast, pregnancy outcome in women with acrodermatitis enteropathica given Zn therapy has been normal to date (Brenton et al., 1981).

Behavioral abnormalities associated with Zn deficiency. Prenatal or early postnatal Zn deficiency can result in a variety of behavioral and learning deficits. In 1972 Warkany and Petering suggested that the microscopic lesions discovered in otherwise normal brains of Zn-deficient fetuses could result in functional postnatal disabilities. Consistent with this idea, there have been numerous reports describing effects of pre- and early postnatal deficiency on behavior. Aggressive behavior, open-field behavior, conditioned emotional responses, avoidance learning and cognitive performance have all been reported to be influenced by the Zn status of an animal (File, 1989). However, as has been pointed out by File (1989), differences in study design from laboratory to laboratory make it difficult at the present time to comment with any degree of confidence on exactly how, and to what extent, Zn deficiency affects behavior.

Manganese

Teratogenic effects of prenatal Mn deficiency. The most prominent effect of Mn deficiency during development is an irreversible congenital ataxia, characterized by lack of coordination, loss of equilibrium, head retraction, and tremor. This effect has been demonstrated in the chick, rat, mouse, and guinea pig (Hurley, 1981). In addition, congenital ataxia occurs in a number of genetic mutants of Mn metabolism, including the pallid mouse and screwneck mink (Hurley, 1981). Erway and co-workers (Erway et al., 1970) have demonstrated that ataxia results from abnormal development of the otoliths, calcified structures in the vestibular portion of the inner ear. The otoliths are made up of otoconia, small crystalline structures embedded in an amorphous, proteoglycan-rich matrix. In the otolithic matrix and in both the cells and matrix of the otic cartilage of a Mn-deficient animal, there is a deficit of proteoglycans. Thus, it is thought that the block in otolith development is secondary to depressed proteoglycan synthesis because of low activity of Mn-requiring glycosyltransferases (Hurley, 1981). The congenital ataxia of Mn deficiency does therefore, seemingly, not to involve a neurological defect. Ataxia in offspring of Mn-deficient animals or Mn mutants can be prevented by Mn supplementation during pregnancy, but postnatal treatment has no effect (Hurley, 1981).

In addition to otolith abnormalities, pre- and early postnatal Mn deficiency can result in shortened and thickned limbs, curvature of the spine, and swollen and enlarged joints (Hurley and Keen, 1987). The basic biochemical defect underlying the development of these bone defects is a reduction in proteoglycan synthesis secondary to a reduction in the activities of glycosyltransferases. These enzymes are needed for the synthesis of chondroitin sulfate side chains of proteoglycan molecules. Stause and Saltman (1987) reported that Mn deficiency in adult rats can result in an inhibition of both osteoblast and osteoclast activity. The implications of this observation in regard to human bone disease needs to be ascertained.

Effects of Mn deficiency on development of the brain. Data on adverse effects of Mn deficiency on the development of the brain are few at present. When offspring of Mn-deficient rat were fed a Mn-deficient diet, their threshold for electroshock-induced seizures was significantly lower than that of controls (Hurley et al., 1961). There were also changes in the maximal electroshock seizure pattern, indicating that brain excitability and convulsability were greater than normal in ataxic, Mn-deficient rats. Later experiments showed that this increase in convulsability was due to Mn deficiency and not the presence of ataxia (Hurley et al., 1963).

It has been demonstrated that prenatal Mn deficiency can adversely affect postnatal carbohydrate metabolism. In the guinea pigs, perinatal Mn deficiency results in severe pancreatic pathology, with animals exhibiting aplasia or marked hypoplasia of all cellular components (Everson and Shrader, 1968). When Mn-deficient guinea pigs are given a glucose challenge, they respond with a diabetic-type glucose tolerance curve. Mn supplementation completely reverses the pancreatic pathology and abnormal glucose tolerance observed in these animals. In addition to its effect on pancreatic tissue integrity, Mn deficiency can directly impair pancreatic insulin synthesis and secretion. In rats, Mn deficiency results in depressed pancreatic insulin synthesis and enhanced intracellular insulin degradation as well as a depression in the insulin secretory process (Baly et al., 1984; 1985). The mechanisms underlying the effects of Mn on insulin metabolism have not been delimited; however, it is clear that abnormal insulin and glucose metabolism may profoundly influence brain development and function in the Mn-deficient animal.

Mechanisms of effects of Mn deficiency. The biological functions of Mn in the brain are not well understood. Mn is thought to be involved in the activation of brain glutamine synthesase (Wedler et al., 1982), UDP-galactose: GN2 ganglioside galactosyltransferase (Yip and Dain, 1970), catechol O-methyl transferase (Tagliamonte et al., 1970), and adenylate cyclase (Katz and Tenenhouse, 1973). None of the above enzyme systems have been studied under conditions of dietary Mn deficiency, so it is not known if a disturbance in any of the above pathways may explain some of the neurological lesions seen with Mn deficiency. Mn may also be directly involved in the metabolism of biogenic amines via complex formation. Thus, Mn may be essential for normal binding, transport, and storage of catechols and ethanolamines (Papavasiliou, 1981).

The activity of Mn superoxide dismutase is significantly lower in tissues of Mn-deficient rats than in controls. In adult animals low activity of the enzyme has been related to an increased rate of tissue lipid peroxidation and cell membrane damage (Zidenberg-Cherr and Keen, 1987). However, these changes have not been demonstrated in very young animals; thus, it is not known whether a reduction in the activity of Mn superoxide dismutase contributes to prenatal and early postnatal brain structural defects. Altered lipid and protein metabolism may also occur as a result of Mn deficiency (Keen et al., 1984), but again this has not been demonstrated to be a factor in the developing brain.

Mn deficiency in humans. The importance of the observations on the effects of Mn deficiency on brain function in experimental animals is underscored by the report by Papavasiliou and coworkers (1979), who found that blood Mn was significantly lower in epileptics than in controls. furthermore, blood Mn concentration correlated with the frequency of seizures. Patients with only a few seizures per year had blood Mn levels similar to those of controls, whereas those with frequent seizures (13 per month) had lower concentrations. Blood Mn levels were not correlated with blood levels of the anticonvulsive drugs taken by these patients, indicating that the low blood Mn was not attributable to drug therapy. Dupont and Tanake (1985) have also reported that one third of children with convulsive disorders of unknown origin had whole-blood Mn concentrations significantly lower than normal. It is not known if the low blood Mn levels found in some epileptics is due to a primary Mn deficiency, which in turn results in the neurological abnormalities, or if the low levels are a consequence of the disease. However, Carl et al. (1986) have reported that whole-blood Mn concentrations tend to be lower in epileptics in whom the cause of the epilepsy is unknown than in epileptics where the disease can be traced to head trauma. This observation suggests that the low blood Mn levels are not a consequence of the seizures, or drug therapy, since they are similar in the two groups. Interestingly, Carl et al. (1990) have also recently reported that the GEPR rat, a genetic model for epilepsy, is characterized by low tissue Mn levels, suggesting that there may be a genetic lesion in Mn metabolism in these animals.

While at the present time Mn deficiency has been implicated in only a few human disorders (Keen and Zidenberg-Cherr, 1990), this may be due in part to lack of a practical method for assessing an individual's Mn status. Whole-blood Mn can be a useful indicator of whole-body Mn status, with low blood levels of Mn-deficient rats reflecting low levels of the element in soft tissue (Keen et al., 1983). These observations support the idea that blood Mn levels are a useful indicator of soft tissue Mn levels, and not just a reflection of recent diet history.

Mn toxicity can also affect brain function. There are numerous reports of the effects of Mn toxicity on brain function in humans who chronically inhale large amounts of airborne Mn, a situation that occurs in Mn mines, steel mills, and some chemical industries. Excess Mn enters the body mainly as oxide dust via the lungs and also via the gastrointestinal tract from the contaminated environment (Keen and Leach, 1988). The lungs apparently act as a depot from which the Mn is continuously absorbed. Mn poisoning is characterized by a severe psychiatric disorder (locura manganica) resembling schizophrenia, followed by a permanently crippling neurological disorder clinically similar to Parkinson's disease. The presence of elevated tissue Mn levels is thus not necessary for the continuance of the neurological manifestations of the disease, and metal chelation therapy is unlikely to secure remission (Cotzias et al., 1968). It has been reported that children living in urban areas can have elevated blood Mn levels (Joselow et al., 1978). The mechanisms underlying the cellular toxicity of Mn have not been firmly identified, although there is evidence that it involves Mn-initiated catechol autooxidation and tissue lipid peroxidation (Donaldson, 1987). Abnormal carbohydrate metabolism may also underlie some of the effects of Mn toxicosis, given the observation that insulin production can be impaired in animals subjected to high amounts of the element (Baly et al., 1985).

It is not clear at the present time if Mn toxicity during early development is a problem in man; however, the observation that the neurological lesions resulting from Mn toxicity are permanent shows the importance of not oversupplying this element to the infant.

REFERENCES

Adeloye A, Warkany J (1976). Experimental congenital hydrocephalus. Child's Brain 2:325-360.
Apgar J (1985). Zinc and reproduction. Annu Rev Nutr 5:43-68.
Baly DL, Lönnerdal B, Keen CL (1985). Effects of high doses of manganese on carbohydrate homeostasis. Toxicology Letters 25:95-102.

Baly DL, Curry DL, Keen CL, Hurley LS (1984). Effects of manganese deficiency on insulin secretion and carbohydrate homeostasis in rats. J Nutr 114:1438-1446.

Baly DL, Curry DL, Keen CL, Hurley LS (1985). Dynamics of insulin and glucagon release in rats: influence of dietary manganese. Endocrinology 116:1734-1740.

Beach RS, Gershwin RS, Hurley LS (1982). Gestational zinc deprivation in mice: persistence of immunodeficiency for three generations. Science 218:469-471.

Brenton DP, Jackson MJ, Young A (1981). Two pregnancies in a patient with acrodermatitis enteropathica treated with zinc sulphate. Lancet 2:500.

Carl GF, Critchfield JW, Thompson JL, Holmes GL, Gallagher BB, Keen CL (1990). Genetically epilepsy prone rats are characterized by altered tissue trace element concentrations. Epilepsia, in press.

Carl GF, Keen CL, Gallagher BB, Clegg MS, Littleton WH, Flannery DB, Hurley LS (1986). Association of low blood manganese concentrations with epilepsy. Neurology 36:1584-1587.

Clegg MS, Keen CL, Hurley LS (1989). Biochemical pathologies of zinc deficiency. In Mills CF (ed): "Zinc in Human Biology," Dorchester: Springer Verlag, pp 129-145.

Cotzias GC, Horiuchi K, Fuenzalida S, Mean I (1968). Chronic mangangese poisoning: Clearance of tissue manganese concentrations with persistence of the neurological picture. Neurology 18:376-382.

daCunha Ferreira RMC, Monreal Marquiegui I, Villa Elizaga I (1989). Teratogenicity of zinc deficiency in the rat: Study of the fetal skeleton. Teratology 39:181-194.

Donaldson J (1987). The physiopathologic significance of manganese in brain: Its relation to schizophrenia and neurodegenerative disorders. Neurotoxicology 8(3):451-462.

Dreosti IE (1987). Zinc deficiency and the developing embryo. Neurotoxicity 8:369-378.

Dreosti IE, Record IR, Manuel JJ (1980). Incorporation of 3H-thymidine into DNA and the activity of alkaline phosphatase in zinc-deficient fetal rat brains. Biol. Trace Element Res 2:21-29.

Dupont CL, Tanaka Y (1985). Blood manganese levels in children with convulsive disorder. Biochem Med 33:246-255.

Dvergsten CL (1984). Retarded synaptogenesis and differentiation of cerebellar neurons in zinc-deficient rats. In Frederickson CJ, Howell GA, Kasarskis EJ (eds): "The Neurobiology of Zinc. Part B: Deficiency, Toxicity, and Pathology", New York: Alan R Liss, pp 17-31.

Erway L, Hurley LS, Fraser A (1970). Congenital ataxia and otolith defects due to Mn deficiency in mice. J Nutr 100:643-654.

Everson GJ, Shrader RE (1968). Abnormal glucose tolerance in manganese-deficient guinea pigs. J Nutr 94:89-94.

File SE (1989). Zinc and behaviour. In Mills CF (ed): "Zinc in Human Biology", Dorchester: Springer Verlag, pp 225-234.

Hambidge KM, Neldner KH, Walravens PA (1975). Zinc acrodermatitis enteropathica, and congenital malformations. Lancet 1:577-578.

Hetzel BS, Mano MT (1989). A review of experimental studies of iodine deficiency during fetal development. J Nutr 119:145-151.

Hinks LJ, Ogilvy-Stuart A, Hambidge KM, Walker V (1989). Maternal zinc and selenium status in pregnancies with a neural tube defect or elevated plasma alpha-fetoprotein. Br J Obstet Gyn 96:61-66.

Hurley LS (1981). Teratogenic aspects of manganese, zinc, and copper nutrition. Physiol Rev 61:249-295.

Hurley LS, Keen CL (1987). Manganese. In Mertz W (ed): "Trace Elements in Human and Animal Nutrition - Fifth Edition", San Diego: Academic Press, Inc, pp 185-223.

Hurley LS, Shrader RE (1972). Conenital malformations of the nervous system in zinc-deficient rats. In Pfeiffer CC (ed): "Neurobiology of the Trace Metals Zinc and Copper", New York: Academic Press, pp 7-51.

Hurley LS, Shrader RE (1975). Abnormal development of preimplantation rat eggs after three days of maternal zinc deficiency. London Nature (London), 254:427-429.

Hurley LS, Swenerton H (1966). Congenital malformations resulting from zinc deficiency in rats. Proc Soc Exp Biol Med 123:692-696.

Hurley LS, Wooley DE, Timiras PS (1961). Threshold and pattern of electroshock seizures in ataxic manganese-deficient rats. Proc Soc Exp Biol Med 106:343-346.

Hurley LS, Wooley DE, Rosenthal F, Timiras PS (1963). Influence of manganese on susceptibility of rats to convulsions. Am J Physiol 204:493-496.

Hurley LS, Gordon P, Keen CL, Merkhofer L (1982). Circadian variation in rat plasma zinc and rapid effect of dietary zinc deficiency. Proc Soc Exp Biol Med 170:48-52.

Iniguez C, Casas J, Carreres J (1978). Effects of zinc deficiency on the chick embryo blastoderm. Acta Anat 101:120-129.

Jameson S (1976). Effects of zinc deficiency in human reproduction. Acta Med Scand Suppl 593:5-89.

Joselow MM, Tobias E, Koehler R, Coleman S, Bogden J, Gause D (1978). Manganese pollution in the city environment and its relationship to traffic density. Am J Pub Health 68:557-560.

Katz S, Tenenhouse A (1973). The relation of adenyl cyclase to the activity of other ATP utilizing enzymes and phosphodieterase in preparations of rat brain: Mechanism of stimulation of cyclic AMP accumulation by adrenalin, ovabain and Mn^{++}. Br J Pharmacol 48:516-526.

Keen CL, Leach RM (1988). Manganese. In Seiler HG, Sigel H (eds): "Handbook on Toxicity of Organic Compounds", New York: Marcel Dekker, Inc, 405-415.

Keen CL, Hurley LS (1989). Zinc and reproduction: Effects of deficiency on foetal and postnatal development. In Mills CF (ed): "Zinc in Human Biology", Dorchester: Springer Verlag, pp 183-220.

Keen CL, Lönnerdal B, Hurley LS (1984). Manganese. In Frieden E (ed): "Biochemistry of the Essential Ultratrace Elements", New York: Plenum Press, pp 89-132.

Keen CL, Clegg MS, Lönnerdal B, Hurley LS (1983). Whole blood manganese as an indicator of body manganese status. N Engl J Med 308:1230.

McKenzie JM, Fosmire GJ, Sandstead HH (1975). Zinc deficiency during the latter third of pregnancy: effects on fetal rat brain, liver, and placenta. J Nutr 105:1466-1475.

Mieden GD, Keen CL, Hurley LS, Klein NW (1986). The effects on whole rat embryos cultured on serum from zinc and copper deficient rats. J Nutr 116:2424-2431.

Oteiza PI, Cuellar S, Lönnerdal B, Hurley LS, Keen CL (1990). Influence of maternal dietary zinc intake on in vitro tubulin polymerization in fetal rat brain. Teratology 41:97-104.

Papavasiliou PS (1981). Manganese in the extrapyramidal system. In Alexander PA (ed): "Electrolytes and Neuropsychiatric Disorders", New York: SP Medical and Scientific, pp 187-225.

Papavasiliou PS, Kutt H, Miller ST, Rosal V, Wang YY, Aronson RB (1979). Seizure disorders and trace metals: Manganese tissue levels in treated epileptics. Neurology 29:1466-1473.

Prohaska JR (1987). Functions of trace elements in brain metabolism. Phys Reviews 67:858-899.

Rogers JM, Hurley LS (1987). Effects of maternal zinc deficiency on development of the fetal rat eye. Development 99:231-238.

Rogers JM, Keen CL, Hurley LS (1984). Maternal zinc nutriture during pregnancy and lactation in the rat: Survivability and growth of offspring. Fed Proc 43:1052.

Rogers JM, Keen CL, Hurley LS (1985a). Zinc, copper and manganese deficiencies in preatal and neonatal development, with special reference to the central nervous system. In Gabay S, Harris J, Ho BT (eds): "Metal Ions in Neurology and Psychiatry" New York: Alan R Liss, Inc, pp 3-34.

Rogers JM, Keen CL, Hurley LS (1985b). Zinc deficiency in the pregnant Long Evans rat: Teratogenicity and tissue trace elements. Teratology 39:89-100.

Strause L, Saltman P (1987). Role of manganese in bone metabolism. In Kies C (ed): "Nutritional Bioavailability of Manganese", Washington DC: American Chemical Society, pp 46-66.

Tagliamonte A, Tagliamonte P, Gessa GL (1970). Reserpine-like action of chlorpromazine on rabbit basal ganglia. J Neurochem 17:733-738.

Warkany J, Petering HG (1972) Congenital malformations of the central nervous system in rats produced by maternal zinc deficiency. Teratology 5:319-344.

Warkany J, Petering HG (1973). Congenital malformations of the brain produced by short-term zinc deficiency in rats. Am J Ment Defic 77:645-653.

Wedler FC, Denmen RB, Roby WG (1982). Glutamine synthetase from ovine brain is a Mn (II) enzyme. Biochemistry 24:6389-6396.

Yehuda S, Youdim MBH (1989). Brain iron: A lesson from animal models. Am J Clin Nutr 50:618-29.

Yip GB, Dain JA (1970). The enzymic synthesis of ganglioside. II. UDP-galactose: N-acetylgalactosaminyl-(CNacetylneuraminyl) galactosyl-glucosylceramide galactosyltransferase in rat brain. Biochim Biophys Acta 206:252-260.

Zidenberg-Cherr S, Keen CL (1987) Enhanced tissue lipid peroxidation - mechanism underlying pathologies associated with dietary manganese deficiency. In Kies C (ed): "Nutritional Bioavailability of Manganese", Washington, DC: American Chemical Society, pp 56-66.

(Chapter by invitation)

(Mal)Nutrition and the Infant Brain, pages 237–248
© 1990 Wiley-Liss, Inc.

THE DEVELOPMENT OF THE MITOCHONDRIAL ENERGY SYSTEM IN MAMMALIAN BRAIN

John B. Clark

Biochemistry Department, St Bartholomew's Hospital Medical College, University of London, Charterhouse Square, EC1M 6BQ

Until birth, brain development and the energy provision for it, are largely dependent upon and regulated by maternal factors. At birth a partially developed and poorly protected organ is suddenly made dependent on external fuel supplies whilst continuing to develop its intricate and complex function in a co-ordinated and competent fashion. Not the best example of biological organisation! Indeed if brain development in a variety of species is considered, it is quite clear that some species, eg horse, cow are much more developed and neurologically better organised at birth than others such as the human or rat. This has given rise to the division of mammalian species into the precocial (neurologically mature at birth) and non-precocial (neurologically immature) by Dobbing and his associates (Dobbing & Sands, 1979) on the basis of whether the brain 'growth spurt' is highest before or after birth. A further complication is that the mammalian brain is functionally heterogenous with each of its regions possessing not only diverse activities but also chronologically different developmental profiles. Thus any change in energy substrate supply that the brain may be subject to as a consequence of its developmental state, may give rise to different responses within the various regions of the mammalian brain. This will have a particular significance for the enzyme systems involved in ATP synthesis since in a situation of great metabolic and synthetic demand such as is found in the developing brain energy provision will be of the highest priority.

A key question is therefore to ask what biological changes/adaptations are processed during brain development to provide the appropriate energy status for the brain to express its full neurological maturity and competence particularly in terms of both substrate supply and enzyme complement.

Substrate Supply

Investigations into substrate supply have been mainly carried out on the whole animal and involve the measurement of arterial - venous differences and blood flow across the vessels supplying the brain (Cremer, 1982). Clearly 2 parameters are important: a) the available circulating substrates, and b) the extent to which these may be accumulated by the brain. In the neonatal period, the former will be dependent on the suckling activities of the young whereas the latter will depend on the development of the blood brain barrier.

The suckling neonate is presented with a very specific and probably unique diet in the form of milk and this is related to the exceptional demands put upon the nutrient source during this period, particularly in the provision of energy (Edmonds et al, 1985). In terms of calorific content, fat seems to be the most important component - around 60%+ in both human and rat milk, although human milk is also quite high in carbohydrate (Edmonds et al, 1985). However, the utilisation of this fat source for energy purposes by the brain seems to be mainly in the form of ketone bodies. It is variously estimated that in children, infant baboons and rats the brain utilises a mixture of glucose and ketone bodies and can tolerate the replacement of one third to one half of its normal glucose needs by ketone bodies (Cremer, 1982). However the total replacement of glucose is not possible with the maintenance of normal functioning. When ketone body utilisation in the developing brain occurs the glucose is usually metabolised only as far as lactate, which itself may under certain circumstances also act as a substrate for brain energy metabolism (Cremer, 1982).

The ability to utilize ketone bodies so extensively by the rat and human neonatal brain is in contrast to the normal adult brain and is related to the fact that the extraction coefficient for ketone bodies by the neonatal brain is some four times greater than that of the adult brain. This in turn is probably related to the relatively poor development of the blood brain barrier in these species at this stage of development (Cremer, 1982). Furthermore, as will be indicated in later sections, it also reflects the relatively low activity of the pyruvate dehydrogenase complex (Land & Clark, 1975; Land et al, 1977) in the neonatal brain of these species. In other species however, dogs, cows, sheep or guinea pigs, ketone bodies are not an energy fuel for the brain, and under hypoglycaemic conditions the glucose extraction coefficient for glucose is increased and lactate may also be used as a fuel, (Cremer, 1982). On a regional basis it is also to be anticipated that variations in substrate supply may change as a function of development, although no specific data is yet available on this.

Glucose Oxidation

For the most part, the activity of the enzymes involved in the complete metabolism of glucose i.e. the glycolytic and citric acid cycle enzymes, in rat brain rise rapidly during the neonatal period and reach adult activities at or shortly after weaning (21-22 days post partum). Data supporting this view is presented in Table 1 where a number of enzymes, both cytosolic and mitochondrial in location, which are involved in glycolysis and the citric acid cycle, are listed with their activites in the neonate and adult rat brain with an estimate of the time after birth that an activity which is 50% of the adult value is attained. Several points of interest emerge from this analysis. Firstly, although there is a general pattern of development for this group of enzymes [constant proportion enzyme groups or clusters (Baquer et al, 1975; Baquer et al, 1977)],

TABLE 1. Enzyme Activities Associated with Energy Metabolism in the Neonatal and Adult Rat Brain

ENZYME	ENZYME ACTIVITY (Units/g.wet wt.)		AGE when 50% Enzyme Activity attained (days)	REF.
	NEONATAL	ADULT		
Hexokinase	3-5	12-18	15	Baquer et al (1975) Booth et al (1980) Kellogg et al (1974) Leong & Clark (1984a)
Phosphofructokinase	6.5-7.2	25-36	11	Baquer et al (1975)
Lactate dehydrogenase	34-35	120-160	10-11	Baquer et al (1975) Booth et al (1980) Leong & Clark(1984a)
Pyruvate dehydrogenase	0.2-0.4	2	13-20	Booth et al (1980) Land & Clark (1975) Land et al (1977) Leong & Clark (1984b)
Citrate synthase	3-9	15-36	10-12	Baquer et al (1975) Booth et al (1980) Land & Clark (1975) Land et al (1977) Leong & Clark (1984b)
Isocitrate dehydrogenase (NAD)	0.7-1	5-6	13-15	Baquer et al (1975) Leong & Clark (1984b)
Pyruvate carboxylase	0-0.06	0.5-0.8	17-18	Land & Clark (1975)
Creatine kinase	31	207	16	Booth & Clark (1978a)
Butyryl-CoA dehy.	1.1	2.3	3	Reichmann et al(1988)
Octanoyl CoA dehy.	14.7	18.5	< 1	"
Palmitoyl CoA dehy.	4	9	7	"
Glutaryl CoA dehy.	0.38	1.2	10	"
Crotonase	4	24	> 22	"
3-HOacyl CoA dehy.	0.2	1	10	"

a number of important differences within the group are apparent.. The development of both hexokinase and creatine kinase, both classically considered to be cytosolically located, appear to have a closer correlation with mitochondrially located members of the citric acid cycle e.g. isocitrate dehydrogenase, than with the cytosolically located glycolytic enzymes e.g. phosphofructokinase. This may be related to the apparent association of both hexokinase and creatine kinase in brain with the mitochondrial fraction as well as the cytosol, and the rapid increase in the activity of the mitochondrially located component of these enzymes during the neonatal period (Booth & Clark, 1978a; Booth et al, 1980; Land et al, 1977; Kellogg et al, 1974). This may relate to the involvement of these 2 enzymes in the establishment of fully functional aerobic glycolysis in the adult rat brain (Bessman et al, 1978: Bessman & Geiger,

1980), a necessary prerequisite for neurological competence. A further indication of the adaptation towards a fully aerobic energy metabolism in brain is the induction of the development of isoforms of lactate dehydrogenase and pyruvate kinase. In the brain of 1 day old rats lactate dehydrogenase is predominantly in the M form (associated with anaerobic glycolysis) and pyruvate kinase in H form. As development progresses the lactate dehydrogenase isoform type becomes mainly the H form and the pyruvate kinase the M form, both associated with a high aerobic glycolytic flux.

The development of the pyruvate dehydrogenase complex in rat brain has been the subject of special interest in view of its key role in linking the glycolytic and citric acid cycle activities and hence the flux through aerobic glycolysis. Furthermore the development of its activity in the neonatal rat brain lags behind other citric acid cycle enzymes such as the citrate synthase, with the major part of the development of pyruvate dehydrogenase complex occurring during the period 10-15 days after birth as compared to 0-10 days for citrate synthase (Land et al, 1977, see also Table 1). This will limit the amount of glycolytic product that will be able to be fully oxidised by the citric acid cycle and hence limit the development of the brains ability to provide full energy potential. Interestingly, this pattern of development of the pyruvate dehydrogenase complex also correlates well with a period of particular significance in the development/of the rat brain. During this period there is the emergence of electrical excitability in the cerebral cortex (Millichap, 1958), a pronounced change in neuromuscular coordination with the acquisition of visual perception and swimming ability of the young rat (Schapiro et al, 1970). Is then the development of pyruvate dehydrogenase activity a necessary prerequisite for neurological competence?

The pyruvate dehydrogenase complex (PDHC) of rat brain, in common with that of other tissues, is regulated by covalent phosphorylation/ dephosphorylation and this occurs in both the neonatal and adult rat brain (Booth & Clark, 1978b, 1981). The increase in rat brain pyruvate dehydrogenase complex activity during development could therefore be due to a) an activation of existing protein (E_1 subunit) b) a change in the subunit composition of the complex eg foetal to adult isoenzyme induction or c) an increase in enzyme protein. The first of these possibilities was ruled out on the basis of studying the reversible steady-state phosphorylation of the pyruvate dehydrogenase complex in neonatal and adult rat brain mitochondrial preparations using $^{32}P_i$ and separating the various subunits of the complex by SDS-PAGE prior to immunoblotting using a polyclonal antibody raised to beef heart pyruvate dehydrogenase complex (Malloch et al, 1986). These studies also indicated that there was no change in subunit composition of the PDHC from neonatal and adult rat brain (Malloch et al, 1986). Using the PDHC antibody the amount of enzyme protein was then estimated by ELISA techniques in both homogenates and mitochondrial preparations from the brains of rats of different ages and compared to that of citrate synthase (Malloch et al, 1986). These investigations indicated a developmental increase in enzyme protein from 2 sources, one of which was related to the increase in mitochondrial numbers, and was shown by both enzymes, PDHC and citrate synthase. The second was a specific increase in enzyme protein per mitochondrion shown only by PDHC, which related closely to the period of the development of neurological maturity. Using a c-DNA probe to the E1 subunit of PDHC developed by means of synthetic oligonucleotides, studies are now well underway to clarify the regulation of the gene expression of the PDHC in the developing rat brain.

If various areas of the rat brain are studied in terms of enzyme development it is clear that different areas show developmental profiles which are consistent with the concept that the development of a fully active aerobic glycolysis is a necessary prerequisite for neurological competence. Details of the developmental patterns of a number of enzymes associated with glycolytic and citric acid cycle activity from 6 different brain areas are summarised in Table 3. Whilst there are differences between the regions with respect to individual enzyme activities, the pattern of the profiles is similar in that they all rise from the neonatal activity to a maximal activity in the adult. What is different however is the time frame in which these areas reach their adult profile. Data on this is summarised in Table 3b where the age (days after birth) at which each enzyme attains 50% of its adult activity has been estimated in each of the regions studied. It is clear that the enzymes fall into a cluster, each of them developing at much the same rate on a regional basis. However it is interesting to note that the medulla oblongata attains its adult profile much earlier (50% adult activity at approx 11 days) than the cortex (13 days) and cerebellum (15 days). This order recapitulates the embryological and neurophylogenetic development of the brain regions, which in its simplest concept proceeds from the medulla forwards and appears consistent with the view that the morphological and neurological maturity in the various brain regions may be correlated with the development of the potential for aerobic glycolysis and in particular pyruvate dehydrogenase activity.

Enzymes of ketone body metabolism

As indicated earlier the other major fuel of the rat and human neonatal brain are the ketone bodies, 3-hydroxybutyrate and acetoacetate. The data relating to the relevant enzymes is summarised in Table 2. The 3 mitochondrially located enzymes of ketone body metabolism, D-3-hydroxybutyrate dehydrogenase, 3-oxoacid CoA transferase and the acetoacetyl-CoA (C_4) thiolase all show similar developmental profiles in rat brain. There is an increase in activity from birth of between 3-5 fold to a maximum just after weaning, with a subsequent fall in the adult brain to an activity broadly comparable to the 1 day old value (Booth et al, 1980; Middleton, 1973; Page et al, 1971). In Table 2 the 1 day old and adult activities have been detailed, together with peak activity and an estimate of the time (post partum) at which that activity has been obtained. The decrease in activity of these enzymes is associated with the change in diet of the rat from high fat milk to laboratory chow and also the establishment of a fully active aerobic glycolytic potential consequent upon the achievement of adult activities of the pyruvate dehydrogenase complex. It is interesting to note that the acetyl CoA acyl (C_{10}) transferase (Reichman et al, 1988) and the carnitine palmitoyl transferase (Bird et al, 1985) also show similar profiles albeit with maximal enzyme activites approximately only twice the 1 day old value.

TABLE 2. Enzyme Activities Associated with Ketone Body and Fatty Acid
Utilisation in the Neonatal and Adult Rat Brain

ENZYME	ENZYME ACTIVITY Units/g.wet wt.)		MAXIMUM ACTIVITY		REF.
	NEONATAL	ADULT	Units/ gm	Age attained (days)	
D-3HO butyrate dehydrogenase	0.4	0.4	1.6	25	Booth et al (1980) Page et al (1971)
3-oxoacid CoA transferase	1.5	2.9	7.5	25	Booth et al (1980) Page et al (1971)
Acetoacetyl - Mit. CoA (C_4)-thiolase	2.1	2.1	5.7	25	Booth et al (1980) Middleton (1973)
- Cyt.	2.4	1.2	> 2.4	< 5	
Acetyl CoA acyl (C_{10}) transferase	0.8	1.3	2.1	15	Reichmann et al (1988)
Carnitine palmitoyl transferase	2	2	3.8	20	Bird et al (1985)

Enzyme activities and units as in Table 1 except for carnitine palmitoyl transferase which is measured as $nmol.min.^{-1}$ per mg. mit. protein.

However the cytosolic acetoacetyl CoA thiolase, associated with fatty acid synthesis rather than ketone body metabolism, does not show this bell shaped profile but rather a general decline in activity from birth to adulthood, characteristic of the fatty acid synthesis enzymes in brain (Baquer et al, 1975). Regional studies on ketone body metabolising enzymes are limited (Leong & Clark, 1984b); the D-3-hydroxybutyrate dehydrogenase however shows a similar profile to that seen in the whole brain, with the maximal increase in activity in the medulla occurring at 5 days, which preceeds other regions by 3-5 days (see Leong & Clark, 1984b + Table 3).

Table 3: Data taken from Leong & Clark (1984a,b,c) and Reichmann et al (1988). Enzyme activities are expressed as units/gm wet wt. where 1 unit = 1 μmole substrate transformed per min. Time values are estimated in days after birth (or, if before birth, as negative numbers). The time estimation is when the enzyme activity is 50% of that in an adult (60d). Where the values were before 10 days post partum for hypothalamus, striatum and mid-brain, they are denoted by <10 days since these regions cannot be differentiated before this time.

TABLE 3. Regional Development of Energy Metabolism Enzymes in Rat Brain

A) Brain regional enzyme activities in adults

ENZYME ACTIVITY (Units/gm. wet wt.)

ENZYME	Medulla & Pons	Hypo-thalamus	Striatum	Mid-brain	Cortex	Cerebellum
Hexokinase	10	16	15	15	18	15
Aldolase	6.6	8.1	8.2	7.2	8.8	7.6
Lactate dehy.	110	143	173	143	106	130
Pyruvate dehy.	1.4	1.6	2.0	1.7	2.2	1.9
Citrate synthase	27	34	36	34	36	34
Isocitrate dehy.	3.7	5.3	5.3	6.3	5.9	5.0
Fumarase	1.8	1.7	1.8	2.1	1.8	2.6
Glutamate dehy.	38.1	33.1	25.6	34.3	24.6	22.7
D-3-HObutyrate dehyd.	0.2	0.24	0.34	0.28	0.38	0.34
C$_4$-thiolase	4.7	-	-	4.5	3.5	3.0
Butyryl CoA-dh.	1.25	-	-	1.6	1.3	1.4
Octanoyl CoA dh.	17.2	-	-	19.9	15.9	15.8
Palmitoyl CoA dh.	4.8	-	-	5.8	4.4	4.5
Glutaryl CoA dh.	0.5	-	-	0.6	0.5	0.5
Crotonase	21.0	-	-	21.5	15.1	19.8
3HOacyl CoA dh.	0.9	-	-	1.00	0.6	0.7
C$_{10}$-thiolase	1.3	-	-	2.00	1.2	1.4

B) Age at which 50% adult regional activity attained

AGE (days)

ENZYME	Medulla & Pons	Hypo-thalamus	Striatum	Mid-brain	Cortex	Cerebellum
Hexokinase	3	11	13	10	16	19
Aldolase	5	< 10	12	11	13	11
Lactate dehy.	1	10	11	10	11	12
Pyruvate dehy.	4	11	12	10	13	17
Citrate synthase	-1	10	11	11	12	17
Isocitrate dehy.	3	11	11	13	13	13
Fumarase	6	12	12	13	13	16
Glutamate dehy.	7	12	10	12	8	10
D-3-HObutyrate	- 1	< 10	< 10	< 10	6	6

Fatty acid oxidation

Whether or not the brain actually utilizes fatty acids as a source of energy during development or other situations is unclear. There has been however a number of reports over the years that various brain preparations can utilize and metabolize fatty acids (Spitzer & Wolf, 1971; Warshaw & Terry, 1970). In the developing rat brain, it has been reported that the oxidation 1-^{14}C-palmitate increases to a peak at weaning and then falls to adult levels (Warshaw & Terry, 1976). Also the activity of the carnitine palmitoyl transferase (Bird et al, 1975) which may be involved in the transport of fatty acids across the mitochondrial membrane and act as the rate limiting step in β-oxidation (Warshaw & Terry, 1976) shows a similar profile. More recently, a detailed study on the activities of enzymes involved in fatty acid oxidation has been carried out in the developing rat and human brain and on a regional basis in the adult rat brain (see Table 1 & 3). The general pattern is similar to that seen for the glycolytic and citric acid cycle enzymes of a general increase in activity from the neonatal brain to adulthood (Table 1), with relatively little differences in the regional activities. The importance of these enzymes therefore to the energy metabolism of the rat brain (or indeed the human brain) is still unclear, although when other species are concerned it is worth noting that it has been estimated that fasted puppies, which rarely become ketotic, can derive up to 25% of their brain energy requirements from circulating fatty acids (Spitzer, 1973).

Species variation

One of the major aims of studying the developing brain is to define the enzyme complement necessary for the provision of energy for the fully functional neurologically competent brain. In terms of our understanding of the human situation, the rat has been a useful model in that it shares with the human the situation in which there is considerable brain development, both morphological and biochemical, occurring post partum ie it is non-precocial (Dobbing & Sands, 1979). However, the study of other species of the precocial variety have also been useful in that with neurolgical competence being achieved much earlier, any necessary prerequisites for it should also be observed earlier. Very few comprehensive studies have been carried to test this hypothesis at least at the biochemical level. Such a study was carried out to compare enzyme development in the brains of the guinea pig (precocial) and the rat (non precocial) with special reference to those enzymes concerned with glucose and ketone body metabolism (Booth et al, 1980). In general terms the enzymes of glycolysis show similar profiles in both species except that in the guinea pig most of the development occurs prenatally and that in the rat postnatally. If the pyruvate dehydrogenase complex activity in particular is considered approx. 90% of the adult activity is present at birth in the guinea pig whereas in the rat the activity is extremely low (Booth et al, 1980), which correlates closely with the development of neurological competence in the two species. This general pattern is demonstrated more clearly in Fig. 1 in which the rate of change in the activities of the key enzymes of glycolysis (hexokinase, lactate dehydrogenase) and citric acid cycle (pyruvate dehydrogenase and citrate synthase) are plotted as a function of time before or after birth. It is quite clear that this group (cluster) of enzymes develops primarily before birth in the guinea pig and afterwards in the rat. This correlates closely with the 'growth spurts' in the 2 species and with the development of neurological competence.

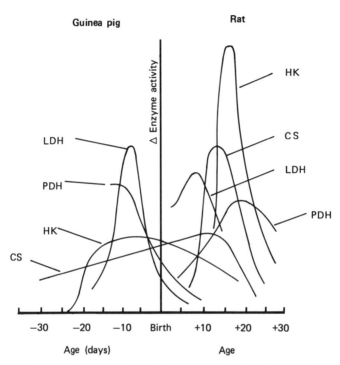

Fig. 1. Relative rate of enzyme activity increase as a function of fetal or neonatal development in guinea pig and rat brain. The enzyme activities are taken from Booth et al (1980) and have been expressed as a percentage of the adult value and the rates of increase over a 5 day period plotted against developmental age. LDH - lactate dehydrogenase: PDH - pyruvate dehydrogenase complex: HK - mitochondrially bound hexokinase: CS - citrate synthase.

Concluding remarks

It has been known for some years now that the developing rat and human brain utilize a mixture of glucose and ketone bodies for their energy fuels, despite the presence of adequate circulatory glucose to satisfy all the energy requirements. The transition to the utilization of glucose alone, characteristic of the adult brain under normal circumstances, appears to be dependent on the development of the full adult activity of the pyruvate dehydrogenase complex. This occurs by the specific synthesis of new enzyme protein in the mitochondria and from regional and species studies appears to correlate closely with the development of neurological competence. Further studies using c-DNAs to the PDHC are needed to understand the regulation of the expression of the PDHC gene and its relationship to neurological activity.

Achnowledgments

This work has been generously supported by MRC, SERC, The British Council, NATO and M W Beer & Son Ltd.

REFERENCES

Baquer NZ, Hotershall JS, McLean P, Greenbaum AL (1977). Aspect of carbohydrate metabolism in developing brain. Dev Med Child Neurol 19:81-104.

Baquer NZ, McLean P, Greenbaum AL (1975). Systems relationships and the control of metabolic pathways in developing brain. In Hommes, FA and Van den Berg CJ (eds): "Normal and Pathological Development of Energy Metabolism." London: Academic Press, pp 109-132.

Bessman SP, Borreback G, Geiger PJ, Ben-Or S (1978). Mitochondrial creatine kinase and hexokinase, two examples of compartmentation predicted by the hexokinase mitocondrial binding theory of insulin action. In Srere, PA and Estabrook, RW (eds): "Microenvironments and Metabolic Compartmentation." New York: Academic Press, pp 111-128.

Bessman SP, Geiger PJ (1980). Compartmentation of hexokinase and creatine phosphokinase, cellular regulation and insulin action. Top Cell Reg 16:55-

Bird MI, Munday LA, Saggerson ED, Clark JB (1985). Carnitine acyltransferase activities in rat brain mitochondria. Biochem J 226:323-330.

Booth RFG, Clark JB (1978a). Studies on the mitochondrially bound form of rat brain creatine kinase. Biochem J 170:145-151.

Booth RFG, Clark JB (1978b). The control of pyruvate dehydrogenase in isolated brain mitochondria. J Neurochem 30:1003-1008.

Booth RFG, Clark JB (1981). Energy metabolism in rat brain: Inhibition of pyruvate decarboxylation by 3-hydroxybutyrate in neonatal mitochondria. J Neurochem 37:179-185.

Booth RFG, Patel TB, Clark JB (1980). The development of enzymes of energy metabolism in the brain of precocial (guinea pig) and non-precocial (rat) species. J Neurochem 34:17-25.

Cremer JE (1982). Substrate utilization and brain development. J Cereb Blood Flow and Metab 2:394-407.

Dobbing J, Sands J (1979). Comparative aspects of the brain growth spurt. Early Hum. Dev. 3/1:79-84.

Edmonds J, Auestad N, Robbins RA, Bergstrom JD (1985). Ketone body metabolism in the neonate: development and the effect of diet. Fed Proc 44:2359-2364.

Kellogg EN, Knull HR, Wilson JE (1974). Soluble and particulate hexokinase in developing neuronal systems. J Neurochem 22:461-463.

Land JM, Booth RFG, Clark JB (1977). Development of mitochondrial energy metabolism in rat brain. Biochem J 164:339-348.

Land JM, Clark JB (1975). The changing pattern of brain mitochondria substrate utilization during development. In Hommes, FA and Van den Berg, C.J. (eds) London: Academic Press, pp 155-167.

Leong SF, Clark JB (1984a). Regional enzyme development in rat brain: enzymes associated with glucose utilization. Biochem J 218:131-138.

Leong SF, Clark JB (1984b). Regional enzyme development in rat brain: enzymes of energy metabolism. Biochem J 218:139-145.

Leong SF, Clark JB (1984c). Regional development of glutamate dehydrogenase in the rat brain. J Neurochem 43:106-111.

Malloch GDA, Munday LA, Olson MS, Clark JB (1986). Comparative development of the pyruvate dehydrogenase complex and citrate synthase in rat brain mitochondria. Biochem J 238: 729-736.

Middleton B (1973). The acetoacetyl CoA thiolases of rat brain and their relative activities during postnatal development. Biochem J 132:731-737.

Millichap JG (1958). Seizure patterns in young animals. Significance of brain's carbonic anhydrase. Proc Soc Exp Biol Med 97:606-611.

Page MA, Krebs HA, Williamson DH (1971). Activities of enzymes of ketone body utilization in brain and other tisues of suckling rats. Biochem J 121:49-53.

Reichmann H, Maltese WA, De Vivo DC (1988). Enzymes of fatty acid-oxydation in developing brain. J Neurochem 51:339-344.

Schapiro S, Salas M, Vokovich K (1970). Hormonal effects on ontogeny of swimming ability in the rat: Assessment of CNS development. Science, 168: 147-150.

Spitzer JJ (1973). CNS and fatty acid metabolism. Physiologist, 16:55.

Spitzer JJ, Wolf EH (1971). Uptake and oxidation of FFA administered by ventriculocisternal perfusion in the dog. Am J Physiol 221:1426.

Takagaki G (1974). Developmental changes in glycolysis in rat cerebral cortex. J Neurochem 23:479-487.

Warshaw JB, Terry ML (1976). Cellular energy metabolism during fetal development. VI. Fatty acid oxidation by developing brain. Dev Biol 52:161.

DISCUSSION

Q (Harper): Is it possible to calculate from the information we have about enzyme activity during the developmental phase and the K_m of the enzyme, what proportion of the total enzyme level is required to meet the metabolic needs of the tissues.

A: I think this is possible. A number of people have, I believe, made these sorts of calculations, either on the back of an enveloppe or in their minds. I think it is fair to say that the general concensus is that the pyruvate dehydrogenase, even in the adult, is working fairly close to its full activity. This is an important point, thank you for raising the question. It does mean that any alterations in its activity could have a marked influence on the flux through the system. It is not like some other enzymes you are aware of, where the activities are well in excess of what is actually required.

Q (Lake): When you are looking at ketone body metabolism. Have you ever tried delaying the weaning time.

A: We have not. Some studies have tried to do this and I think it would be fair for me to say that there are varying results. I am not quite sure why that is, whether it is because the control of dietary intake has been difficult. But it would be an interesting experiment to do and I think J. Edmonds in UCLA has now set up a system, whereby he can study neonatal pups on a formula milk. He therefore can vary the dietary input through that formula. There may therefore now be a way of looking at this.

As I recall, last time I spoke to him, he had not found any variations in the developmental profile of pyruvate dehydrogenase. I am sure he would not mind me sharing this with you. If that is the case (no enzyme development change), it rather looks that the development of this enzyme is, as we say, pre-programmed. This would in itself be very fascinating.

Q (S. Hashim): There is some evidence, I believe, that the starved adult brain can utilize short-chain fatty acids. And perhaps also the brain during development. Are there corresponding changes in the oxidative enzymes for such fatty acid metabolism.

A: Yes. There is evidence, mainly from enzymatic profiles. I think Jean De Vellis has done some studies on the development of the enzymes of β-oxidation. In the brain they do tend to develop in a comparable profile to the enzymes of glycolysis. They do not show the peak that the enzymes of ketone body metabolism show. I think the evidence for the brain actually using fatty acids - although it appears to have the capability - is somewhat more tenuous.

Q (Hamberger): I would like to ask a question with respect to the differences between the rat and the guinea pig. Is this difference unique for the brain, that you have the early development of enzymes in the guinea pig and a delay in the rat. And, secondly, do you see any permanent differences between the rat brain and the guinea pig brain, or are they quite similar after a couple of months.

A: I actually don't know of any studies. We certainly have not done them. I am answering your second question. I am not aware of studies which have carried out a sort of an enzyme profile of the adult guinea pig brain. Again, I do not know of any developmental studies on other organs in the guinea pig versus the rat. Suffice to say that the guinea pig is pretty well up and going at birth, so one presumes that its other organs are quite well organized. But then, of course, the guinea pig may well have a very different metabolism. There is evidence for that in connection with its different diet, from the rat. In some respects, the guinea pig, in terms of gluconeogenic activity reflects the human better. I really do not think I can tell you more.

Q (Hamberger): Can you see any advantage for the guinea pig to be so highly developed at birth versus the rat. From an evolutionary point of view. After all, they are both rodents, what would be the advantage.

A: I don't know. It is an interesting point which bears some thought. We don't have an immediate answer however.

Section IV: NURTURE AND ENVIRONMENT IN INFANT DEVELOPMENT

Frank food insufficiency (starvation) while still occurring occasionally in certain areas of the world, is today nevertheless becoming an increasingly exceptional and isolated phenomenon. Outward migration and massive international emergency aid usually limit these appalling insults to humanity to a rather restricted period and region. When it does occur, the existing infant population is rapidly decimated. Moreover, under these conditions sexual drive and fertility drop sharply, thus assuring that such incidents are self limiting. The human grief factor and individual tragedies are scientifically irrelevant and therefore of little interest, or so it seems.

In contrast to starvation, however, chronic caloric insufficiency (undernutrition) and imbalanced food intake (malnutrition) is encountered throughout the entire global population, in industrially developed and underdeveloped countries alike. Whithin almost every community there exists a subpopulation of uneducated, economically disadvantaged, and disease prone individuals or families which, seemingly, are genetically defined since this population perpetuates itself from one generation to the next. Birth rates are usually high to offset (anticipated) high infant mortality, and because of the need to pool the efforts of many individuals to maintain the survival of the family.

The size of this subpopulation varies enormously among different communities; it may represent anywhere from a few percentage points to over 80% of the individuals in recognized social units. A figure of 10-15% appears to cause little alarm and seems acceptable as a norm. As discussed in the preceding sections, the biochemical and anatomical consequences of chronic malnutrition and undernutrition may lead to intellectual stunting and poor sociality, which in turn has a disruptive effect on the social fabric of the community.

In this final section, the problems of impairments of intellectual development and growth are discussed in terms of the community - how environmental or nutritional insufficiencies within a social group affect the individual in terms of his or hers neurological and social maturation. The report by Roeder demonstrates that even in the richest of nations, chronic (generational?) intellectual underdevelopment is a quite pervasive threat in specific subpopulations, even though preventable and not inevitable. While, for obvious reasons, the socioeconomic disadvantaged are most affected and at risk, other social factors such as drug abuse, inadequate education, emotional stress, and mother-child relationships can sharply influence the outcome of development. These factors do not only touch the poor.

Stress levels in industrialized nations are high because of working conditions, mental and environmental pollution, and increasing expectations for social success. The daily interaction between mother (or parents) and the infant tend to be far shorter than is often the norm in so-called underdeveloped nations. Mass education, conceived to provide maximum intellectual stimulation, in many communities are yielding opposite results. Teen-age pregnancies and parenthood bring their own special problems: Emotional relationships are more labile and stressful, economic power is often uncertain, physical health is more threatened because of still incomplete growth, and nutritional education is in many cases inadequate; social dislocation from the peer group is a common occurrence.

Hence, for many reasons, intellectual and social underdevelopment of the child may be far more prevalent in any community than official socioeconomic statistics would predict. The data presented by Roeder indicates that poverty may be only one of a number of predictors which influence the optimum development of the child.

Project Venezuela is gathering population data which clearly demonstrate that socioeconomic factors in a community do play an important role, through nutrional availability and quality, in the physical and intellectual maturation of entire groups of children. These factors thus eventually may not only shape the biological characteristics of a regional population, but they may also prevent or resist rapid reversal. The biological parameters can therefore appear to assume inherited biological traits whereas in reality they mostly reflect socioeconomic and regional conditions which have become indigenous.

Mendez Castellano and Angulo de Rodriguez report variations in physical growth, protein-calorie intake, neurological maturation, and blood cholesterol levels between children in various geographic or administrative regions of a country. To a large extent such variations can be attributed to differences in socioeconomic status and agro-industrial development. The authors point out that these variables and their causes need to be properly defined and regionally delineated, in order to formulate adequate restorative measures. Statistical data gathering must be uniform and comparable and their interpretation must take into account cultural differences, regional industrial and/or agricultural diversity, and socioeconomic as well as educational opportunities within the child's immediate social structure. Such massive data accumulation involves large numbers of adequately trained censors and by necessity therefore, the criteria and tests which define the developmental level of the child must be unequivocal, yet easy to amass by workers after only a short period of special instructions.

Based on such biological and socioeconomic criteria the data by Roeder, Mendez Castellano and Angulo Rodriguez, while still being accumulated, already leads to an unambiguous and frightening conclusion: It would appear that thousands, if not millions, of infants never are able to reach their genetic intelligence potential because of adverse social and nutritional circumstances. That this potential can be so profoundly influenced by diet and environment, reinforces the need to stipulate that the acquisition of intelligence and of knowledge constitutes an inalienable right of an individual. Indeed, these are the essential attributes that define a human being.

Unfortunately, even if all the causes for mental and social underdevelopment were known, intervention in the form of government policies are not always easy to implement nor, if implemented, are they always properly formulated.

This is the subject broached by Harper who discusses the establishment of dietary guidelines and government dietary advise, principally as it pertains to the U.S.A. His report suggests that even in a highly industrialised and prosperous nation with a vast and efficient methodology for data gathering and statistical analysis, national standards for minimum and maximum nutritional requirements do not necessarily lead to a concensus as to what should constitute an optimum (essential) diet for proper child development; the social requirements at this time are even less understood or definable.

In certain instances, despite available scientific data, the standards adopted may strongly reflect current popular interest for a prevalent disease, which nevertheless is restricted to only particular subpopulations of a community. Cardiovascular diseases and high blood cholesterol levels may serve as one such example.

High cholesterol levels may or may not be the cause for such type of illnesses, but it is quite evidently strongly associated with these disease entities as well as having a predictive value for the development of cardiovascular anomalies. However, aside from the arguable premise that blood cholesterol levels are dominantly influenced by dietary cholesterol, in a heterogeneous population, the advocacy of low cholesterol diets for the entire population may seriously jeopardize the development of the fetus and the growing infant. If, as Project Venezuela and other studies show, a more advantageous socioeconomic status is accompanied by (average) higher blood cholesterol levels in children, it may be pointed out that the infants in this privileged population, as a group, grow faster, achieve more rapid and more efficient neurological integration, are psychologically more robust and are less disease-prone; their scholastic achievement scores also are higher. Although none of these characteristics may be directly attributed to the availability of blood cholesterol, it would be highly surprising, given the importance of myelination and hormone metabolism during growth, if low cholesterol levels during this period might not cause far more harm to an individual than is posed by the future potential for cardiovascular disease.

Clearly many other examples can be cited: the addition to foods of preservatives or antioxidants, growth promotors in the agro-meat industry, iodine in salt, fluoride in water, mass vaccinations, etc. All such measures represent permissible, if not actively promoted practices sponsored by government supported agencies and health advisory groups. While possibly commendable, they nonetheless can harm a substantially large subpopulation with special allergic sensitivities or other somewhat unusual genetic or environmental health problems.

Do critics of these policies then demand that government sponsored advise and regulations are abolished. As Harper indicates, the answer is clearly a resounding no. The plea of the participants to this symposium is, rather, that guidelines are more specifically targeted for only certain subpopulations with special health needs, and that they are formulated according to firm scientific principles before being implemented for the entire community. In this respect, the minimum and maximum dietary requirements guidelines may merit special attention for possible redefinition.

As to overeating and overweight, these are problems of a special subpopulation and belong, like any other type of overindulgence, in the domain of medicine together with other diets designed to alleviate particular health problems. It is here, when dealing with specific health problems, where scientific nutritional research is probably most deficient. There is a commonly held believe that special nutrition and a positive mental attitude may influence the onset or progress of a disease and, in very rare cases, may bring about a remission. Medical treatment of even the most serious disorders-cancer, multiple sclerosis, epilepsy or AIDS, for example - now includes at least some nutritional and psychological counseling. How effective these measures are in supplementing the "proven" benefits of drug therapy is still hard to judge, but at least the concept is no longer rejected out of hand. Perhaps the observation of a lower incidence of disease in children receiving loving parental care in a positively integrated community may try to tell us something. Nevertheless, not withstanding that "psychic" cures are part of community folklore world wide and that the practice of ritualistic or nutritional medicine is popularly considered to be an important adjunct to coventional drug (herbal) therapy, a scientific justification for these claims or practices were until recently very uncertain and have met with considerable scepticism.

It is a particular pleasure therefore that the work presented by Madden and collegues clearly points to one scientific principle which explains a possible joining of cerebral activity (hence emotion) to the immune system. Their investigations indicate that the fibers of the sympathetic nervous system early in life begin to innervate specific compartments of the splenic white pulp; there they become associated with lymphocytes and macrophages. Such nor-adrenergic innervation, together with reports by others of a similar type of innervation in the thymus leaves little doubt that neuroimmunomodulation is a true biological phenomenon (J Neurosci Res 1987:18). The "modern" medical ethos of a point source or single cause for disease may therefore require some revisions, to incorporate possibly some of the most ancient methods of treating illnesses. This may similarly apply to our concepts of idealized conditions for optimizing neural integration and intellectual development. One may debate whether the malnourished child living on the street in close companionship with its peers is worse off than that child in an efficient but sterile surroundings of certain institutions. If we are to give such a child an alternative to the street, it may require greater investments in care facilities than most communities at this time are willing to afford.

In human societies and even among many sub-human species, the process of food gathering, preparation and eating is accompanied by intense socialization. From breast feeding to the preparation of (gathered) food, these daily periods provide the most propitious moments for the infant to become a member of his or her society. While taking nourishment it learns at the same time to interact with other individuals of the community, to restrain certain asocial impulses, and to assimilate the extremely complex and varied guidelines which are in place to maintain a stable social unit. These learning periods are reinforced by the sense of well being which accompanies the process of feeding. Thus, nurture and learning represent mutually reinforcing influences which help to integrate and merge the individuality and sociality of a human infant.

Nico M. van Gelder

(Mal)Nutrition and the Infant Brain, pages 253–265
© 1990 Wiley-Liss, Inc.

THE SOCIAL INFLUENCE: DIET, CHILD CARE AND INTELLECTUAL
PERFORMANCE

Lois M. Roeder

Department of Pediatrics, University of Maryland
School of Medicine, Baltimore, Maryland 21201, USA

Nutrition in early life is one component of a host of complex environmental factors that, in interrelationship with each other, may have a profound impact on the child's intellectual performance. This chapter will emphasize the identification of long-term impairments in intellectual performance observed in children who experienced episodes of malnutrition in their early years; it will highlight a few studies that focus particularly on the role of the social milieu in the etiology of the behavioral or mental deficits, and/or that have developed models which seem especially helpful in understanding this very complex situation.

In evaluating the effects of malnutrition on mental development and intellectual performance, distinctions must include the timing of the evaluation relative to the episode of malnutrition (Galler, 1984). Behavioral assessments obtained concurrent with the presence of malnutrition, during recovery from malnutrition, or in later years, may yield quite different results, depending at least in part on environmental factors that can either interfere with, or facilitate, recovery. Galler and colleagues (1983) conducted a longitudinal study of Barbadian school children at age 5 to 11 years on whom they had documentation of episodes of severe protein-energy malnutrition i.e., marasmus, in the first year of life. Their aim was to determine the long-term consequences of early malnutrition on IQ, classroom behavior and school performance, The controls were classmates with similar social background, but no history of malnutrition. The criteria for the Index group included birth weight of at least 5 lb. in order to rule out fetal growth retardation. There were 129 children (77 boys and 52 girls) in each group. The IQ's were assessed using an adaptation of the Wechsler Intelligence Scale for Children and the results showed lower values for the previously malnourished children than controls. Overall, there was a 12 point difference between the 2 groups, re-flecting a larger percentage of the Index group having low scores; 17% of the controls and 50% of the malnourished group scored less than 90.

Since it has frequently been proposed that socioeconomic factors and the home environment influence IQ, the data were analyzed after controlling for several of these factors. The effect of malnourishment was still evident as shown in Table 1. Each group was divided into 2 sub-groups, representing high or low socioeconomic status (SES) on the basis of household items, housing or type of job the father held. The scores of the previously malnourished children were still consistently and significantly (P<0.001) lower than those of the controls.

TABLE 1. Relationship Between Socioeconomic Factors and Full IQ. Adapted from: Galler et al, 1983.

Intelligence Score

	High SES		Low SES	
	Malnourished	Control	Malnourished	Control
Household Items	91.36	104.45	89.98	100.37
Housing	93.83	103.46	88.95	103.49
Father's Work	91.30	103.71	89.26	102.92

Assessment of grades achieved in school showed that previously malnourished children received marks an average of 1 point lower than controls in 8 of 9 subjects (they did not differ in writing).The grades were significantly correlated with IQ. Thus, children with histories of severe malnutrition perform less effectively in school. Classroom behavior was evaluated on the basis of questionnaires completed by teachers who were not informed of the nutritional history. In 4 of 7 categories of behavior, the malnourished group were impaired relative to controls; e.g., 60% of this group evidenced Attention Deficit Disorder compared to 15% of controls. The Index children were also less emotionally stable. There were 21 boys and 16 girls in this group who were below expected grade level; the difference in emotional stability disappeared when they were excluded. Reduced social skills and poor physical appearance were also found in the previously malnourished children. School marks were more highly correlated with classroom behavior than with IQ. When classroom behavior was controlled, the difference in nutritional history had no further effect on school grades. Thus, the probability of school failure seems to be predicted by classroom behavior and poor classroom behavior is prominent in previously malnourished children. The impairments in academic performance of these children persisted into the later teen years (Galler et al, 1986).

In a later study (Galler et al, 1987b), this group compared children with histories of infantile kwashiorkor with those who had episodes of marasmus, using as controls children of similar socioeconomic background but no early malnutrition. Fig.1 shows the distribution of IQ scores for these 3 groups and demonstrates that the 2 previously malnourished groups were very similar but were both shifted to the left of the controls. In this study they found that certain current environmental conditions were significantly associated with IQ, but the effects of early malnutrition were still significant when these factors were controlled.

There are other studies which showed that intervention following an early episode of malnutrition, such as food supplementation (Evans et al, 1980)

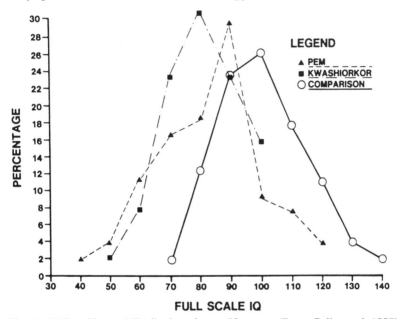

Fig. 1. Malnutrition and distribution of mean IQ scores. From: Galler et al, 1987b.

or change in environment (Winick et al, 1975) can support catch-up growth and even support improvements in IQ score. However, if the malnutrition is severe, or the age at intervention delayed, the deficits in performance may persist (Lien et al, 1977).One of the most striking observations of the longitudinal study in Barbados was that deficits in intellectual performance persisted long after the nutritional insult, whereas impairments in physical growth disappeared during this interval (Galler et al, 1987a). Thus, although measures of physical growth are important and useful immediately after acute episodes of malnutrition, evaluation of behavioral function would be more relevant for assessing long-term outcome. Such tests should focus particularly on adaptive functions, i.e., those behaviors that permit the individual to respond appropriately to the demands of the environment (Galler, 1984).

Stein and Susser (1985) reviewed a number of studies focusing on the role of early nutrition on mental competence, including their own analyses of the results of the Dutch Famine during World War II. They concluded that, except for deficiencies in early pregnancy, undernutrition at other young stages of development was accompanied by depressed cognitive performance only when social deprivation was also present. In addition, the response to food supplementation following malnutrition was itself mediated by the quality of the social environment. These findings point to a further implication of Galler's work which, although it revealed effects of early malnutrition after controlling for variations in socioeconomic status, was based on a population that was mostly lower middle class and relatively homogeneous (Galler et al, 1983). Where poverty is more extreme, and health care and education less available, malnutrition may be expected to have an even greater impact on the child's development.

Unfortunately, lags in development may have a cumulative detrimental effect, since failure of the child to master specific developmental tasks at one age is likely to interfere with later stages of development. Thus, this recovery phase is a critical time for intervention. Studies on children with non-organic failure to thrive have also concluded that environmental factors are important predictors of the child's cognitive development, and that, unless intervention is powerful enough to modify the the influence of these risk factors, cognitive development of the child may actually deteriorate with time (Drotar and Sturm, 1988).

However, Galler (1984) makes an important point in noting that clinical malnutrition is not uniformly distributed among the poorest of families, or even among siblings in the same family. Thus, socioeconomic deprivation alone cannot explain the effects of childhood malnutrition. The very occurrence of malnutrition appears to be a function of home conditions that are not accounted for by inadequacies in the usual host of basic needs. Cravioto and De Larcardie, (1975) in their systematic study of home situations in Mexico, focused especially on the interactions between mother and child and described conditions that were antecedent to the development of malnutrition.

Rush (1984) has emphasized that malnutrition is "not a random event, but surely occurs in the most deprived, disrupted and unstimulating families, those least likely to nurture their children"; by "nurture" he meant more than just supplying food. Dobbing has pointed out (1984) that the components of social background (including quality of family life, and parental care) may each contribute to later achievement by the child, with no one factor predominant, even nutrition. What may count most is that there be a sufficient number of positive factors relative to negative ones.

The factor that does keep emerging as a critical component of this social milieu impacting on mental development, this "nurturing" factor, or parenting skill or quality of maternal care, defies quantitation. Certain aspects of mother-infant interactions appear to play a major part of this nurturing or care. A considerable degree of mutual adaptation and social learning is apparently required from both mother and infant to support appropriate emotional, behavioral and intellectual development of the child. A model for the relationship of this system to malnutrition (Fig.2) proposes that a disturbance or dysfunction in the mother-infant relationship is a condition antecedent to the malnutrition. Once malnutrition develops, these conditions may persist and result in maladaptive responses of both mother and child.

Malnutrition can affect the physical and behavioral attributes of the child and changes in these attributes will in all likelihood influence both the child's response to others and the response of others to the child. Given a mother disadvantaged to begin with by virtue of impoverishments in a constellation of environmental factors, her preparedness to respond to such a child with appropriate learning and adjustment on her part may be quite inadequate. If the mother herself experienced early childhood malnutrition, her own intellectual capacity and educational attainment may make her even more unable to participate in the required mother-infant interaction. She may become apathetic and even reject the child. The child then does not receive the needed support and stimulation, and development is impeded. This simultaneous dysfunction serves to solidify the barrier to social and intellectual advancement and may lead to long-term impairment of function for the child.

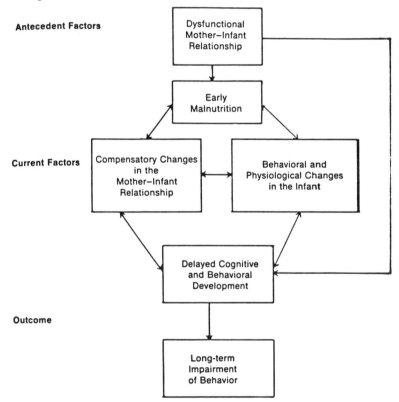

Fig. 2. Possible relationships between mother-infant interaction and malnutrition. From: Galler et al, 1984.

Given how critical the nature and timing of this mother-infant interaction appears to be, it can be predicted that additional factors that further impair the mother's ability to respond to the child will strengthen the possibility of developmental deficiency for the infant. Figure 3 summarizes some of the sources of these other influences.

One of these, the specific family environment, may include a life style that impacts adversely on both mother and child, such as drug use. It is clear from the study of Zuckerman et al (1989) that fetal growth measured by birth weight and length is compromised by the use of marijuana or cocaine by the mother during pregnancy; cocaine use was also accompanied by reduced head circumference of the infant. Their multiple regression analysis of the data indicated that the use of cocaine, which is an appetite suppressant, was associated with lower pre-pregnancy weight and decreased weight gain, and thus may have an indirect effect mediated by maternal undernutrition, as well as an independent, direct negative effect on birth weight. Women with multiple risk factors in this study (low weight gain, smoking and drug use) gave birth to infants weighing 416 grams less than a control group. It will be very important to assess the mother-infant interactions in such a family situation and to determine the long-term effects on the child's development.

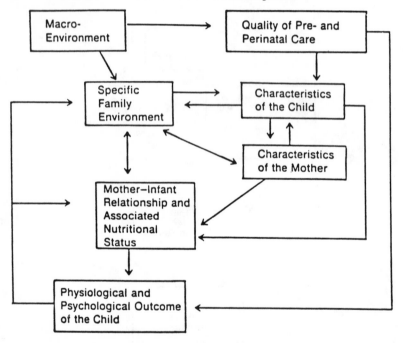

Fig. 3. Sources and directions of influences affecting mother-infant relationship. From: Galler et al, 1984.

Among the characteristics of the mother that would have an important impact is young age. Teenage mothers have been shown to have less than optimal nutrition and prenatal care and are more likely to have an infant with low birth weight than are older mothers. National statistics for the U.S. have shown that 13.8% of infants born to women under 15 years of age weighed less than 2500gm compared to 9.3% for 15 to 19 year old mothers and 5.8% for 25-29 year olds (McAnarney, 1987).Thus, very young mothers have a much higher chance of their infant dying than older mothers, since low birth weight infants are 40 times more likely to die during the neonatal period than infants weighing more than 2500 gms. Maternal weight gain is an important predictor of infant birth weight (Niswandwer and Jackson, 1974) and this is especially true for adolescents (Garn and Petzold, 1983), reflecting probable poor nutritient intake (Hampton, 1967). It has been shown that for the same weight gain during pregnancy, teenage mothers have smaller infants than older mothers (Stevens-Simon and McAnarney, 1988). Part of the explanation for this may be the need for the mother to complete her own growth. Teenage mothers are also at risk for more emotional stress during pregnancy than older mothers (McAnarney, 1983), and it is possible that such stress may impair the young mother's participation in the cognitive development of her child. Whitman et al (1987) developed a model to analyze causes and developmental consequences of adolescent parenting (Fig. 4).

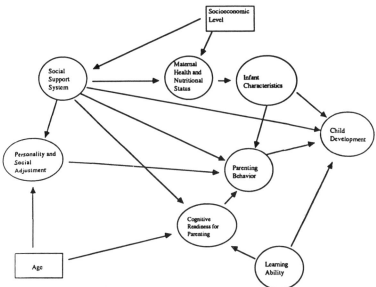

Fig. 4. Model of teenage parenting and child development. From: Whitman et al, 1987.

The model has many similarities to that in Fig. 2 based on information on older mothers. Figure 4 specifically predicts that an adolescent mother's personality and cognitive readiness for parenting are age-related variables and that both are influenced by her social-support system. The latter also influences the mother's health and nutritional status, in turn a major influence on the infant's physical characteristics at birth. The infant's development reflects the mother's learning ability, her parenting skills, the infant's own characteristics and the social support system.

Recommendations for intervention to prevent adverse outcome in teenage pregnancies include the ideal of avoiding such pregnancies with emphasis on education about the risks involved. A more general focus on education should also contribute toward this same goal since statistics verify that children who have early experiences of success in school are less likely to become pregnant as teenagers (Hansen et al, 1978), and Felice et al (1987) suggest that withdrawal from school may be a precipitating factor for, rather than a social consequence of, pregnancy. Strategies to improve outcome for teenagers who have become pregnant include that used at the University of Maryland Hospital (Fig. 5) which provided a program of prenatal care within the Division of Adolescent Medicine in the Department of Pediatrics as an option for teenagers under 15 who came for obstetrical care.

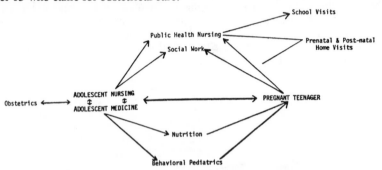

Fig. 5. Schema for interdisciplinary care of pregnant teenagers. From: Felice et al, 1981.

This was a very staff-intensive program and included home and school visits by the public health nurse. Outcome of pregnancy was evaluated on the basis of the distribution of birth weights and the rate of prematurity, compared to outcomes for teenagers who opted for the regular obstetrical clinic. Outcome was significantly improved by this program, although it may be argued that those who chose the program were a self-selected, lower risk group. One of the points made in presenting these findings was the marked saving in cost of intensive care in the nursery by preventing low birth weight. The reduction in cost for care of low birth weight infants achievable by prenatal care was also addressed by the Institute of Medicine (Report, 1985) and their conclusions are summarized and discussed by Behrman (1985).

The importance of social factors in the incidence of malnutrition and in the survival and well-being of children has been increasingly recognized by national and international agencies whose mission is to provide assistance for development in Third World countries. Malnutrition exists on a very large scale in some of these countries. However, it is no longer held that most childhood malnutrition is caused by lack of food in the home (Grant, 1989). Major contributing factors that have been identified are illnesses, parental ignorance of children's nutritional needs or of how to monitor the child's growth and development, and poor maternal health. Efforts are being made to confront these issues; UNICEF in particular has set for itself certain goals for changing the level of well-being of children and will use a set of social indicators to evaluate progress (Grant, 1989). These include Under 5 Mortality Rate (U5MR) and Illiteracy Rate (especially of females). UNICEF and other organizations have determined that these measures, rather than Gross National Product, reflect a real shift in the quality of life for large segments of the population. The relationship of U5MR to a variety of factors related to quality of life are shown in Table 2. As U5MR increases, there are concomitant increases in maternal mortality and in the incidence of low birth weight, and decreases in the percentage of children immunized, the percentage of the population with health services or drinking water, and the percent who are literate. Thus, U5MR reflects the nutrition, health and health knowledge of mothers, the level of immunization and use of oral rehydration therapy, the availability of maternal and child health services, income and food availability in the family, availability of clean water and safe sanitation, and the overall safety of the child's environment.

TABLE 2. Relation of Under Five Mortality Rate (U5MR) to Measures of Nurtirional Status and Health. From: World Bank, 1988.

Measure	Under Five Mortality Rate			
	Low (<30)	Middle (31-94)	High (95-170)	V.High (>170)
Maternal Mortality	11	91	140	420
Percent Low Birth Weight	6	9	13	15
Percent Immunized	90	59-75	55-72	27-46
Percent With Health Services	80-100	60-97	26-97	15-90
Percent With Drinking Water	86-100	36-93	9-96	6-92
Literacy Rate Male/Female	97/90	87/80	68/49	43/22

In the area of literacy, the emphasis has been on educating women, because of their key role in providing nutrition and early education for the children. The World Bank (1980) has stated that "Maternal education is clearly related to child health, whether measured by nutritional status or infant and child mortality". They propose that by increasing female literacy, a cascade of positive effects is stimulated, including better birth spacing, fewer pregnancies, better child care, improved maternal and child health, better school attendance and performance, increased productivity and income, better diets, child health and survival. Attention to these aspects of health and well-being for the world's people, especially children, plus some significant advances in vaccine availability, implementation of immunizations, and development of technologies such as oral rehydration therapy, were accompanied by a steady improvement in child survival and health. However, severe economic problems in the 1980's produced international recession and rising debt, and with them, a marked reversal of this progress in child health. In economic terms, the net flow of money between developed nations (primarily in the Northern Hemisphere) completely changed from a level of $40 billion going toward development in the Southern Hemisphere in 1979 to debt payments amounting to $20 billion going in the opposite direction in 1989. The resulting economic climate for the developing countries has been one of increasing debt and decreasing prices for goods, leading to economic adjustment policies that included cuts in expenditures for health. This is reflected in increased infant mortality rates (IMR). For example, in Brazil, after a steady decline from 1977 to 1982, there was a sharp rise in IMR, especially in the northeast region (Fig. 6).

Worldwide in 1988, 1/2 million child deaths were related to reversal or slowing down of development; 2/3 of these occurred in Africa. This sober note is repeated in other statistics (World Bank, 1988). For example:

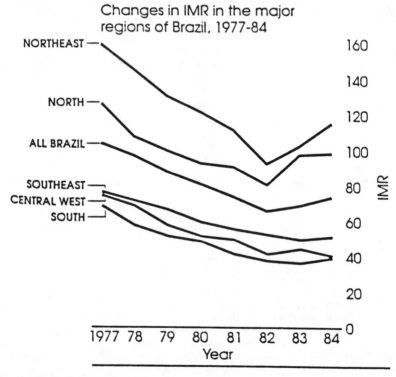

Fig. 6. Rising infant deaths. From: Grant, 1989.

In 21 of 35 low income developing countries, the daily calorie supply per capita was lower in 1985 than in 1965.

Between 1979 and 1983, life expectancy declined in 9 Sub-Saharan African countries.

In Zambia, deaths from malnutrition among infants and children doubled during 1980-1984, and in Sri Lanka, the calorie consumption of the poorest 1/10 of the population fell 9% between 1979 and 1982.

In Costa Rica, falling real wages during 1979-1982 increased the incidence of poverty by more than 2/3.

In some of the low income countries, the number of physicians per capita decreased and enrollment ratios for primary education declined between 1965 and 1981.

The challenge, then, in supporting optimal development for children is not only to identify and shift the social milieu so that a favorable outcome is facilitated for the individual child at risk, but also to confront the host of political and economic issues that threaten survival and impede development for large populations at risk.

REFERENCES

Behrman RE (1985). Preventing low birth weight: A pediatric perspective. J Ped 107: 842-854.

Cravioto J, DeLicardie ER (1975). Mother-infant relationship prior to the development of clinically severe malnutrition in the child. In White PL, Selvey N (eds): Western Hemisphere Nutrition Congress IV Acton, MA, Publishing Sciences Group, pp 126-137.

Dobbing J (1984). Infant nutrition and later achievement. Nutr Rev 42:1-7.

Drotar D, Sturm L (1988). Prediction of intellectual development in young children with early histories of non-organic failure-to-thrive.J Ped Psychology 13:281-296.

Evans D, Bowie MD, Hansen JDL, Moodie AD, van der Spuy HIJ (1980). Intellectual development and nutrition. J Ped 87:355-363.

Felice ME, Granados JL, Ances IG, Hebel R, Roeder LM, Heald FP (1981). The young pregnant teenager. Impact of comprehensive prenatal care. J Adol Hlth Care 1:193-197.

Felice ME, Shragg GP, James M, Hollingsworth DR (1987). Psychosocial aspects of Mexican-American, White, and Black teenage pregnancy. J Adol Hlth Care 8:330-335.

Galler JR (1984). Behavioral consequences of malnutrition in early life. In Galler JR (ed): "Nutrition and Behavior", New York: Plenum, pp 63-117.

Galler JR, Ramsey FC, Salt P, Archer E (1987a). Long-term effects of early kwashiorkor compared with marasmus. I. Physical growth and sexual maturation. J Ped Gastroenterol 6:841-846.

Galler JR, Ramsey FC, Forde V, Salt P, Archer E (1987b). Long-term effects of early kwashiorkor compared with marasmus. II. Intellectual performance. J Ped Gastroenterol 6: 847-854.

Galler JR, Ramsey F, Forde V (1986). A follow-up study of the influence of early malnutrition on subsequent development.4. Intellectual performance during adolescence. Nutr Behav 3:211-222.

Galler JR, Ramsey,F, Solimano G, Lowell WE (1983). The influence of early malnutrition on subsequent behavioral development. I. Degree of impairment in intellectual performance. J Am Acad Child Psychiatry 22:8-15.

Galler JR, Ricciuti HN, Crawford MA, Kucharski LT (1984). The role of the mother-infant interactions in nutritional disorders. In Galler JR (ed): "Nutrition and Behavior", New York: Plenum, pp. 269-304.

Garn SM, Petzold AS (1983). Characteristics of the mother and child in teenage pregnancy. Am J Dis Child 137:365-368

Grant JP (1989). "The State of the World's Children", Oxford: Oxford University Press, 116pp.

Hampton MC, Huenemann RL, Shapiro LR et al. Caloric and nutrient intakes of teenagers. J Am Diet Assoc 50:385-396.

Hansen H, Stroh G, Whitaker k (1978). School achievement: Risk factor in teenage pregnancies. Am J Publ Hlth 68:753-759.

Lien NM, Meyer KK, Winick M (1977). Early malnutrition and "late" adoption: A study of their effects on the development of Korean orphans adopted into American families. Am J Clin Nutr 30:1734-1739.

McAnarney ER (1983). "Premature Pregnancy and Parenthood". New York: Grune and Stratton, 1983.

McAnarney ER (1987). Young maternal age and adverse neonatal outcome. Am J Dis Child 141:1053-1059.

Niswander K, Jackson EC (1974). Physical characteristics of the gravida and their association with birth weight and perinatal death. Am J Obstet Gynecol 119:306-313.

Rush D (1984). The behavioral consequences of protein-energy deprivation and supplementation in early life: An epidemiological perspective. In Galler JR (ed): "Nutrition and Behavior", New York: Plenum, pp. 119-157.

Stein Z, Susser M (1985). Effects of early nutrition on neurological and mental competence in human beings. Psychological Med 15:717-726.

Stevens-Simon C, McAnarney ER (1988). Adolescent maternal weight gain and low birth weight: A multifactorial model. Am J Clin Nutr 47:948-953.

Whitman TL, Borkowski JG, Schellenbach CJ, Nath PS (1987). Predicting and understanding developmental delay of children of adolescent mothers: A multidimensional approach. Am J Mental Defic 92:40-56.

Winick M, Meyer KK, Harris RC (1975). Malnutrition and environmental enrichment by early adoption Science 190:1173-1175.

World Bank (1988). "World Development Report". Oxford: Oxford University Press.

World Bank Staff (1980). The effects of education on health. Working Paper #405.

Zuckerman B, Frank DA, Hingson R, Amaro H, Levenson SM, Kayne H, Parker S, Vinci R, Aboage K, Fried LE, Cabral H, Timperi R, Bauchner H (1989). Effects of maternal marijuana and cocaine use on fetal growth. N.Engl, J Med 320:762-768.

DISCUSSION

Q (van Gelder): I have a physiological question. Why is labor so much more difficult in undernourished women.

A: The small stature of the mother due to undernutrition or chronic malnutrition during their development. There may also be other factors such as hormones.

Q (Jhaveri): Is low birth weight as damaging in the case of young girls (smaller birth canal).

A: This is controversial right now. The trend has been to encourage automatic weight gain, that produces healthier babies. But this is all based on data for older women. So there is now a reluctance on the part of some physicians to recommend a large weight gain just for that purpose because in this instance you are dealing with a person (young girls) whose own growth is not yet complete. So there is not a concensus of opinion for this.

Q (Jhaveri): But you base the data of undernourishment on the low birht weight of the child. This therefore may not (only) relfect poor nutrition or nursing on the part of the mother, it may simply mean that the mother is small or young.

A: That could be. But the data have been interpreted in association with documented poor nutrient intake and, also, assessments of poor nutritional status.

Q (Rassin): Two other factors, particularly in the U.S., may account for low birth weight. One is race, particularly in teenagers. There is increasing evidence that there is a (natural) tendency for Afro-American teenagers to have small babies. The other factor is smoking. It is probably the single most significant factor in reducing birth weight and size. It probably has an effect of several hundred grams, and that is not the mother.

A: No doubt that would be one of the factors which has an impact. But even beyond race, it is poverty. When they take race into consideration (in examing the data), poverty is an issue that remains.

Q (Audience): How successful are you in education. Does the cultural background make a difference.

A: Well, there has not been a lot of studies in this regards but I have seen some, where they have offered opportunities to, say, teenage mothers at the time of delivery to enrole in educational programs. They do find them quite receptive. Now, what the long term impact is remains to be seen, but at least they are receptive to participate.

PROYECTO VENEZUELA: Fundación "Centro de Estudios Sobre Crecimiento y Desarrollo de la Población Venezolano" (**Fundacredesa**).

Project Venezuela was established in 1976 when, by Presidential Decree, a 7 membered commission was formed to oversee a national effort to examine in depth the socioeconomic and health factors which shape the growth and development of the Venezuelan child. It is an ongoing project coordinated by Fundacredesa, with as a final goal the formulation of national standards relevant and applicable for all levels of society. Such standards can then be used as guidelines to set policies which will assure the health and wellfare of the population so that social conditions give children the opportunity to grow up in a cultural environment which permits their intellectual and physical abilities to develop fully according to their natural endowment.

In order to reach this ambitious target, a large number of academic and health professionals are engaged in investigations at three levels: (i) the gathering of data on the current psychological and physical development of the population; (ii) comparisons between various populations with different life styles (rural vs urban), socioeconomic levels, and nutritional habits; and (iii) the clinical health of these various subpopulations. Among the principal investigators are Hernan Méndez Castellano (director) and Nancy Angulo de Rodriguez, whose reports are included here.

Thus, starting with the individual efforts in the early forties, such as the studies by Manuel Sánchez Carvajal (1939), Méndez Castellano and Barrera Moncada (1948), Fermin Vélez Boza (1963), Project Venezuela has grown into a series of investigations aimed at providing a scientific and social data bank on which future governments and health professionals can draw to initiate policies for the promotion of population wellfare. Fundacredesa represents the answer to a recommendation made at the meeting of the International Biology Program (1964), namely that each country supports an Institute dedicated to the study of the population and its adaptation to existing environmental and cultural conditions.

A first pilot program was initiated in 1978 under the auspices of the National Research Council for Science and Technology (CONICIT), as a priority project. Today, the Foundation continues to be financially supported by this organization as well as by special funds from the government of Venezuela and by certain private donations. Project Venezuela is considered so important to the nation that it has retained a priority classification since its inception despite changes in political administrations and the economic fortunes of the country. With the acquired knowledge and government initiatives it is hoped to provide better information to the population for proper child care, to improve the general standards of health and nutrition, as well as to provide greater access to an education. By means of such measures the country intends to give each child the intellectual and physical resources needed to meet his/her future with competence and confidence.

Boris D. Drujan

Instituto Venezolano de Investigaciones Cientificas
Laboratorio de Neuroquimica, Carretera panamericana Km 11
Aptdo 1827, Caracas 1010 A, Venezuela

(Mal)Nutrition and the Infant Brain, pages 269–284

THE SOCIAL IMPACT ON CHILD GROWTH AND DEVELOPMENT IN VENEZUELA

Hernan Méndez-Castellano, Mercedes López-Blanco, Maria Mendéz, Marlene Fossi, Maritza Landaeta-Jimenez, Virgilio Bosch

FUNDACREDESA: Center for Studies on Growth and Development of the Venezuelan Population, Post Office Box 61660, Chacao - Caracas 1060-A, VENEZUELA.

Around the middle of the XVIII century, the Carol School in Germany pointed out for the first time the relationship between social and biological factors, when it published a paper showing the differences between nobles and middle class adults. Later on, the works of Villarme (France, 1812), Quetelet (Belgium, 1831), Stanway (England, 1836) and finally Pickering (USA, 1831), showed the difference in height between children of the lower classes and those of the more favoured social strata. In this century, the "Centre International de L'Enfance", in Paris, coordinated 340 investigations in various countries, using a social stratification method proposed by M. Graffar. These studies have been revised and published by Eveleth and Tanner in the book, "Worldwide Variation in Human Growth" (1977).

According to this source, European children from the highest social strata grow more rapidly than those from the lower strata, as do children living in cities in comparison to children from rural areas. Also, in general, children from Northern Europe are taller than those from Central Europe, while these last are heavier. In Asia they reported the lowest heights, even in children belonging to upper social strata.

In Venezuela, the health of our people depends not only on biological factors such as infections caused by parasites, bacteria and virus, but also on the quality of life of the family. This in turn is conditioned by family income, housing, air pollution, drinking water and, finally, stress derived from social pressure which influences interpersonal human behaviour. In this difficult "modern" milieu, the human organism has to make use of all the genetic mechanisms available to adapt successfully to its surrounding. Nevertheless, these mechanisms are insufficient and man must make use of science and technology to compensate for this biological inadequacy in a manner that could be defined as an artificial and dependent pseudo-adaptation process.

All this is due to the fact that not enough generations have passed to produce a human being genetically adapted to the present environment. In other words, biological survival is no longer achieved by natural selection procedures.

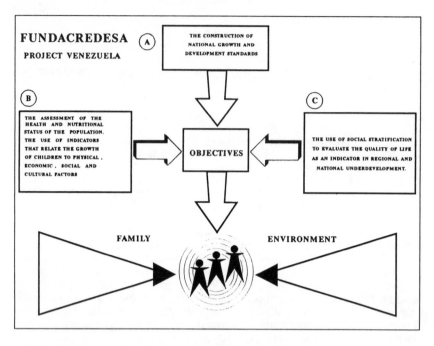

Fig. 1. Objectives of Project Venezuela (Mendez-Castellano, 1985)

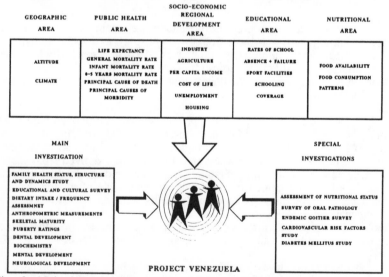

Fig. 2. Main investigation and special investigations of Project Venezuela; interrelationship with geographic, public health, socioeconomic, educational and nutritional factors (Mendez-Castellano, 1985)

A Venezuelan child suffers multiple and severe aggressions from his milieu, some related directly to the environment, but most - the most important - are consequences of situations related to nutrition, housing and culture. We consider our biological characteristics to be the result of a combination of our genetic potential and favourable or unfavourable influences during growth. Among these last, nutrition is one of the most important factors, for it is this variable influence which seems highly correlated with the observed differences in growth and development among Venezuelan children.

The biological and social needs of communities must be taken into account when formulating policies of economic planning. Therefore, investigations of health in the country, through the analysis of the growth and development of Venezuelan children, should help to establish integrated improvement policies on behalf of the entire population.

PROJECT VENEZUELA, the national Human Growth, Nutrition and Family Survey, directed and coordinated by FUNDACREDESA, was initiated to examine how the growth and intellectual performance of an individual, especially in the Venezuelan population, is influenced or affected by his or her biological potential, socio-economic status and cultural or tribal affiliation. Fig. 1 shows that the project aims to establish:

(I)   The construction of National Standards for Growth and Development, taking into account biological constraints of any particular genetically "homogeneous" population.
(II)   Public Health Indicators, reflecting (child) growth rates in terms of the physical, economic and "cultural" population affiliation of the infant.
(III)   Standards in evaluating the quality of life by defined social status stratifications.

The hypothesis to be tested by PROJECT VENEZUELA are the following:
a. Genetic variability among individuals does not exert a dominant constraint on the average growth and development of Venezuelans.
b. Nutrition is the main factor that limits growth and development in Venezuela
c. The economic and cultural status of the Venezuelan family can influence and limit normal growth and development.
d. The growth and development data derived from upper middle class Venezuelan families can be used as a national standard of reference.

Taking into account that overall development is determined by a complex interaction between the environment and the biology of the individual and, also, that any parameter of development chosen as a measure of development needs to be quantified, FUNDACREDESA decided to perform the following studies (see Fig. 2.):
1. Social Environment: The family
    - Socio-economic and cultural survey
    - Personality survey of adolescents
    - Nutritional survey
    - Epidemiological survey

- Special survey of Indian families

2. Infant and Adolescent Growth Study
   - Growth variables (auxological data)
   - Biochemical development
   - Cognitive development
   - Neuropediatric development
   - Dental examination and development
   - Skeletal development
   - Pubertal development

It is well known that the many factors implicated in arriving at a stable social community (strata) within a population are difficult to isolate or to quantify individually. PROJECT VENEZUELA therefore decided not to concentrate their studies on single Venezuelan families or individuals. Rather, the project attempts to analyze social and biological development within the framework of the social hierarchy or stratum to which the family or person belongs.

One of the main objectives of this project is the assessment of the health and nutritional status regionally. For this purpose the country was divided into seven geographic regions, distinguishable by their differing political and economic character. The geographic distinctions will aid in the eventual formulation of policies and priorities in health, nutrition and welfare and will also serve as a basis for evaluating government programs both nationally and regionally; only four of the seven regions are discussed in this paper:

(i)   The Caracas Metropolitan Area (CMA) contains 20% of the country's population and is totally urbanized; 12.5% of its inhabitants are immigrants principally from South America and Southern Europe (Spain and Portugal), and 40% are migrants from other parts of the country. The birth rate is 32.6 per thousand. Infant mortality is 18.5 per thousand, the lowest in the country, and the social unit averages 4.5 inhabitants per household.

(ii)   The Zulia Region (ZR), has 12% of the nation's population and is 84% urban. It is the main producer of oil in the country and its capital, Maracaibo, is the second largest city in Venezuela; 8% of the population are immigrants, mainly from Columbia. The birth rate is 33.5 per thousand. Infant mortality is 27.6 per thousand and a household averages 5.7 inhabitants.

(iii)   The Northeastern Region (NER), has 12.8% of the country's total population, 80% urban, with 3.6% immigrants. Birth rates are 35 per thousand, infant mortality 24.9 per thousand, average inhabitants per household is 6.5.

(iv)   The Midwestern Region (MWR) contains 7.3% of Venezuela's population. It is 75% urban, and immigrants represent only 1.4%: mainly South Americans, Portuguese and Spanish. Birth rate is 35.4 per thousand. Infant mortality is 44.9 per thousand, the highest in the country. Inhabitants per household average 5.6.

Preliminary results of immunogenetic frequency studies, performed as part of PROJECT VENEZUELA by FUNDACREDESA and the National Center for Clinical Inmunology, demonstrate that the genetic composite of the Venezuelan population is derived from the mixing of a number of human races. As is well known, three races have contributed to this genetic composite: Caucasoid (Spaniards), Mongoloid (Amerindians) and Negroid (Africans). The major histo-compatibility antigens characteristic of these races are identified, in various proportions, in all parts of the country, allowing us to argue that the genetic factor is not the most determining factor for the differences found in growth and development, and that the socio-economic and cultural characteristics of the environment are mostly responsible for such differences.

To verify these assertions, we used the Social Stratification Method proposed by M. Graffar, from Belgium, which is based on multiple variables, and which was modified and adapted for Venezuela by H. Mendez-Castellano. This method is considered more reliable to arrive at a quantifiable social grouping than relying on a single social-economic parameter such as income. The classification used in the present studies has three distinct advantages in that: 1) The data lend themselves better to detect temporal (i.e. progressive) changes, as well as to perform geographic comparative analysis; 2) The information on which the classification is based is less biased by the intentional or unintentional prejudicies or omissions by the person interviewed; 3) Finally, and perhaps most important, the classification takes into account the cultural variables which are a key determinant in the management of the family budget and of other social factors contributing to a family's "quality of life".

The variables used by PROJECT VENEZUELA to arrive at a reliable and quantifiable social classification are:

1. Profession of the head of the family
2. Mother's level of instruction
3. Main source of income
4. Housing conditions

Each of these variables consists of five items, with each being accorded an increasing numerical importance, from 1 to 5, as the (judged) quality becomes less. According to a scale previously designed, the sum of these items will determine the social stratum of the family investigated, with the highest score representing the lowest socio-economic quality.

The social stratification classifies families according to the following score:

STRATA	SCORE
I	4,5,6
II	7,8,9
III	10,11,12
IV	13,14,15,16
V	17,18,19,20

Scores 4,5 and 6 correspond to Stratum I, with the maximum conditions for a high quality of life. This quality decreases progressively, and thus we find stratum IV with a score of 13,14,15 and 16, which we call "relative poverty" and culminates in what has been called "critical poverty" in stratum V, which has scores of 17,18,19 and 20. In general, one should take into consideration that borderline classification scores between groups can change, depending on whether the economy of the country is in recession or in a growth phase.

SAMPLE:

Height was used as the basis for establishing the sample size for each age group. This variable was chosen because of its relative stability. For instance, only in cases of severe and prolonged malnutrition is it affected. Thus it can be used as an independent variable for designing a model (within the context of Venezuela).

The size of the sample was estimated considering the height at age 7, where growth is typical and stable. The sample size had to be sufficiently large to obtain a 95% confidence level and was determined, using as a reference model, random sampling that defines de following formula:

$$e^2 = \frac{K^2 \cdot S^2}{n}$$

where:
- e : maximum accepted error
- K : Confidence coefficient
- S : Standard deviation
- n : Sample size

For the selection of the age group samples, growth increments were considered, using data from Tanner, Whitehouse & Takaishi (1966) which are similar to those of Barrera Moncada & Mendez-Castellano (1969).

The value of K was chosen for a confidence level of 95%, that is 1.96. The value for the variance was taken from previous studies in Cuba (Jordan, 1972), the United Kingdom (Tanner, 1966) and Venezuela (Barrera & Mendez, 1969); the value chosen was 5.26 cm. The error chosen was 3 mm, which means a confidence interval of 6 mm. The sample size for age and sex was 1156.

The total sample size encompassed 67548 children, and their corresponding families. This sample size is considered sufficient to discriminate height differences, within 95% confidence limits, between the following groupings:

1. Social Strata (five stratum)
2. Regional Levels (seven regions)
3. Urban and Rural Areas (two)

The purpose of this paper is to present a part of the results from PROJECT VENEZUELA. The data demonstrate the relation between social factors and the growth and development of Venezuelan children in terms of the following parameters:

Growth differences according to social strata.

Differences in consumption patterns according to social strata.

Correlation between blood cholesterol levels and fat consumption according to social strata.

A brief analysis of overall trends in average growth.

The assessment of the nutritional status of Venezuelan children by Weight/Age, Height/Age and Weight/Height indicators.

Differences in Growth According to Social Strata

Venezuelan children who belong to the upper social strata are similar, from birth and throughout growth, in height and weight to the upper strata children in Europe, America and Asia. For instance, growth is the same as the growth of children in London, Helsinki, Amsterdam and Prague (Fig. 3). This demonstrates that Venezuelans are not predetermined genetically to be short in stature and that they reach a growth and development similar to children of industrialized countries when their environment is adequate.

Differences up to 5 cm are evident between children from the upper strata (I+II+III), whose growth is similar to those of the industrialized countries, and the children of stratum IV and V (Fig. 4.). The main problem lies in the fact that the children of upper socio-economic strata (I+II+III) represent only 20%, and that the children from strata IV and V represent 80% of the population; they belong to families with low socio-economic and cultural status, which thus represent a very large percentage of the total Venezuelan households.

Furthermore, age at menarche of girls belonging to the upper social strata (I+II+III) averages 12 years and 3 months; this contrasts with the girls belonging to stratum IV, whose mean age at menarche is 12 years 6 months, and those from stratum V with an average of 12 years 8 months.

Diffferences in the Consumption Patterns, According to Social Strata

Results from Carabobo State, characterized as a region with a high level of industrial and agrarian development in 1987, show an average consumption of meats that differs according to social strata: Cattle = 146.62 gm per person/day

----

Fig. 3. Venezuelans's weight and height from high social strata ses (I+II+III) compared with values in industrialized countries (Mendez-Castellano , 1985).

Fig. 4. Venezuela: Weight and height according to socioeconomic strata (Mendez-Castellano , 1985).

Fig. 5. Feeding habits according to social strata. Carabobo state (Grams per person per day; Fundacredesa, 1987).

Fig. 6. Feeding habits according to urban - rural source. Carabobo state (Grams per person per day; Fundacredesa, 1987).

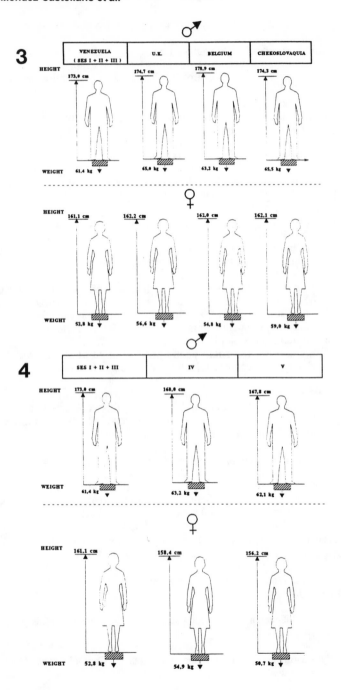

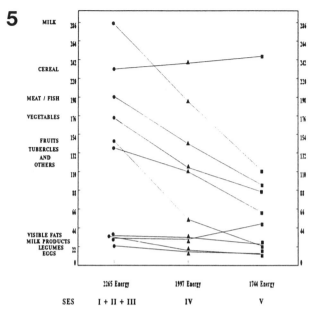

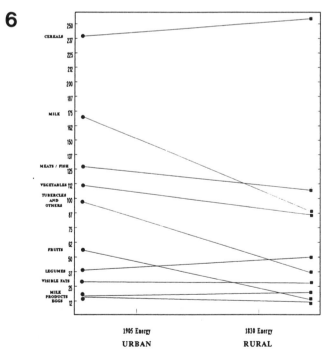

in social strata I=II+III; 57.78 gm in stratum IV and 38.10 gm in stratum V; pork = 18.9 gm per person/day in social strata I=II=III, 12.11 gm in stratum IV and 8 gm in stratum V (Fig. 5.).

This gradient is also evident in the consumption of milk and its derived products: 72.47 gm per person/day for social strata I+II+III, 43 gm for stratum IV and 27.9 gm for stratum V; as well as in fruit, which was consumed as follows: 145.8 gm per person/day for strata I+II+III, 53.8 gm for stratum IV and 23.3 gm for stratum V (Fig. 5.).

The intake of calories averaged 2265 calories per person/day for social strata I+II+III, 1997.7 for stratum IV and 1830 calories for stratum V. It is important to point out that caloric intake in the rural areas is highly deficient and very similar to that of stratum V   (Fig. 6.).

Correlations between Cholesterol Levels in Plasma, and Fat Intake According to Social Strata

In Tables 1 and 2, cholesterol levels in children's plasma are presented for both sexes and for ages 5 to 11 and 11 to 15 years. These tables show the mean values of cholesterol concentrations in boys and girls and that of the three socio-economic levels: strata I+II+III, IV and V.   A clear tendency for a decrease in the average plasma cholesterol is observed as one descends from the priveleged strata (I+II+III) to stratum IV and finally to the level of the critically poor (V). This data is in accord with fat consumption in the following manner: Intake of total fats is 34.8 gm per person/day for socio-economic strata I+II+III, 32.6 gm for stratum IV and 23 gm for stratum V.

These results allow us to propose that the study of plasma lipids in children, besides its specific interest as a screening device of hyperlipidemias, might be used to observe the effect of environmental factors in a population. Accordingly, FUNDACREDESA plans to perform serial determinations of this variable in the whole population for its use as a public health indicator.

Brief Analysis of Secular Growth Trend

In industrialized countries in the last hundred or more years, a positive trend in growth and maturity has become apparent, more evident in adolescents than in adults. These secular changes are correlated with urbanization, a smaller family, the improvement in sanitation and especially, with a better nutrition. In some of these countries this process has stopped due, presumably, to the fact that the environmental conditions are now optimal and/or that the population has reached its genetic growth limitation.

An analysis of the growth studies performed in Venezuela between 1936 and 1976, revealed a positive general growth trend in all socio-economic strata, both in urban as well as rural populations. The increase in growth is of a greater magnitude in males, and higher in weight than for height. These results reflect the great socio-economic transformations that have occurred in Venezuela in the last 50 years.

The importance of these results lies in the fact that for the first time in Venezuela the general trends between social strata was determined in two samples of the same sub-population, using the same methodology both for the

TABLE 1. Plasma Cholesterol Concentrations in Boys (mg/dl)

| region | N | age years | socioeconomic strata | | | difference high-low |
			high I+II+III	medium IV	low V	
Lara	312	5-11	*160	154	137	23
		11-15	147	149	145	2
Northeastern	714	5-11	*163*	148	145	18
		11-15	*152	153	145	7
Metropolitan Caracas	913	5-11	*162*	145	147	15
		11-15	*153*	146	143	10
Zulia	317	5-11	*159*	148	136	23
		11-15	*151*	144	131	20
TOTAL	2256					

* Left of value: *high-low* significantly different (p < 0.01)
* Right of value: *high-medium* significantly different (p < 0.01)
Standard errors of means 2 to 4 mg/dl

TABLE 2. Plasma Cholesterol Concentrations in Girls (mg/dl)

| region | N | age years | socioeconomic strata | | | difference high-low |
			high I+II+III	medium IV	low V	
Lara	378	5-11	*162*	152	137	25
		11-15	*158*	152	147	11
Northeastern	873	5-11	*162*	153	153	11
		11-15	154	159	145	0
Metropolitan Caracas	950	5-11	*159	155	148	11
		11-15	*163*	153	156	7
Zulia	295	5-11	148	145	143	5
		11-15	141	145	153	-12
TOTAL	2496					

* Left of value: *high-low* significantly different (p < 0.01)
* Right of value: *high-medium* significantly different (p < 0.01)
Standard errors of means 2 to 4 mg/dl

data collection and for the analysis. These samples represented boys and girls measured by PROJECT VENEZUELA in Carabobo State from birth to 19 years: 3170 in 1978, and 2710 in 1988.

Means of height and weight are presented by age groups according to sex, taking the mean point of the yearly interval. The data of both samples were interpolated for the exact age and thus used in the analysis. The trend found in the different social strata are differentiated by sex and age and expressed as centimeters (cm) and kilograms (kg) per decade. The comparison of the growth in height and weight of the two unstratified samples has just been published (Lopez-Blanco et al, 1989). Differences in boys were larger, especially with respect to weight (Fig. 7. and 8.); these differences are more evident when one studies the stratified sample.

The overall trend in the height of boys belonging to the upper strata (I+II+III) is analyzed from 6 years of age on, because there is not sufficient data for the previous ages in the 1978 study. A positive growth trend of approximately 3.4 cm by decade is observed at six years of age; it increases with age and reaches its maximum values: 4 to 6 cm by decade between 8 and 11 years, decreasing to 1.6 cm per decade in adulthood (Fig. 7.). In contrast, in upper strata girls (I+II+III) the trend is negative until age 8, becomes positive at 9 years of age, and reaches 2 to 3 cm per decade during puberty. At the end of growth, the average decreases to less than 1 cm per decade (Fig. 8.).

In stratum IV, the trend in boys is negative or very small until age five; at 6 years of age it is 2 cm per decade, increasing progressively and reaching 3 to 4 cm per decade between 9 and 13 years of age. From that age on, it decreases to approximately 0.5 cm per decade at the end of growth. In the girls of this stratum, the growth before 5 years is inconsistent, since it is negative in some ages and positive in others, with values less than 1 cm per decade. Starting at 6 years it becomes positive and progressively increases until puberty, where it reaches almost 5 cm per decade. From then on, the trend decreases in magnitude and it is approximately 1.4 cm per decade in young adults.

In the boys of stratum V, growth is also less than 1 cm per decade or negative before 5 years of age, and becomes positive at 7 years of age, remaining around 2 to 3 cm per decade until adulthood. In the girls of this stratum, the trend before 6 years of age is negative or almost non-existent. Starting at 6 years it is above 1 cm per decade and progressively increases until it reaches between 3 and 4 cm per decade during puberty, after which it decreases to only 1 cm per decade in adulthood.

Nutritional Assessment

The results of the nutritional assessment in Venezuelan children, with the anthropometric indicators weight for age (WA), height for age (HA) and weight for height (WH) using the international reference standards recommended by WHO (NCHS) with a cutoff point of ± 2 S.D. in the total sample, between 0 to 96 months, show that the overall deficits defined by the three indicators varied between 2 and 6 %. These percentages, especially the ones corresponding to the

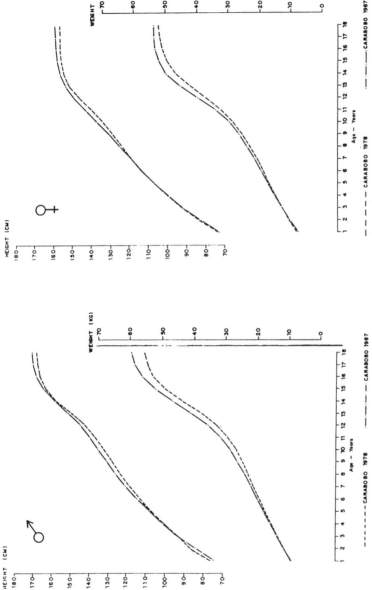

Fig. 7. Median curves obtained by fitting the PB1 model to cross-sectional data (height and weight) of boys - from Carabobo state in 1978 (N: 1296, ----) and - 1987 (N: 1242,-·-·-).

Fig. 8. Median curves obtained by fitting the PB1 model to cross-sectional (height and weight) of girls from Carabobo state in 1978 (N: 1405, ----) and 1987 - (N: 1345,-·-·-).

indicator HA are significantly greater than the expected values (2.3% above and below 2 standard deviations in the reference population).

Again, these values are greater in the stratified samples: stratum V results show a nutritional deficit in all the indicators, especially in HA, with a prevalence from 4% to 14%. It is important to point out that the greatest deficits are found in children less than 3 years of age. Hence, it is the youngest age group which is the most vulnerable to critical situations such as the socio-economic crisis of the country in the last few years. These findings indicate that in Venezuela, stunting due to past or chronic malnutrition, is more prevalent than wasting (actual or acute malnutrition).

The overall prevalence of overweight in the sample of strata IV and V is between 2 and 3%, similar to the reference population. In contrast, the upper strata pervalences are in the order of 5% which duplicate those of the reference population.

Severe malnutrition was negligible, but of the children who presented moderate malnutrition, up to 30% belonged to strata IV and V. Undernutrition was particularly high in Zulia and the Midwestern and Northeastern regions. Overweight was most prevalent in social strata I+II+III, with the highest incidence in the Caracas Metropolitan Area and in the Zulia Region.

SUMMARY

PROJECT VENEZUELA, through immunogenetic methods, has found evidence in Venezuelan blood for an admixture of the Caucasoid (white), Mongoloid (asiatic) and Negroid (black) races, independent of social level.

To obtain the population's social stratification, Graffar's Method modified by H. Mendez-Castellano for Venezuela was used. This method was validated through a "Rutinat" program for a " Stepwise Regression Analysis" in order to verify the weight of the variables plus their combination. Furthermore, the method was standardized in the Pilot Study of 3000 families in Carabobo State. This stratification has shown the differences in the growth of children according to their social level and also in their physical, neurological and biochemical development as well as in their nutritional and health status.

With regard to nutrition, the most important deficit at a national level was energetic, reaching up to 30% in certain areas and also with regard to Vitamins A and B12 as well as Calcium. These deficits are more evident in stratum IV and especially in stratum V. In contrast, protein intake proved adequate, although this consumption is derived mostly from proteins of vegetable origin. The worstoff areas are the Midwestern and Northeastern regions.

It can be asserted that the genetic endowment of the Venezuelan child is substantially modified by the economic, social and cultural variables and differs according to the social stratum in which he/she lives and grows.

We recommend the systematic use of Social Stratification by our standardized method in all the underdeveloped countries and, also, the multidisciplinary methodology that permits a correlation to be made between childrens' growth and the characteristics of their particular environment.

REFERENCES

Bielicki T (1986). Physical growth as a measure of the economic well being of populations: The twentieth century. In Falkner F, Tanner JM (eds): "Human Growth: A Comprehensive Treatise." New York: Plenum Press, pp 285-305.

Boyden SB (1970). "Adaptation Cultural al Malajuste Biologico". Canberra: Nat. Press.

Eveleth PB, Tanner JM (1976). Worldwide Variation in Human Growth - International Biological Programme 8. Cambridge University Press.

Eveleth PB (1986). Population differences in growth environmental and genetic Factors. In Falkner F, Tanner JM (eds): "Human Growth: A Comprehensive Treatise." New York: Plenum Press, pp 221-239.

Fundacredesa-Corpozulia (1985). Estado Zulia, Proyecto Venezuela (Editorial Servicio Grafico de Caracas)

Fundacredesa (1987a). Area Metropolitana. Proyecto Venezuela (in press)

Fundacredesa (1987b).Region Centroccidental. Proyecto Venezuela (in press).

Graffar M (1956). Une méthode de classification sociales d'échantillons de population. Courrier VI: 445-459.

Graffar M (1957). "Cinq Cents Familles d'une Commune de l'Agglomération Bruxelloise.". Université Libre de Bruxelles. Editions de L'Institut de Sociologie. Solvay.

Graffar M (1974). Reflextions sur l'évaluation des méthodes de classification sociales. In "Compte Rendu de la XII Réunion des Equipes Chargée des Etudes sur la Croissance et le Dévelopment de l'Enfant Normal." Paris.

Graffar M (1976). Reflexiones sobre la evaluacion de los methodos de estratificacion social. In "Traduccion del Frances por la Lic Maria Cristina de Mendez, UCV." Facultad de Humanidades y Educacion. Instituto de Investigaciones Literarias.

Laxague G, Noguera G, Mendez-Castellano H (1986). Investigaciones sobre la consistencia de las variables utilizadas en el metodo Graffar modificado. Aplicacion del "Stepwise Regression Analysis". Arch Venez Puer Ped 49 (3-4):105-110.

Lopez Contreras-Blanco M, Izaguirre-Espinoza I, Macias-Tomei C (1986a). Estudio longitudinal mixto del area metropolitana de Caracas Arch Venez Puer Ped 49 (3-4):156-171.

Lopez Contreras-Blanco M, Landaeta-Jimenez M, Izaguirre-Espinoza I, Macias-Tomei C (1987) Crecimiento y maduracion de los Venezolanos de las regiones Zuliana, Centroccidental, Nororiental y del Area Metropolitana de Caracas. In Mendez-Castellano H (ed): "La Familia y el Nino Iberoamericano y del Caribe." 1er Simposio, Caracas: (in press).

Lopez Contreras-Blanco M, Landaeta-Jimenez M, Mendez-Castellano H (1989) Secular trend in height and weight: Carabobo, Venezuela, 1978-1987. In Tanner JM, Smith-Gordon (eds): "Perspectives in the Science of Growth and Development." Auxology 88:207-210.

Mendez-Castellano H et coll. (1978) Manual de Procedimientos del Proyecto Venezuela.- FUNDACREDESA.

Mendez-Castellano H, Lopez-Blanco M, Landaeta-Jimenez M, Gonzalez-Tineo A, Pereira I (1986) Estudio transversal de Caracas. Arch Venez Puer Ped 49 (3-4):111-115

Mendez-Castellano H (1982) Metodo Graffar Modificado para Venezuela.- Manual de Procedimientos del Area de Familia. FUNDACREDESA.

Mendez-Castellano H (1985) Aproximacion a la Salud de la Venezuela del Siglo XXI.- Cuadernos Lagoven Serie Siglo XXI, impreso en Venezuela por Refolit C.A., Set.

Mendez-Castellano H, Mendez de MC, Mateo de L, Fontaine R, Manrique de B et coll (1970). Investigacion Sobre el Patron Educativo de la Familia Venezolano. Memorias Conferencia Internacional de la Educacion de los Padres. Tomo I, Lig Venezolana de Higiene Mental. Caracas.

Mendez-Castellano MC de, Carrera GL, Proyecto Venezuela (1979) Una Muestra de Aspectos Socioculturales de la Familia en Venezuela-Trabajo presentado ante el Congreso Iternacional de Auxologia, La Habana, Cuba.

Ossowsky S (1969). Estructura de Clases y Conciencia Social.-Editorial Peninsula, Barcelona.

Tanner JM, Whitehouse RH, Takaishi M (1966). Standards from birth to maturity for height, weight, height velocity and weight velocity: British children 1965, part II. Arch Dis Child 41:454-471.

Tanner JM, Hayashi T, Preece MA, Cameron N (1982). Increase in length of leg relative to trunk in Japanese children and adults from 1957 to 1977: Comparison with British and with Japanese Americans. Ann Hum Biol 9:411-423.

Vallois RH (1964). Les races humaines, Paris, 1944. In Pierre Morel (ed): Cit Antropologia Fisica, Argentina Eudeba: Cap. IV, p 81.

Villerme LR (1829). Memoires sur la taille de l'homme en France. Annales d'Higiene Publique et de Medicine Legale 1:351-399.

Warner W, Meeker M, Fells J (1949). Social Class in America-Chicago, Science Research Associates, Inc.

Wolf E, Clyde R, Mitchell J et coll (1980). Antropologia Social de las Sociedades Complejas - Alianza Editorial S.A., Madrid.

(Mal)Nutrition and the Infant Brain, pages 285–299
© 1990 Wiley-Liss, Inc.

NEUROLOGICAL DEVELOPMENT AND NOURISHMENT IN VENEZUELAN CHILDREN

Nancy Angulo-Rodriguez, Armando Sanchez, Yudieth Alizo, Marilyn Cabedo

Special Research Division of Pediatric Neurology. Family Nutrition Research Division. FUNDACREDESA, P.O. BOX 61660. Chacao, Caracas. Venezuela. Mailing Address: Dra. Nancy Angulo de Rodriguez, Apartado 80474. Codigo 1080-A Caracas, Venezuela.

This paper analyzes the neurological development of an apparently healthy population of Venezuelan children in relation to family group characteristics, and their socioeconomic class , within the context of geographical and cultural affiliation. The report forms part of Project Venezuela, a multidisciplinary national health study of how biological, social and cultural variables influence growth and development patterns of children.

The hypothesis postulates that genetic variations (if any) *are not* the major factor in observed differences in normal child growth and development, whereas the environment together with nutrition or food intake, *are* important variables in determining the final outcome. The problem is complex because the interaction between man and the environment is multifaceted. Thus when considering nutrition, the degree of interaction depends on food availability, in general, as well as on the specific patterns of consumption dictated by socioeconomic differences between groups within any one region.

Since ancient Greek times, the phenomenon of growth and development has been a subject of study. Although we still do not have all of the answers, updating of 19th century theories has led to a consensus that the DNA directs the overall (similar) pattern of development of each child and that it is programmed as an age- related sequence of events which changes as a function of time. Materialistic determinism as an explanation for differences in functional development has been proposed by some authors (Prechtl, 1978; Connoly 1981). Nevertheless, the concept of probability (opportunity) has come to play an increasingly important role in theories of child development; this concept has been interpreted by Waddington (1977) in his idea of rheostasis. Rheostasis refers to the existence of a guide for the initiation of change; one which is restricted by genetic predetermination but which is also variable by chance in the course of development. The concept of probalibity, as opposed to functional predetermination, offers a point of view which may provide a better understanding of the many complex, yet subtle, influences which affect development.

This study attempts to uncover the relative importance of some of the variables which are implicated in the process of neurological maturation. At least in part, such maturation is defined by the degree of neurophysiological integration achieved during the various stages of perinatal to adult development. Neurological maturation was determined by a series of simple finger/hand coordination tests, and the achievement score for each test group was compared to a previously determined norm of performance within specified age groups. This permitted the establishment of criteria for average maturation, slow maturation or underdevelopment (suspect or pathological responses).

METHODOLOGY

The sample groups were drawn from the Venezuelan population under forty years of age. Venezuelan children of foreign mothers were excluded in order to control for culturally influenced food and life-style habits. Geographically, it includes the entire country except for the forest-dwelling indigenous population.

The sample design for Project Venezuela is a probabilistic multistage cross-sectional study with socioeconomic stratification (Graffar's method modified by H. Mendez, 1978). The selection of the stages followed the politic-territorial division of the country as established during the 1971 census. This design guaranteed inclusion of all age groups of each sex, and permitted to control for differences between administrative regionalities as well as for urban and rural areas.

The nationwide sample comprised 75000 individuals, divided into groups in proportion to the estimated population of each geographic region and/or Federal District, according to the figures provided by the Central Statistical and Data Processing Office (O.C.E.I.). The single research unit is defined by the individual within the family, thus ensuring that the subject is considered within the context of his or her environmental conditions. In consequence, an individual-home relationship classification is established which provides a basic focal point for both the project and its fundamental hypothesis.

The neuropediatric sample used for this report was chosen from the Mid-Western (WCR) and North-East (NER) Regions of the country. A total of 6 184 children of both sexes, between the ages of three (3) and fourteen (14) years were examineted. Forty two percent (42%) of the sample came from the North-East region and fifty eigth percent (58%) from the Mid-Western region (Table 1).

The sample for the nutritional part of the study is represented by 1213 families in the Mid-Western region and 1013 families from the North-East, 54.6% and 45.4% of the total sample respectively (Table 2).

TABLE 1. Sample Size of Individuals Subjected to Neuropediatric Examination, Classified According to Socio-Economic Status (Resources)

Socio-Economic Resources	I-II-III	IV	V	Total
North-East	316 (12%)	802 (31%)	1505 (57%)	2623
		Fraction of total sample:		42%
Mid-West	508 (14%)	1388 (39%)	1665 (47%)	3561
		Fraction of total sample:		58%

TABLE 2. The Number of Families Within Various Socio-Economic Classes Interviewed to Ascertain Nutritional Status

Socio-Economic Resources	I-II-III	IV	V	Total
North-East	116 (12%)	348 (34%)	549 (54%)	1013
		Fraction of total sample:		45%
Mid-West	187 (15%)	499 (41%)	527 (44%)	1213
		Fraction of total sample:		55%

In the North-East region a group of thirty-three subjects from socioeconomic groups IV and V were suspected to have minor neurological pathologies. The sub-sample was matched to a control group of thirty two apparently healthy subjects, selected from the same area by a multistage sampling procedure. This was done in order to measure the degree of relationship between the variables being analyzed (Table 3).

With reference to the neuropediatric research data we have classified children between three (3) and fourteen (14) years of age as "school children" in order to obtain age related information from responses to the test protocol. This methodology was adapted and standardized for research by N.Angulo-Rodriguez (1976-1980).

The variables discussed in this report were defined by the three following procedures:

TABLE 3. Classification of a Small Group of Children with Some Neurological Dysfunction, and Matched Control Group.

Soc. Econ. Status	IV	V	n
Neurol. dysfunction	39%	61%	33
No dysfunction	38%	62%	32

Motor coordination

(i)   Fingertip Touching Test
(ii) Finger Opposition Test
(iii) Mirror Movements

The norm for the age at which a perfect score for the fingertip touching test can be achieved was set at 5 years, while a delay until 5-7 years to obtain such a score was considered to indicate slowed maturation. This criterion was selected based on data from two previous appraisals (Rebollo, 1973; Lefevre, 1972) which established that 3 years is the earliest age at which this test can be successfully executed, irrespective of perfection achieved. Moreover, another preceding study of children in the "high" socioeconomic group, showed that already 80% were able to perform the test correctly by 4 years of age (Conicit-Fundacredesa Study, 1977; in press). [It should be noted that of the total number of children tested in the NE region during this study, only 75% could perform the exercise at the age of 5 years].

Nutrition

To measure the food intake, field workers visited the home in the morning to weigh the food expected to be consumed. They then returned in the afternoon to evaluate how much of that food was consumed by the subject. This methodology was conceived and standardized for Project Venezuela (Manuales de Procedimientos, 1976).

Survey Control

To assure proper and uniform executions of procedures, periodic reviews were made in both regions to maintain the quality of field workers and their performance. These reviews, in turn, were subjected to careful further appraisal at the Research Center.

RESULTS

NEUROPEDIATRIC EXAMINATION

(i) Fingertip Touching Test

The analysis of the responses in the North-East region revealed that almost fifty percent (50%) of the three and one-half years old subjects completed the test correctly. Thirty five percent (35%) of the subjects made one or two mistakes, and fifteen percent (15%) showed lack of coordination. By age 5 years, 75% demonstrated a perfect or near perfect response, with only 5% being judged to have impaired coordination.

In the Mid-Western region only twenty five percent (25%) of the subjects at 3.5 years responded optimally. Forty nine percent (49%) fell into the intermediate range while the incidence of lack of coordination was twenty five percent (25%). The mean age of the group achieving a perfect score was just over five (5.25) years. The age at which 75% of the children scored a perfect response was 6 years, when 20% still made one or two mistakes; the mistakes were suspected to be due to minor neurological impairment. Five percent of this sample continued to demonstrate impaired coordination, even at 7 years.

Among the 10 years old children, in the North-East region an imperfect coordination response was found in one percent (1%), and was also found in the Mid-Western region (Figs. 1, 2). There is thus a two years difference in the distribution of the responses between the North-East region and the Mid-Western region, with children in the North-East region developing faster until the age of eight than in the Mid-Western region.

When based on behavioural parameters, in the Mid-Western region significant statistical differences by social class exist between the three and four years old, in their ability to perform the test correctly at an early age, even when taking into account the more rapid maturation in the upper social classes: ($chi^2 =$ 17.03 between groups I-II-III and IV; between groups I-II-III and V, chi^2 (95%) = 16.02).

The results classified according to the socioeconomic status showed differences in the quality of response and in maturation, with group IV in the North-East region between three and four years demonstrating the fastest development (Fig. 3; % mistakes). Thirteen percent (13%) of the group V subjects at eight (8) years of age showed minor neurological disorders. Nevertheless, even in the I, II, III classes still 4% showed signs of neurological deficits (Fig. 4; % mistakes).

(ii) Finger Opposition Test

This test, compared with the fingertip touching test, can be considered to demonstrate a more advanced stage of neurological maturation. In the North-

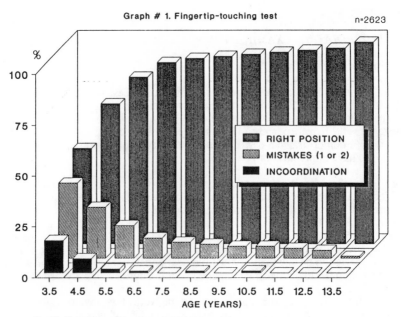

Graph # 1. Fingertip-touching test

n=2623

North-Eastern region. Neurological Maturation

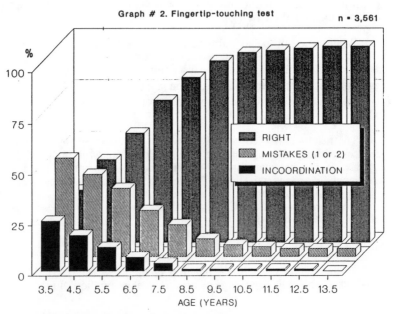

Graph # 2. Fingertip-touching test

n = 3,561

Mid-Western region. Neurological Maturation

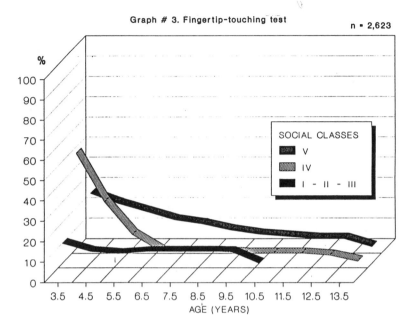

Graph # 3. Fingertip-touching test   n = 2,623

North-Eastern region.Differences by socio-economical classes

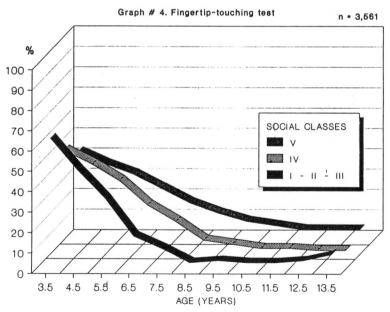

Graph # 4. Fingertip-touching test   n = 3,561

Mid-Western region. Differences by socio-economical classes

Graph # 5. Finger opposition test

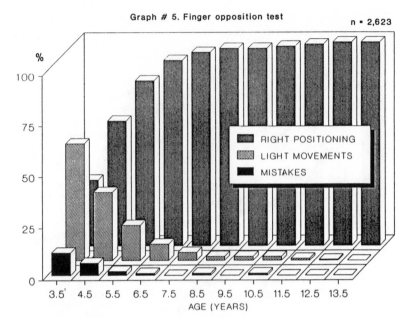

North-Eastern region. Neurological Maturation

Graph # 6. Finger opposition test

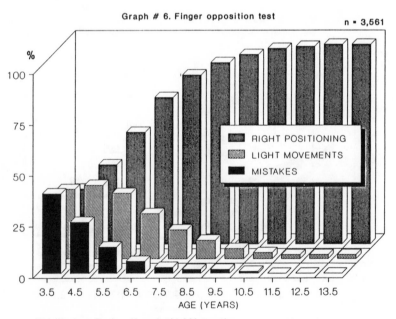

Mid-Western Region. Neurological Maturation

East region 50% of 4.25 years old children performed the test correctly, while in the Mid-Western region this mean score was only reached at 5.25 years. The seventy fifth percentile was reached at five and one-quarter (5.25) years in the NER, and at six and three-quarter (6.75) years in the WCR.

A wavering trajectory showed up in 22% of the six years old children, decreasing to 2% in eleven years old. In the North-East region mistakes were present in 1% of the subjects between six and ten years of age, while in the Mid-Western region it appeared in 5% of the six and three-quarter years old subjects; in both regional samples the score progressively improved until by age 10 it reached 99% . Regional differences were no longer apparent at this age (Figs. 5, 6).

(iii) Mirror Movements

The median age in the North-East region was five and one-half (5.50) years for the existence of moderate mirror movements, while 25% of nine and one-half years old (9.50) reached a perfect score. These findings contrasted with those of the Mid-Western region where the 25% perfect score was reached only at 11 years median age was 9 years (Fig. 7; % mistakes).

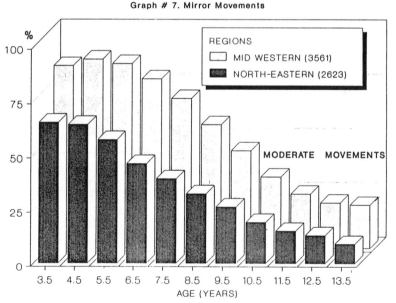

Graph # 7. Mirror Movements

Compared differences among regions

ANALYSIS OF A SUB-SAMPLE OF NORMAL AND PATHOLOGICAL CASES

In the North-East, a sub-sample from groups IV and V demonstrated suspected or obvious neurological pathology. Only two children (3, 4 years) in this group were classified as slow maturers; the four year old subject was diagnosed as moderately retarded. The rest of the subjects were classified as having Minor Neurological Dysfunction (MND), defined by a lack of fine motor coordination. A subgroup classified as having Minimal Brain Dysfunction (MBD) showed changes in behavior and may have had some poorly defined laterality problems (laterality refers to right or left sided preference to perform a task). The majority of individuals also showed minor anatomical abnormalities such as changes in the ear lobe, low placement of the ears, or epicanthal irregularities. Cases of flat feet and scoliosis were also found. The selection of the normal subjects was governed by the socioeconomic distribution of the pathological cases (See Table 3).

The data shows that in 25% of children belonging to the lowest socio-economic group (V) protein intake is inadequate, whereas only 8% of group IV children demonstrated such malnutrition. In contrast, over 65% of these children had an insufficient caloric intake; the incidence of caloric undernutrition was even higher in the least privileged group (Table 4).

NUTRITIONAL DATA

In the appraisal of daily dietary intake, both the child as well as the other members of its family group were included.

Differences were found in the caloric deficit in the underpriviliged social classes. There was an adequate intake of the protein in both regions,although it was lower in group V of the North-East region. Daily caloric intake varied inversely with socioeconomic status (Table 5). There was a deficit of twenty-four percent (24%) in the North-East region and of seventeen percent (17%)

TABLE 4. Undernutrition[1] in NER Population of Children with Neurological Impairment, and a Matched Control Group (65 total).

Soc. Econ. Status	IV	V
PROTEIN	8%	25%
CALORIES	68%	75%
Group size	25	40

[1] Less than 80% dietary requirement

in the Mid-Western region. Vitamin intake was lower in the Mid-Western region. Thus, there are important differences between the middle and the lower status groups, and this difference is even more accentuated when comparing the two extreme groups on the socioeconomic distribution curve. However, protein intake appeared nevertheless not a limiting factor in the growth process (Figs. 8, 9).

TABLE 5. Daily Caloric Intake (Kcal) According to Socio-Economic Status

Socio-Economic Resources	I-II-III	IV	V
North-East	2 083	1 927	1700
Mid-Western	2 245	2 137	1855

Observation of the eating habits revealed that in the North-East region, fish was eaten instead of beef and there was a larger intake of rice and a kind of bean known as Cajanus *indicus spreng* from the leguminous family. In the lowest social classes of the Mid-Western region most of the protein was derived from vegetable sources, more corn than rice and less fruit was consumed. No other differences in types of food were noted. In both regions, group V showed a significant deficit of vitamin A, some of the B complex, and calcium.

DISCUSSION

The use of a developmentally-oriented neurological examination permitted an evaluation of neurological maturation, appropriate for a specified age, according to three variables. Thus, the fingertip touching test can be achieved at an early age (5 years) whereas the ability to correctly score on the mirror movement test is reached only around 9 years; the finger opposition test defines an intermediate age of maturation (7 years).

Differences in neurological competence with age reflect important differences in regional and socioeconomic conditions. In the North-East region correct responses were obtained two years earlier than in the Mid-Western region. In groups I, II, III (high to middle status) maturation arrives at five (5) years of age; it is delayed in the lower socioeconomic children, where a greater number of suspected neuropathologies were found on all tests. (Project Venezuela - Neuropediatric Area 1976-1988)

The tests described here have been shown to be sensitive to variations with age, although they have not yet demonstrated the limits of sensitivity to denote chronological maturation; they do however appear to distinguish between differences in the rate of maturation as a function of social and economic factors

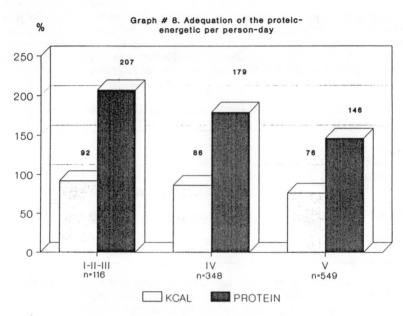

Graph # 8. Adequation of the proteic-
energetic per person-day

North-East region. Differences by socio-economical classes

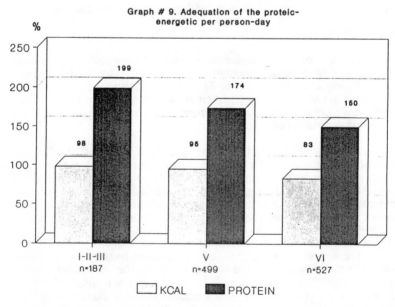

Graph # 9. Adequation of the proteic-
energetic per person-day

Mid-Western region. Differences by socio-economical classes

and they may also be indicators of child health. The tests appear to evaluate short-term developmental changes quite well, especially in the earlier years. Since the tests are relatively simple, non specialized personel can also interpret the results, to obtain an index of overall development of the nervous system in relation to age. The responses used for each variable were developmentally-related which permits the establishment of the normal range of neurological competence for each age group.

An Index of Neurological Maturation

The index was elaborated by assigning a value of 1 to each variable which is used to judge maturation for each age group. Thus, perfect comprehension of the commands (i.e. "intellectual maturation") plus the execution without error of the 3 neurological tests was assigned a theoretical score of 4. Table 6 shows the scores actually obtained during normal development.

TABLE 6. An Index of Neurological Maturation: Age-Related Ability to comprehend and to Perform 3 Neurological Tests Perfectly (= score of 4).

AGE	SCORE
3-3.99	1.20
4-4.99	1.82
5-5.99	2.34
6-6.99	2.69
7-7.99	2.96
8-8.99	3.15
9-9.99	3.33
10-10.99	3.45
11-11.99	3.55
12-12.99	3.60
13-13.99	3.64

Differences in maturation found between the two regions studied can be explained in the first place by geographic characteristics. The North-East has an extensive, largely inhabited, coast line; an abundance of sea food permits easy access to protein from an early age on. Thus, even children of group V (the marginal economic group) in the North-East come from families of fishermen or of people with easy access to low-priced fish. Not only is this region a highly valuable fishing zone but, in the past few years, there has been an important development of the petroleum industry in some of the states that make up the region. In general then, group V in NER nutritionally and (perhaps) economically appears less underpriviliged when compared to similar groups in certain other parts of Venezuela, for example the Mid-West.

Although the Mid-Western region has an extensive coast line, it is mainly uninhabited; its principal economy is agriculture. The major part of the protein consumed by the social group V comes from vegetable sources.

In our judgement it is important to consider the growth, neurological integration and emotional development of the child in the context of its total environment: nutrition, educational opportunities, environmental pollution, available health services, and the mental health of its immediate community. Only by appraising all these factors and their interaction, will it be possible for the government to establish social and medical guidelines which permit optimal development of the child while yet respecting cultural and traditional values by which success is measured. It is the eventual goal of Project Venezuela to develop easy-to-perform and universally applicable methods to appraise child development, so that adequate measures can be taken to prevent permanent damage. This report illustrates one example of the efforts now under way to reach these goals in Venezuela.

ACKNOWLEDGEMENT

Recognition to the Social Nutrition and Statistical and Computer Departments of Fundacredesa, and special thanks to M Fossi, M Alvarez, R Colmenares, D Espejo and L Swartz.

REFERENCES

Angulo-Rodriguez N (1978). Metodología para Evaluar el Desarrollo Neurológico. Fundacredesa: Manual de Procedimientos del Proyecto Venezuela. Tomo II, pp 235-251.
Angulo-Rodriguez N (1976). Evaluacion Neuropediatrica del Pre- Escolar. Monografía de las Jornadas Nacionales de Neurología. Sociedad Venezolana de Neurología. Capitulo VIII, pp 1-16
Barrera MG (1958). Desarrollo psicomotriz del nino Venezolano. Archivos Venezolanos de Puericultura y Pediatría 68:131-143.
Bax Martin (1976). Developmental assessment is a necessity. Proc Roy Soc Med 69: 378-388
Connolly KJ (1981). "Maturation and Development. Biological and Psychological Perspectives". S.I.M.P. C.M.D. 77/88, pp 216-230.
Constanti M (1979). Fallas y peligros del uso de los modelos importados en los países sub-desarrollados del Tercer Mundo. Acta Científica Venezolana 30 : 4-6.
Eveleth PR, Tanner JM (1979). "Worldwide Variation in Human Growth." Cambridge: University Press, pp 222-240
Lefevre AB (1972). Examen Neurológico Evolutivo del Pre-Escolar Normal. Monografías Médicas. Serie Pediátrica 5. Brasil (Sao Paulo)
Mendez-Castellano H (1978). Método de Graffar Modificado. Fundacredesa: Manual de Procedimientos del Proyecto Venezuela, Tomo I, pp 198-213.
Prechtl H (1978). Minimal brain syndrome and the plasticity of the nervous system, Adv Biol Psych 1: 96-105.
Rebollo MA, Cardies S (1973). "Semiología del Sistema Nervioso en el Nino." Montevideo: Editorial Delta, pp 139-248.

Touwen BCT (1980). "Examination of the Child with Minor Neurological Dysfunction", 2nd. Edition. SIMP. C.D.M. 71.

Waddington CH (1957). "The Strategy of the Genes." London: George, Allen and Unwin.

DISCUSSION

Q (van Gelder): This is more a congratulation than a question. The data offers all kinds of possibilities to obtain some hard answers. The results are also rather frightening, to see how clear the differences are. I do have a question also.

The privileged group, I, II, III of the Mid West and of the North East, is there (nevertheless) a difference in the diet. Because you showed in one of your figures that children at a young age of even the most privileged group of the Mid Western Region were still performing poorer than those in the North East. I wonder what this is due to.

A: Yes, there is a striking difference. In this age group (3-5.5 years). It may be the difference in diet.

Q (Rassin): You have not much addressed the early feeding history of these children. I know that in many countries with large degrees of malnutrition, formula feeding is presenting a real problem. Because the cost of formula is usually such that these families cannot afford to properly feed the children, so you get a real exacerbation of the situation with respect to malnutrition. I am just curious whether you have looked at your populations in terms of the types of feeding during the first year of life and what kind of impact that had on later outcome. Do you know what the distribution is (in these groups) with respect to breast versus bottle feeding, especially among the various different socioeconomic groups.

A: Only 3% in the population are fed exclusively by breast feeding. The majority of the mothers give formula or other nutrition (milk?) once or twice a day, and mixed with formula.

Q (Rassin): But can they (all) afford the formula. Can they buy it?

A: Actually many can't, but there is a maternity program for those in the lower socieconomic classes. The formula is given free to the mothers (also vaccination); but now it (the program) is less efficient.

(Mal)Nutrition and the Infant Brain, pages 301–311
© 1990 Wiley-Liss, Inc.

ROLE OF GOVERNMENT IN NUTRITIONAL ADVICE

Alfred E. Harper

Departments of Nutritional Sciences and Biochemistry, University of Wisconsin, 1415 Linden Drive, Madison, WI 53706

Protection of natural resources, at least from foreign encroachment, has been an accepted function of governing authorities from time immemorial. Those in power recognized early that armed forces were an essential resource for the protection of other resources and that, to function effectively, such forces required an adequate supply of food. It should not be surprising, therefore, that concern over the food needs of the armed forces has been a major impetus for involvement of governments in nutritional advice (Leitch, 1942; Harper, 1985).

Despite early recognition of the importance of food and diet in maintaining an effective fighting force, governing bodies seem, until recently, to have viewed the population as a whole as an expendable and renewable resource. This view changed only slowly over time. The shift from an agrarian to an industrial society led to the realization that maintenance of some tolerable state of nutrition of working people had economic value as a means of maintaining productivity and social stability. The steadily increasing complexity of social organization and the vast expansion of knowledge that have occurred since the beginning of the industrial revolution in the 18th century, forced governments to assume increasing responsibility for many aspects of life that earlier were left to individual initiative and action. Also, as political institutions have become more democratic, governments have accepted greater and greater responsibility for ensuring the well-being of the individual and, thereby, of the population as a whole. Nowhere is this more evident than in the area of health and medical care of which nutritional advice is a part.

Since the end of World War II, most industrialized nations have established comprehensive programs of medical care for their entire populations, the USA and South Africa being notable exceptions. Even where national medical coverage has not been implemented, health care programs have become extensive; but, with costs of medical care rising steadily, governments have begun to search for ways of curtailing these costs. One approach for accomplishing this, that has attracted the attention of politicians and government officials, is the idea of instituting programs of diet modification for the prevention of major diseases (U.S. Senate Select Committee, 1977; U.S. DHEW, 1979; U.S. DHHS, 1988). This represents a marked change in the role of government in nutritional advice. It has led to controversy and adversarial exchanges over the appropriate role of government in offering nutritional advice (Ahrens et al., 1979; Harper, 1981a; Truswell, 1987).

My approach in dealing with this topic will be to: outline briefly the evolution of the role of governments in providing nutritional advice; discuss changes that have occurred in the state of health and major disease problems during this century; and then, comment on the dilemma this has posed in establishing what is appropriate nutritional advice.

Evolution of dietary advice

The beginning of a role by government agencies in nutritional advice can be traced to the action of British naval authorities in 1796 to include "lime" juice in naval rations to protect sailors from scurvy. Leitch (1942) has identified the first formal action to institute a dietary recommendation as passage of the Merchant Seaman's Act in Britain in 1835 by which provision of lime juice in the rations of the mercantile service was made compulsory. Involvement of government in nutritional advice was expanded when starvation and malnutrition became prevalent among the unemployed during the economic recession of the early 1860s. The Privy Council at that time sought information about the amount of food that would be needed to relieve the problem at least cost. Using the best scientific knowledge then available, Dr. Edward Smith responded with the advice that it could be done by providing each person daily with food yielding about 3000 kcal of energy and 80 g of protein (Leitch, 1942; Harper, 1985). The U.S. Department of Agriculture (U.S. DA), in 1895, proposed that foods be evaluated for their contribution to nutrition on the basis of the amounts of energy and protein they provided per unit cost. Dietary advice by governments during the 19th and into the early part of the 20th century seems to have been directed mainly toward advice on how to preserve the working capacity of the armed services and the labor force at least cost.

New directions in nutritional advice evolved from the discoveries made during the period between 1910-1920 that many minor constituents of foods were essential nutrients and from efforts to solve the problems of providing a nutritionally adequate supply of food for the populations of European countries during and immediately following World War I. A Food Committee of the British Royal Society that examined human nutritional requirements during that time recommended that "protective foods," such as fruits and vegetables, be included in all diets and that milk be included in the diets of all children (Leitch, 1942). In the USA, a Cooperative Extension Service was established during this period and given the responsibility of providing nutritional advice to the public. The first publication of the Service dealt with "Food for Young Children" (1916); and, in 1917, it made recommendations for avoiding nutritional deficiency diseases by selecting a variety of foods from among 5 different food groups (U.S. DHHS, 1988). In 1924, in the state of Michigan, iodine was added to the salt supply as a means of preventing goiter. This was a highly successful program in that the incidence of goiter fell from 38% to 9% within 5 years. Also during this time recommendations were made for adding vitamin D to milk to prevent rickets. These actions extended government involvement in nutritional advice to programs for prevention of dietary deficiency diseases in the entire population (Sebrell, 1974).

Efforts to relieve food and health problems created by the severe depression of the 1930s, and concern about meeting nutritional needs of both the armed forces and the civilian population after the outbreak of World War II, provided the impetus for further involvement of governments in nutritional advice. The Health Organization of the League of Nations had begun to compile information about human nutritional needs and the nutritional status of populations after the end of World War I. These efforts were intensified after 1929 when the effects of the depression in reducing the availability of food became evident. The League transmitted the information it had compiled to member nations and encouraged them to establish national councils on nutrition and health.

During the 1930s, the U.S. DA, in conjunction with its food distribution programs, devised a dietary standard based on known nutritional needs to evaluate the nutritional quality of foods and diets. Also, it was advising the public to consume a diet that included a variety of foods selected from among 12 different food groups in a pattern designed to provide adequate quantities of the various essential nutrients, not just amounts needed to prevent deficiency diseases (Stiebling and Clark, 1939). Governments had thus assumed responsibility for providing advice to the public for improving the state of nutrition of the population as a whole.

In 1940, as part of the national defense effort, the U.S. government initiated action to form a Committee on Food and Nutrition. This Committee, which later became the Food and Nutrition Board, proposed a set of standards - Recommended Dietary Allowances - for appropriate intakes of essential nutrients. In May of 1941, this standard was accepted as the basis for developing programs of nutritional advice for the nation at a National Nutrition Conference called by President Franklin Roosevelt. The U.S. DA translated the scientific information about nutrient needs into the easily understood language of foods. This was done by grouping foods into four major groups according to their nutrient content so that selection of appropriate numbers of servings from among these groups would ensure that the quantities of essential nutrients recommended in the dietary standard (Recommended Dietary Allowances) could be met without consuming an excess of energy (calories) (Harper, 1987a). This represented involvement of government in providing advice for meeting nutritional needs for health for the entire population. Nutritional advice of this type evolved in parallel in Canada, the United Kingdom, several other countries, and the Food and Agriculture and World Health Organizations (FAO/WHO). This approach has now been adopted by nations throughout the world (Truswell, 1983, 1987).

To recapitulate, dietary guidance by governments underwent extensive transformation during the period between 1800 and 1950 from: 1) recommendations for preventing scurvy, and malnutrition associated with food deprivation; to, 2) recommendations for maintaining the working capacity of the armed services and the labor force; 3) preventing various nutritional deficiency diseases; 4) improving the state of nutrition of the population; and finally, 5) to providing nutritional advice directed toward ensuring that the genetic potential of the individual for growth, development, reproduction, and health generally, would not be jeopardized by nutritional inadequacy (NRC, 1980).

The current guidelines for a nutritionally adequate diet represent the main type of nutritional advice that has been offered to the public by governments during the past 50 years. They were based on scientific knowledge of human requirements for essential nutrients and of the nutrient content of foods and have been used as the basis for programs to improve the nutritional quality of the food supply. The process by which the guidelines were developed represents an example of the evolution of sound health policy based on scientific principles. It has provided the basis for an effective solution for a health problem, nutritional inadequacy, to which the entire population is susceptible and which can be prevented in the entire population by consumption of a nutritionally adequate diet. It is a highly appropriate role for governments.

During the past 20 years, however, new directions in nutritional advice have been evolving (Harper, 1987a; Truswell, 1987). The reason for this is related to the changes that have occurred in the state of health during this century (Harper, 1987b).

Changing health status

At the turn of the century in the industrialized nations, infant mortality exceeded 100/1000 live births, less than 40% of the infants born lived to 65 years of age, life expectancy was less than 50 years, infectious diseases were major causes of death, and in the U.S., as recently as the 1930s, several thousand people died each year from nutritional deficiency diseases such as pellagra.

As knowledge of nutrition expanded, and as infectious diseases were brought under control through advances in sanitation and immunization, health in the industrialized nations improved steadily (U.S. DHEW, 1979; Harper, 1987b). Infant mortality has declined until it is now about one-tenth of what it was; height at maturity has increased until children now appear to be approaching their genetic potential for growth; close to 80% of newborn infants can now be expected to live for at least 65 years; death rates at all ages have declined steadily; life expectancy has risen from less than 50 years to 75 years (72 for males and 79 for females); and, as a result, the proportion of elderly people in the population has increased from about 4% in 1900 to 12% at the present time.

As these improvements in health have occurred, the major causes of death have changed. Mortality from infectious diseases, which take their highest toll among the young, has declined. Mortality from chronic and degenerative diseases and disorders, diseases mainly of people living to old age, has risen.

Cardiovascular diseases and cancer now account for about two-thirds of all deaths in most industrialized countries (Harper, 1987b).

During the period of time over which these changes occurred, the proportion of fat in the diet rose from less than 30% to about 40% of total energy (calories). Although the rise in the fat content of the diet has been associated with steadily improving health, increasing life expectancy and an increase in the proportion of people living to old age, these relationships seem to have attracted little attention. Epidemiologic studies in the 1950s of the populations of several countries in which associations between a high fat intake and high mortality from heart disease and some major cancers were observed, have attracted much more attention. The association is not nearly as strong as is usually claimed (Feinstein, 1987); nonetheless, in experimental studies on animals and human subjects, associations have been observed between saturated fat intake and serum cholesterol concentration, and between serum cholesterol concentration and increased risk of developing atherosclerosis.

This type of information provided the basis for claims that changes in diet during this century were responsible for an epidemic of chronic and degenerative diseases, especially heart disease and cancer. This in turn led to a series of proposals for dietary guidelines for prevention of chronic and degenerative diseases (US Senate, 1977). Seventeen sets of such guidelines have been summarized by Truswell (1987). The emphasis in all of them is, in the main, on dietary advice to reduce consumption of fat (to 30-35% of total energy), saturated fatty acids (to 10% of total energy), cholesterol (to 300 mg/day), and salt (to about 5 g/day).

Such guidelines have proliferated as if mortality from these diseases were the only meaningful measure of the state of nutrition and health of the population. Last year the US Surgeon General published a 700 page report on "Nutrition and Health" (USDHHS, 1988) and the US National Research Council has released a summary of an equally voluminous report on "Diet and Health" soon to be published (NRC, 1989). The conclusions and recommendations of these reports differ insignificantly from those of the previous reports (Truswell, 1987). Government agencies in several countries have adopted dietary guidelines resembling these, but usually less specific and quantitative, as part of their health policy.

Chronic and degenerative diseases in pespective

Such guidelines represent a change in the underlying basis for nutritional advice offered by governments to the public, and a shift in the approaches that have been used in developing public health programs. Problems encountered in applying a public health approach to medical problems have been discussed by Ahrens (1979), Oliver (1986), Olson (1986), James (1981), Harper, (1987b) and Simopoulos (1987).

For diseases to which the entire population is potentially susceptible, e.g. nutritional deficiency and infectious diseases, public health programs have been directed toward instituting measures that will protect the entire population.

Guidelines for a nutritionally adequate diet for the entire population, together with programs for fortification of the food supply with iodine to prevent goiter, vitamin D to prevent rickets, and niacin to prevent pellagra, represent examples of this approach which have been highly successful.

For diseases and disorders that are basically medical or clinical problems of individuals or segments of the population, not of the population as a whole, public health programs have been directed toward identification of individuals who have the disease, or are at high risk of developing it, and encouragement of those who are identified to undergo appropriate treatment by following guidelines designed specifically for them. Tuberculosis is an example of such a disease in which specific tests, chest x-rays, tuberculin tests, have been used to identify individuals who have been exposed to the disease. A similar approach is being used widely now to identify, through blood pressure measurements, individuals with, or susceptible to, hypertension so they can be encouraged to accept specific treatment.

Recommending general dietary guidelines as measures for controlling chronic and degenerative diseases and disorders - heart disease, hypertension, stroke, cancer, osteoporosis, diabetes - resembles the approach used successfully to control dietary deficiency diseases to which the entire population is susceptible. There are, however, major differences between these two types of health problems: first, in the adequacy of the base of knowledge about causes, treatment and prevention of them; second, in the extent to which the population is susceptible to them.

Dietary deficiency diseases, like infectious diseases, have specific, readily identifiable causes. Preventive measures for them are, therefore, specific and highly effective. Chronic and degenerative diseases are not single disease entities; they are highly heterogeneous. They do not have specific, readily identifiable causes; they are multifactorial. Programs to control them must, therefore, focus on controlling "risk factors" - personal and environmental characteristics associated with an increased incidence of the disease - of which there are many, and which may or may not be causative agents.

The known risk factors for heart disease taken together account for only about half the "risk" of developing the disease. Also, although diet modification may reduce serum cholesterol concentration in experimental and clinical tests, in intervention trials it has not proven to be a highly effective preventive measure; it has not been shown to reduce total mortality even in trials with high risk individuals in which modest reductions in infarcts and mortality were observed (Olson, 1986; Oliver, 1986). This suggests that decreased mortality from one chronic disease may be accompanied by increased mortality from another. Also, a high proportion of those susceptible to such diseases require, not just simple dietary advice, but comprehensive medical care including drug treatment. In addition, despite great differences in mortality from various chronic and degenerative diseases and in the types of diets consumed in different countries, life expectancy differs little from one to another (e.g. Japan vs The Netherlands; France vs the US; Harper, 1987b).

Secondly, the entire population is susceptible to dietary deficiency diseases and the entire population can be protected from them by following a set of dietary guidelines. Chronic and degenerative diseases affect only segments of the population. Most, if not all, of these diseases have a strong genetic component. In a study in Utah, over half of the deaths from heart disease in individuals under 55 years of age occurred among only 2-5% of families (Williams, 1988). Individual variability in susceptibility to them is great. The increasing proportion of deaths from heart disease and cancer is associated closely with the increase in the proportion of elderly people in the population. At least half of the deaths from heart disease, for example, occur among people 75 years of age or older and 35% or more among those over 80. Predictions of who will and who will not develop them are neither accurate nor reliable and after the age of 65 years, an age to which 80% of newborn infants survive, even major risk factors, such as serum cholesterol concentration, are not reliable predictors (Olson, 1986; Oliver, 1986).

All of this should make us pause to consider whether simple dietary guidance for control of these diseases, with its implied promise of effectiveness, is appropriate public health policy or an appropriate type of advice for governments to offer.

Dietary Guidelines for Health

It is important, nonetheless, that we have a set of dietary guidelines for maintenance of health; it is appropriate for the government to offer such advice as part of its effort to protect the health of infants, growing children, pregnant women, and the population as a whole. The major guidelines needed are for meeting essential nutrient needs, and how to accomplish this through appropriate selection of foods, and for moderation in intake in order to maintain appropriate body weight. In the US and several other countries, additional dietary guidelines have been proposed (U.S. DA/U.S. DHHS, 1985). These usually include recommendations to reduce fat, saturated fat, cholesterol, sugar and sodium consumption and increase starch and fiber consumption. This has been influenced by pressures to institute guidelines for disease prevention, but the recommendations have usually been less specific, with claims for disease prevention being modest (Truswell, 1987). It is not inappropriate for governments to include with the advice for meeting essential nutrient needs without exceeding energy needs, a recommendation to consume fat, the major source of energy in the diet, only in moderation; and to consume a variety of fats in order to ensure that the supply of essential fatty acids will be adequate and that the balance of fatty acids will be appropriate. To recommend curtailing cholesterol intake, I consider to be a therapeutic recommendation, needed only for individuals who have defects of lipid metabolism.

Recommendations for consuming a substantial amount of starch and a moderate amount of fiber are, in essence, recommendations for variety in carbohydrate consumption. They represent an extension of the recommendation for consumption of a diet in which a substantial part of the energy needs come from fruits, vegetables and grain products. These foods provide bulky carbohydrates and fiber which are helpful for maintaining efficient gastrointestinal function; they are also sources of several important essential nutrients. A recommendation for maintaining sodium intake within the safe and adequate limits as established by the RDA is also appropriate, especially for the elderly for limiting the load on the kidney, as is a recommendation to avoid an excessive intake of any individual nutrient, some of which may be toxic when consumed in excessive amounts.

These recommendations can all be accepted as guidelines for maintenance of health. They tend to be oversimplified but, when supplemented with advice for appropriate modifications for young children, pregnant women and the elderly, provide safe and effective guidelines for healthful diets for the entire population. There is no sound scientific basis, however, for promoting them as measures for controlling specific chronic and degenerative diseases.

In my judgment, it is deceptive and misleading for governments to propose general dietary guidelines for the nation with the implication that following them will prevent chronic and degenerative diseases unless there is convincing scientific evidence of the effectiveness and safety of the recommendations. Despite the pressures from many professional health organizations and the conclusions of consensus conferences that dietary guidelines for disease prevention should be instituted, there is deep disagreement over the adequacy of the evidence to support such action.

In making decisions about public policy, factors other than scientific knowledge often take precedence (Harper, 1981b). Sanford Miller (1982), former Director of the Bureau of Foods of the Food and Drug Administration, noted: "when there is conflict, Congress attempts to determine public perception and, as a result, does not necessarily accept the dominant scientific view if it conflicts with public desire." It would be refreshing if government agencies would follow the suggestions of Thomas James (1981), former President of the American Heart Association, and make clear when they are using established knowledge, when they are depending on extrapolation to imply knowledge not established, and when they are speculating about solutions to health problems. It would then be more likely that the advice of Paul Kurtz (1976): "where we do not have sufficient evidence, we ought, if possible, to suspend judgment," would be followed. Philip Handler (1979), late past-president of the US National Academy of Sciences, in expressing his concern about implementation of public policy without adequate scientific evidence, stated: "the necessity for scientific rigor is even greater when scientific evidence is being offered as the basis for formulation of public policy than when it is simply expected to find its way in the market place of accepted scientific understanding."

General dietary guidelines for disease prevention are actually guidelines for reducing the consequences of disease in individuals and specific susceptible populations, not in the general population. The assumed effectiveness of such guidelines is based on assumptions that have not been firmly established but have been reached through extrapolation and speculation and, in some instances, by ignoring certain sets of data. I would suggest that the appropriate approach in dealing with the problem of chronic and degenerative diseases and disorders is that currently being used to control hypertension despite the general advice to reduce salt intake. That is, to focus efforts on identifying the susceptible population, targeting dietary and other advice to those identified, and encouraging them to participate in programs of medical centers that can provide the comprehensive care they need.

Also, guidelines for disease prevention have created what Passmore (1986) has called "trophophobia" - fear of food. Guidelines for chronic and degenerative diseases result in foods being classified as "good" or "bad," depending upon whether they are assumed to be disease-preventing or disease-promoting. Little if any attention is given in such guidelines to the nutritional needs of the most nutritionally vulnerable groups, the young, the pregnant, and the elderly. Guidelines that do not focus on the total diet and on nutrition for health, but instead, on nutrition as therapy for disease can lead to chaos in nutrition education.

In conclusion, it is most appropriate for governments to be intimately involved in promoting soundly-established, scientifically supportable advice for maintenance of health that applies to the population as a whole. It is most inappropriate for governments to be involved in offering general dietary advice for prevention of diseases that are not primarily dietary diseases, and advice, the efficacy of which has not been convincingly established, especially when it creates apprehension about diet and health among a large part of the population, and when there are more appropriate, scientifically more sound, approaches for dealing with the problem.

A statement from the Food and Nutrition Board publication "Toward Healthful Diets" (1980) might serve as an appropriate concluding statement for general dietary guidelines offered by governments for the public. "A nutritious diet is essential for general health and for vigorous defense mechanisms against disease - but - sound nutrition is not a panacea --. Good food that provides appropriate proportions of nutrients should not be regarded as a poison, a medicine, or a talisman. It should be eaten and enjoyed."

REFERENCES

Ahrens EH Jr (1979) Dietary fats and coronary heart disease. Unfinished business. Lancet 2:1345-1348.

Ahrens EJ Jr, Connor WE, Bierman EL et al (1979) The evidence relating six dietary factors to the nation's health. Am J Clin Nutr 32:2621-2748.

Feinstein AR (1987) Scientific standards and epidemiologic methods. Am J Clin Nutr 45:1080-1089.

Handler P (1979) Dedication address, Northwestern University Cancer Center, May 18, 1979.

Harper AE (1981a) Dietary goals. In: Ellenbogen L (ed) Controversies in Nutrition. New York: Churchill Livingstone, pp 63-84.

Harper AE (1981b) Human nutrition - its scientific basis. In Selvy L, White PL (eds): "Nutrition in the 1980s. Constraints on Our Knowledge." New York: Alan R. Liss Inc, pp 15-28.

Harper AE (1985) Origin of recommended dietary allowances - an historic overview. Am J Clin Nutr 41:140-148.

Harper AE (1987a) Evolution of recommended dietary allowances - new directions? Ann Rev Nutr 7:509-537.

Harper AE (1987b) Transitions in health status: implications for dietary recommendations. Am J Clin Nutr 45:1094-1107.

James TN (1981) Sure cures, quick fixes, and easy answers. Nutr Today 16:19-21.

Kurtz P (1976) The scientific attitude vs antiscience and pseudoscience. The Humanist 36:27-31.

Leitch I (1942) The evolution of dietary standards. Nutr Abstr Rev 11:509-521.

Miller SA (1982) The implementation of public health policy: Science and reality. In Fregly MJ and Kare MR (eds): "The Role of Salt in Cardiovascular Hypertension." New York: Academic Press, pp 443-449.

National Research Council (1980) Toward Healthful Diets. Washington, DC: National Academy of Sciences.

National Research Council (1989) Diet and Health. Implications for Reducing Chronic Disease Risk. Washington, DC: National Academy of Sciences.

Oliver MF (1986) Prevention of coronary heart disease - propaganda, promises, problems, and prospects. Circulation 73:1-9.

Olson RE (1986) Mass intervention vs screening and elective intervention for the prevention of coronary heart disease. J Am Med Assoc. 255:2204-2207.

Passmore R (1986). Food propagandists - The new puritans. Nutr Today 2:17-20.

Sebrell WH Jr (1974). Past experience in fortification of processed foods. In Nutrients in Processed Foods. "Vitamins and Minerals." Acton, MA: Publishing Sciences Group Inc, pp 95-100.

Simopoulos A (ed) (1987) Diet and Health: Scientific Concepts and Principles. Am J Clin Nutr 45:1015-1414 (supplement).

Stiebling HK, Clark F (1939) Planning for good nutrition. In Food and Life (eds): "Yearbook of Agriculture USDA", Washington, DC: US Govt Printing Office, pp 321-340.

Truswell AS (1983). Recommended dietary intakes around the world. Nutr Abstr Rev 53:939-1015 and 1075-1119.

Truswell AS (1987). Evolution of dietary recommendations, goals, and guidelines. Am J Clin Nutr 45:1060-1072.

US Dept. of Agriculture/US Dept. Health and Human Services (1985) Dietary Guidelines for Americans. Washington DC: US Govt Printing Office.

US Dept. Health, Education and Welfare (1979) Healthy People - The Surgeon General's Report on Health Promotion and Disease Prevention. Washington, DC: US Govt Printing Office.

US Dept. Health and Human Services (1988) The Surgeon General's Report on Nutrition and Health. Washington, DC: US Govt Printing Office.

US Senate Select Committee on Nutrition and Human Needs.(1977). Dietary Goals for the United States, 2nd Ed. Washington, DC: US Govt Printing Office.

Williams RR (1988). Knowing your family history: to avoid an early heart attack. Proc Ann Fall Meeting, Food Res Inst, Madison, WI. (See also Hopkins PN and Williams RR (1989) Human genetics and coronary heart disease. Ann Rev Nutr 9:303-345).

DISCUSSION

Q (S. Hashim): It is fair to point out, in the US at least, that 50% of the
population after age 60 years has an abnormal (low density lipid) LDL level.
Number two, 80% of all heart attacks (in the U.S.) occur after 65 years, and 50%
of that population is obese. So when we talk about, as you call it, a susceptible
population, this is a population which is getting older. Now we call it "the
eldery" above age 60.

Since records have been kept in Britain for the last 200 years, we know that
for the first time we are pushing the age limit for survival or long-livity to 75.
Big deal! We have never really exceeded the absolute long-livity, because 200
years ago people were reported to have also lived to 100 years. With other words,
the real age, the absolute limit of long-livity has not changed but the proportion of
people living above age 70 is alarmingly high.

A: Not alarmingly, pleasantly high.

Q (S. Hashim): In the U.S. we are talking about 2% of the population in the year
2000 (10 years from now) who will be living above 80! There won't be enough
nursing-homes to go around, therefore, I plead (ask) with you, what do we do with
this population.

A: Ah, that is my point. This (the advise) is not at all going to do anything to solve
that problem. Even, if this were to work. I am not convinced it will, although a
number of other people are - you are not going to improve the situation (quality of
life) for these people. The cost of medical care is primarily during the last two
years of life, sometimes even only the last 6 months of life. So I think that there
is an exageration. There has been a tendendy to move the standard of what is
abnormal down lower and lower and lower. We have done this with hypertension;
we can now see that 25% of the (U.S.) population has hypertension. But if you
reexamine the figures, only 5% have real (essential?) hypertension, while there are
a lot of people which have moderately high blood pressure but who may or may
not have (pathological) hypertension. I think the same is true for our serum lipids.
In fact, one of the beauties of the Cholesterol Program for the NIH is that they
finally have gotten serum cholesterol concentration abnormalities down from 260
to 200 (mg/dl). So now, today, the majority of heart attacks occur within the
normal range of cholesterol levels.

If you are going to look at the statistics, that such a high proportion of a
population is dying of heart disease, as representing the population as a whole, you
have to stop to think. This may represent a whole variety of diseases. Probably a
third of those people demonstrate no real abnormality of serum lipids. Some of
them have a type of abnormality about which you cannot do a thing with diets, or
very, very little. And we got a whole range of diseases that are all being classed
together.

(Mal)Nutrition and the Infant Brain, pages 313-325
© 1990 Wiley-Liss, Inc.

THE DEVELOPING RAT SPLEEN: NORADRENERGIC INNERVATION AND THE ONTOGENY OF IMMUNOLOGICAL REACTIVITY AFTER NEONATAL DENERVATION

Kelley S. Madden, K.D. Ackerman, S.Y. Felten, D.L.Felten

Department of Neurobiology and Anatomy. University of Rochester Medical Center. 601 Elmwood Ave. Rochester, New York 14642, USA

Recent studies have demonstrated both hormonal links and direct autonomic nerve fiber connections between the nervous system and the immune system. These endocrine and neurotransmitter communication channels may regulate the immune system under resting and activated conditions throughout the lifetime of the animal, and are presumed to provide the substrate for behavioral influences, such as stressors and conditioned responses on immunologic activity. In addition to neural-immune connections, cytokines produced by lymphocytes and monocytes can influence brain activity and behavior and may provide a molecular substrate for communication from the immune system to the nervous system.

Our laboratory has studied extensively the noradrenergic (NA) and peptidergic innervation of lymphoid organs in adult, neonatal, and aging animals, and the potential functional role of that innervation in modulating immune responses. NA nerve fibers are in position to provide norepinephrine (NE) and co-localized transmitters to nearby immunological cells of primary and secondary lymphoid organs in a variety of mammalian species examined, including mouse, rat, human, dog, cat, and sheep (reviewed by Felten et al., 1987; Felten et al., 1988). Lymphocytes and macrophages bear ß-adrenoceptors permitting signalling of these cells by catecholamines (Motulsky & Insel, 1982; Brodde et al., 1981; Abrass, O'Connor, Scarpace & Abrass, 1985). Antibody and cell-mediated immune responses generated by lymphocytes and macrophages are modulated by catecholamines *in vivo* and *in vitro* (reviewed by Livnat et al. 1985; Sanders & Munson, 1985), suggesting that, in adults, the release of NE and perhaps other co-localized peptides from NA nerve terminals in lymphoid tissue may represent an important mechanism underlying central nervous system (CNS) modulation of immune function (Ader, Felten, & Cohen, 1990).

The significance of age-related changes in NA innervation of lymphoid organs has been assessed by examining sympathetic neurotransmisson, postsynaptic effector mechanisms, and lymphocyte activity in these tissues throughout the lifespan of the animal. In the neonatal spleen, we have investigated the relationships between NA nerve terminals and lymphoid compartments, NE turnover, and ß-adrenoceptor density to explore the dynamic interactions between nerve fibers and cells of the immune system in developing lymphoid tissue. We have also used neonatal chemical sympathectomy to explore the potential impact of sympathetic innervation on lymphocyte function *in vivo*. This chapter presents findings from these studies which suggest that NA innervation may be a vital constituent of the splenic microenvironment, promoting cellular organization and functional maturation. Interactions between the nervous system and the immune system in the neonatal spleen also may be critical in determining the host's ability to detect and eliminate infectious agents and tumors throughout its life time.

Anatomy and Function of the Spleen

The spleen is a secondary lymphoid organ composed of two anatomically and histologically distinct types of tissue, the white pulp and the red pulp. One of the functions of the spleen is to monitor the bloodstream for foreign substances or antigens, such as virus or bacteria. The white pulp is organized into T and B cell-dependent regions to facilitate activities important for detecting and eliminating the foreign agent, such as antigen recognition, lymphocyte activation and proliferation. Lymphocyte and monocyte precursors from primary lymphoid organs (the thymus and bone marrow in mammals) seed developing secondary lymphoid tissue, where they mature to become functional T and B lymphocytes and macrophages. T cells are located primarily in the inner portion of the white pulp, forming the periarteriolar sheath (PALS), where they serve multiple functions. Cytotoxic T cells lyse infected cells and some tumor cells, T helper cells regulate lymphocyte activation, proliferation, differentiation, and T suppressor cells inhibit immune reactivity. B lymphocytes, the antibody producing cells, are present in the bulging follicles in the outer perimeter of the PALS and in the marginal zone, the border between the red and the white pulp (Fig. 1). Migrating cells enter the parenchyma of the spleen at the marginal zone, via the marginal sinus. Macrophages are also found in the marginal zone, where they phagocytose bacteria and other foreign matter, and along with B cells, serve as antigen presenting cells. They process and display antigen on the cell surface in such a way that enables T cell recognition of the antigen. The other distinct anatomical compartment of the spleen, the red pulp, consists of red blood cells, venous sinuses, macrophages, natural killer cells (important in killing certain tumors and virus-infected cells), and plasma cells (fully differentiated, antibody secreting B cells). Circulating cells exit the spleen through the venous sinuses of the red pulp.

Innervation of the adult rat spleen

To selectively detect NA nerve fibers in the rat spleen, we have used fluorescence histochemistry, a highly sensitive method for directly detecting catecholamines, and more recently, immunocytochemistry, with antibodies specific for the rate-limiting enzyme in the synthesis of NE, tyrosine hydroxylase (TH) (Ackerman et al., 1987; Felten et al., 1985; Felten, Ackerman, Wiegand & Felten, 1987). In the adult spleen, NA innervation is associated with the arteriolar system and with distinct parenchymal regions, generally T lymphocyte-containing areas (Fig. 1). Branches from dense NA varicosities innervate the central artery and its arterioles and distribute through the inner PALS in T cell-dependent regions where they arborize among T lymphocytes. NA nerve fibers also travel adjacent to macrophages and B cells lining the marginal sinus, and branch within the inner portion of the marginal zone. Occasional fibers enter the B cell-containing follicles, although the surrounding area, the parafollicular zone, is innervated. Innervation of the red pulp is restricted principally to the venous system and associated trabeculae.

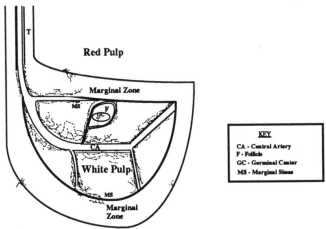

Fig.1. Schematic drawing of NA innervation of the white pulp of the adult spleen. NA varicosities are associated with large plexuses associated with the trabeculae (T) and the central artery (CA) of the splenic white pulp. NA fibers branch away from the central arteriolar system into the inner portion of the PALS where T lymphocytes are abundant, travel along the marginal sinus (MS) where macrophages are clustered, and form a plexus in the parafollicular zone surround B cell-containing follicles (F). Occasional fibers arborize from the parafollicular plexus to branch within the follicle near the germinal center (CG). Not all the follicular regions of a typical white pulp are drawn in this schematic illustration. (From K. D. Ackerman: Noradrenergic Sympathetic Neurotransmission in the Adult and Neonatal Rat Spleen, PhD. Thesis, University of Rochester, 1989).

Electron microscopy combined with immunocytochemistry for TH has revealed direct contacts between TH+ nerve terminals and lymphocytes in the PALS and marginal zone, where they form direct appositions via a neuroeffector junction of approximately 6 nanometers (Felten & Olschowka, 1987). These contacts occur deep in the parenchyma of the PALS, distant from smooth muscle, and also are found at the outer edge of the adventitia of the central artery. They may serve as sites where very high concentrations of NE are released for interactions with lymphocytes and monocytes, and may permit locally-released cytokines to modulate NE release.

The distinct pattern of NA innervation suggest multiple functions for NE and other co-localized peptides released from NA nerves. In addition to the control of blood flow and vasoconstriction, resulting from vascular smooth muscle innervation (Reilly, 1985), innervation of the PALS may provide a modulatory signal for lymphocyte proliferation and differentiation. The presence of nerve fibers in the region of the marginal sinus, the parafollicular zone, and the venous system suggest a NA influence on antigen processing and presentation, and on circulating cells entering and exiting the spleen.

The role of catecholamines in modulating lymphocyte and monocyte function in the adult has been studied *in vitro* and *in vivo*. ß-adrenoceptor-stimulation *in vitro* inhibited proliferation (Hadden, Hadden & Middleton, 1970; Johnson, Ashmore & Gordon, 1981), but enhanced antibody responses (Sanders & Munson, 1984a; Sanders & Munson, 1984b), and cytotoxic T lymphocyte activity (Hatfield, Petersen & DiMicco, 1986; Livnat et al., 1985). Other reports showed that effector functions, such as antibody synthesis and cytolytic activity, were reduced by ß-adrenergic stimulation (Melmon et al., 1974; Strom et al., 1973). *In vivo* studies using chemical sympathectomy in adult animals reduced delayed hypersensitivity, cytotoxic T lymphocyte activity, and antibody production (Madden, Felten, Felten & Livnat, 1989; Livnat et al., 1985; Hall et al., 1982; Kasahara, Tanaka, Ito & Hamashima, 1977). Lymphocyte trafficking was influenced by infusions of adrenergic agonists and by chemical sympathectomy (Ernström & Sandberg, 1973; Ernström & Sandberg, 1974; Felten et al., 1987). Thus, in the adult NE may act at several phases of an immune response, influencing several immunological activities, depending on the cell type and its state of activation. The complexity of the responses elicited by NE stresses the importance of determining its compartmental availability at specific time points during the immune response.

Ontogeny of NA Innervation in the Neonatal Spleen

The anatomical and functional relationships between NA nerve fibers and lymphoid compartments in the adult spleen suggested that NA innervation in the neonatal spleen could play a special role under conditions where stem cell migration and lymphocyte maturation are critical for proper immune system development. Double-label immunocytochemistry for TH and specific markers on lymphoid cells was used to determine when NA nerve fibers appeared, what cell types they arborized among, and their location in the splenic architecture throughout development (Ackerman et al., 1989). At birth, splenic TH+ nerve fibers (NA fibers) were exclusively detected in the parenchyma, adjacent to IgM+ B cells and ED3+ macrophages forming the outer portion of the PALS, at the site of the future marginal sinus. These nerve fibers were distant from the central artery, and clearly were not associated with vascular smooth muscle, which was not present at this time (Fig. 2a). At the EM level, direct contacts between TH+ nerves and lymphocytes were found in the outer PALS, as in the adult spleen (Felten et al., 1988). During the first week, the number and density of NA fibers increased rapidly. Innervated regions in the 7 day old spleen include the arterioles, the PALS (consisting at this time of both T and B cells), and the marginal sinus, populated by ED3+ macrophages (Fig. 2B). NE concentration (mg/wet weight), measured by liquid chromatography coupled with electrochemical detection (LCEC), increased to approximately 50% of adult levels during this time period (data not shown). Between 7 and 14 days of age, the white pulp expanded into an inner PALS, consisting of T cells, and an outer PALS, containing both T and B cells. From day 10-14, B cells began to form follicles. During the second week, NA nerve fibers were observed associated with the central artery and its branches, the inner portion of the PALS, the marginal sinus surrounding the PALS, and the parafollicular zone, with scattered fibers entering the follicles (Fig. 2c). By 14 days of age, NE concentration was equivalent to that in adult. From days 14 to 28, the inner PALS became thinner and more elongated, while the follicles and the marginal zone continue to expand. Compartmentation of NA innervation was maintained during these shifts in the relative size of the compartments. From days 21 to 28, the trabeculae and venous system of the red pulp expanded rapidly, along with the associated NA innervation. From 28 days of age to adulthood, all compartments expanded, the growth of NA innervation and splenic NE paralleled the increased cellularity, but maintained the same precise compartmental patterns of innervation.

Evidence for NE Release and Availability in the Developing Rat Spleen

Although NE concentration in the neonatal spleen was equivalent to the concentration in adult as early as 14 days after birth, definitive evidence for NE release from nerve terminals in the spleen is not yet available. The studies we have presented here have established that NA sympathetic nerve fibers are present in the spleen early in ontogeny and innervate specific anatomical compartments prior to the morphological maturation of these regions. These fibers contain the neurotransmitter NE as demonstrated by fluorescence histochemistry for catecholamines and analysis of splenic NE by LCEC. Studies in intact and neonatally sympathectomized animals have demonstrated that the NE content of the spleen is at least 90% neural throughout development (see below) similar to the neural localization of NE in adulthood (Williams et al., 1981). These observations suggest that NE in the developing spleen is present in nerve terminals among putative target cells, and may function as a neurotransmitter with lymphoid and non-lymphoid cells as targets, provided that NE is released and available for interactions with the surrounding cells, and that the putative targets cells possess receptors capable of recognizing the neurotransmitter.

We approached the issue of NE availability through NE turnover studies. The rate limiting enzyme, TH, was blocked by treatment with alpha-methyl-tyrosine, and the disappearance of NE was measured over time as a putative index of release. In general, the rate of turnover paralleled the growth of cellular compartmentation and NA innervation in the developing spleen, suggesting that NE availability increases in parallel with compartmental expansion (Ackerman, Bellinger, Felten & Felten, 1990). However, the concentration of NE to which lymphocytes are exposed depends on their location relative to the nerve terminals, the presence of any physical barriers, and the means of NE degradation at that site. These issues have yet to be addressed experimentally.

Presence of β-adrenergic Receptors on Neonatal Spleen Cells

The ability of NE to serve as a regulator of developmental processes at the postsynaptic level was assessed by determining spleen cell β-adrenoceptor

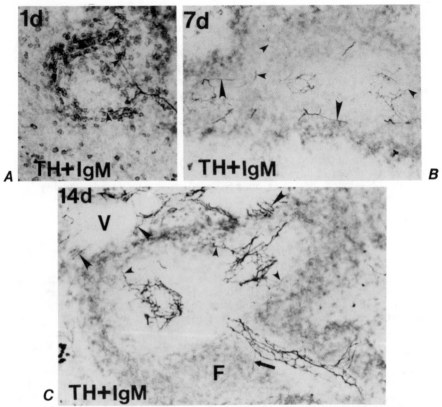

Fig. 2. Neonatal rat spleen stained for TH[+] NA nerves and sIgM[+] B lymphocytes.

A) 1 day old (1d). TH[+] fibers (arrowheads) course among sIgM[+] B lymphocytes at the external portion of the PALS. Double-label ICC. x275

B) 7 day old (7d). Long linear profiles of TH[+] nerves (large arrowheads) separate lightly stained sIgM[+] cells of the PALS from the darkly stained B cells of the marginal zone. Additional TH[+] fibers form a dense plexus within the PALS, arborizing among B lymphocytes within the inner portion of the PALS (small arrowheads). Double-label ICC. x200

C) 14 day old (14d). TH[+] fibers form a dense, tangled plexus within the inner PALS, an area devoid of B lymphocytes. sIgM[+] cells are located within the outer PALS, marginal zone, and follicles. B lymphocytes of the outer PALS and inner marginal zone lie adjacent to TH[+] fibers at the marginal sinus (small arrowheads), while additional TH[+] fibers (large arrowheads) supplied by an adjacent vein (V) arborize among B lymphocytes of the outer marginal zone. A delicate TH[+] profile (arrow) is found within the follicle (F). Double-label ICC. x175

From K.D. Ackerman: Noradrenergic Sympathetic Neurotransmission in the Adult and Neonatal Rat Spleen, PhD Thesis, University of Rochester, 1989.

density and affinity. Binding studies were conducted, using the ß-adrenoceptor radioligand, $(\pm)^{125}$ I-cyanopindolol (^{125}ICYP). Saturable and specific ^{125}ICYP binding to unfractionated, intact spleen cells was detected throughout the postnatal period into adulthood. Spleen cells from rat pups 1 to 10 days of age exhibited approximately 400 sites per cell, which increased to adult density, 800-1000 sites per cell, by 21 days of age (Ackerman, Bellinger, Felten & Felten, 1990). Affinity ($k_d=8$-12×10^{-12} M) remained constant throughout development, equivalent to that of typical high affinity ß-adrenoceptors on other tissues, such as heart and kidney (Sundaresan, Fortin & Kelvie, 1987; Sundaresan, Sharma, Gingold & Banerjee, 1984). The increase in receptor density may represent shifts in spleen cell subpopulations, from a non-lymphoid to lymphoid cell population, or from an immature lymphocyte population to a more mature lymphocyte population. They may also represent a programmed development of receptor expression of lymphoid cells. The presence of ß-adrenoceptors on the surface of spleen cells from birth to adulthood indicates that lymphocytes are capable of receiving specific signals from catecholamines. However, their presence does not tell us is whether intracellular signal transduction through ß-adrenoceptors is intact. Studies measuring the second messenger, cAMP, after ß-adrenoceptor stimulation will be necessary determine the efficiency of receptor-effector coupling in neonatal spleen cells. The functional changes in lymphocyte reactivity following neonatal sympathectomy (see below) suggests that such a second messenger transduction system is present and functional.

Functional alterations following neonatal treatment with 6-hydroxydopamine

Very few studies have examined sympathetic neural-immune interactions in the neonate. We have taken a pharmacological approach to assess the impact of NA innervation on the ontogeny of lymphocyte function in the spleen by using the neurotoxin 6-hydroxydopamine (6-OHDA) to selectively destroy NA nerve terminals. Fischer 344 rat pups were injected subcutaneously with 6-OHDA the first three days of life. This treatment depleted splenic NE more than 90% relative to vehicle controls through 56 days of age (the last time point examined). Spleen cells from sympathectomized rats were tested for their *in vitro* proliferative response to T or B cell selective mitogens, as measured by ^{3}H-thymidine incorporation. This assay provides a measure of the functional capabilities of a large proportion of T or B cells in the spleen.

From the earliest ages examined, neonatal 6-OHDA treatment altered the pattern of responsiveness to varying doses of the T cell mitogen, concanavalin A (Con A; Ackerman et al., 1990). Fig. 3a, illustrating lymphocyte reactivity at 10 days of age, demonstrates the effect of 6-OHDA through the first 14 days of age. After 6-OHDA treatment, the spleen cell proliferative response to Con A shifted such that the response to lower doses of Con A appeared suppressed. However, at intermediate levels of Con A, the cells from sympathectomized animals exhibited ^{3}H-thymidine uptake equivalent to the maximal response elicited at lower Con A doses by control spleen cells. Thus, spleen cells from sympathectomized animals required higher doses of Con A to stimulate a response that in magnitude was equivalent to controls. From 21 to 28 days of age, an adult-like spleen cell proliferative response to Con A began to emerge in control animals, as indicated by increased ^{3}H-thymidine incorporation at higher mitogen doses (2.5-5 µg/ml; see Fig. 3b). At this time, Con A-induced proliferation was greatly reduced in spleen cells from sympathectomized female

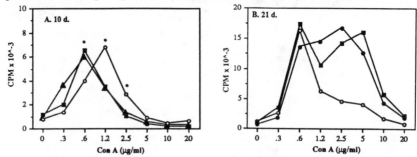

Fig. 3. Spleen cell proliferative response to the T cell mitogen, Con A. F344 rats were injected at postnatal ages 1, 2, and 3 days with 100 mg/kg 6-OHDA, 0.1% ascorbate vehicle, or 10 mg/kg DMI 45 min prior to 100 mg/kg 6-OHDA (DMI + 6-OHDA). Spleen cells from A) 10 day old or B) 21 day old animals were cultured for 72 hours with varying doses of Con A. Results are expressed as the combined mean of three separate experiments (n>6 for each treatment group). Asterisk indicates 6-OHDA different from vehicle and DMI + 6-OHDA by simple effects analysis (p<0.01). At d. 21, there was a trend towards decreased spleen cell Con A responsiveness in the 6-OHDA group relative to vehicle and DMI + 6-OHDA treated animals. However, due to the great variability in Con A reactivity at this time point, the ANOVA was not significant (p=0.18)

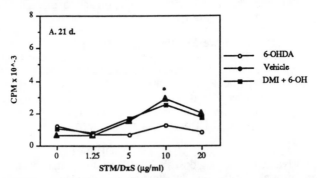

Fig. 4. Spleen cell proliferative response to the B cell mitogen, STM/DxS. F344 rats were injected at postnatal ages 1,2, and 3 days with 100 mg/kg 6-OHDA, 0.1% ascorbate vehicle, or 10 mg/kg DMI 45 min prior to 100 mg/kg 6-OHDA (DMI + 6-OHDA). Spleen cells from 21 day old animals were cultured for 72 hours with varying doses of STM/DxS. Results are expressed as the combined mean from three separate experiments (n>6 for each treatment group). Asterisk indicates 6-OHDA different from vehicle and DMI + 6-OHDA by simple effects analysis (p<0.01)

(Fig. 3b) and male rats. Spleen cell Con A reactivity in 6-OHDA-treated female rats were no longer suppressed after 28 days, while male rats exhibited this pattern of suppression through 42 days of age.

In control animals, spleen cell proliferation induced by the B cell mitogen, Salmonella typhimurium and dextran sulfate (STM/DxS), was suppressed below background (proliferation in the absence of mitogen) through 14 days of age across a broad range of STM/DxS doses (data not shown). This suppression was not altered by sympathectomy (Ackerman et al., 1990). By day 21, ^{3}H-thymidine incorporation above background was detectable, although compared to an adult B cell proliferative response, was greatly reduced. Like the Con A response, spleen cells from 6-OHDA-treated rats exhibited diminished B cell proliferation at 21 days of age (Fig. 4), which was no longer apparent after 28 days of age in the females and 42 days of age in the males. Paralleling the sympathectomy-induced changes in B cell proliferation, another measure of B cell function, polyclonal antibody production, stimulated by STM/DxS, was also inhibited by neonatal sympathectomy at these ages (data not shown).

To determine that these effects were a function of sympathectomy and loss of NA innervation, we used the catecholamine uptake blocker, desipramine, to block the high affinity catecholamine uptake carrier on NA nerve terminals. Desipramine hinders the uptake of 6-OHDA into these terminals, thereby completely preventing sympathectomy. NE levels and histofluorescent nerve profiles in neonates treated with desipramine prior to 6-OHDA were indistinguishable from vehicle controls (data not shown). Spleen cells from animals pretreated with desipramine exhibited proliferative responses to Con A and STM/DxS equivalent to controls (Fig. 3,4). We can conclude, then, that the effects of 6-OHDA treatment are a consequence of sympathectomy, and cannot be attributed to direct toxic effects of 6-OHDA or its oxidative by-products.

The diminished lymphocyte reactivity in vitro following sympathectomy suggests that NA innervation assists or promotes the development of lymphocyte function in the spleen. This influence may be exerted at many functional levels, through many cell types, lymphoid and non-lymphoid. One testable hypothesis is that NE, possibly in conjunction with co-localized peptides, inhibits neonatal suppressor cell activity, a short-lived (up through 21 days of age) inhibitory activity contained in an ill-defined spleen cell subpopulation. Neonatal suppressor cells inhibit the proliferative responses to stimulatory mitogen concentrations in the adult (Middleton & Bullock, 1984). Removal of a signal which normally inhibits neonatal suppressor cell activity (e.g. through sympathectomy) would suppress immune responsiveness. Alternatively, by acting on the vasculature, NA innervation may indirectly influence stem cell migration into the spleen through changes in blood flow and vascular permeability, although at very early ages, before smooth muscle develops, this regulatory mechanism in unavailable. NE may also directly support lymphocyte and monocyte migration, differentiation, and proliferation. Caution must be used, however, in the interpretation of experiments using neonatal sympathectomy. In the absence of a fully developed blood-brain barrier, 6-OHDA can enter the brain, and alter developing CNS catecholaminergic circuitry (Kostrzewa & Jacobwitz, 1974). Altered central catecholamine neurons or pituitary hormone production may be partially responsible for the observed effects of sympathectomy.

There is a limited number of studies examining the effects of neonatal sympathectomy on the ontogeny of immune function. One report demonstrated reduced antibody production to a T cell-independent antigen in sympathectomized females, but not males (Dempsey, Ross & Taylor, 1987). Miles et al., (1984) showed that neonatal sympathectomy enhanced antibody production to a T cell independent antigen. In adults sympathectomized at birth, antibody responses to a T-cell dependent antigen, SRBC, were enhanced (Williams et al.,1981; Besedovsky et al.,1979). Williams et al., (1981) demonstrated that the increased antibody response was further enhanced by alpha-methyl-tyrosine treatment, a blocker of adrenal catecholamine production, suggesting that both sympathetic and adrenal catecholamines may play a role in modulating immune responses in ontogeny, with the sympathetic predominant. Besedovsky et al., (1979) found that alpha-methyl-tyrosine was necessary to observe the 6-OHDA-induced enhancement. Both studies suggest that adrenal catecholamine production following sympathectomy may provide a compensatory mechanism to counter the loss of NA sympathetic innervation following 6-OHDA treatment.

In our studies, the inhibitory effects of neonatal sympathectomy on T and B cell proliferation *in vitro* were not detectable at later ages in rats of either sex (data not shown). One argument is that sympathectomy caused a general delay in development, which gradually recovered over time. We do not believe this to be the case, since body and organ weights from 6-OHDA treated animals were not different from vehicle controls at any age. Instead, compensatory mechanisms in sympathectomized animals may restore the deficit in lymphocyte reactivity, through increased NE and EPI synthesis by the adrenal medulla or through changes sex hormone production, as suggested by the failure to demonstrate effects of sympathectomy after puberty. These possibilities can be tested by determining if the 6-OHDA-induced effects are maintained when catecholamine or sex hormone production are prevented through surgical or pharmacological intervention.

Conclusion and Discussion

In the developing rat spleen, we have begun to assess the structure-function relationship between sympathetic NA innervation and cells of the immune system, by following splenic anatomical development, sympathetic activity, and lymphocyte function throughout ontogeny. The emerging picture is that compartmentation of NA innervation and NE turnover develop concurrently or just prior to morphological maturation of lymphoid compartments. In contrast, NA innervation of other non-lymphoid elements in the spleen, the venous and trabecular systems, does not appear until relatively late in development. For example, it may be significant that NA innervation of the 1 day old spleen is found in the parenchyma among T and B cells. The presence of these nerve fibers appears to demarcate the future marginal sinus; a trophic role for these fibers in attracting appropriate cell types to the marginal sinus is possible. The formation of B cell follicles at day 10 may be accomplished by the exclusion of B cells from the inner PALS, or the aggregation and proliferation of

B cells, which NE (depending on concentration) can influence. In conjunction with the existence of spleen cell ß-adrenoceptors, these results suggest that NA innervation may contribute to the formation of lymphoid architecture.

The chemical denervation studies suggest that the absence of NA innervation influences lymphocyte function, and imply that the presence of NA nerve terminals has a positive or promoting influence on lymphocyte activity. NE concentration and turnover were equivalent to adult levels prior to an adult-like lymphocyte proliferative response, supporting the notion that NE contributes early in ontogeny to lymphocyte functional development, by modulating neonatal suppressor cell activity, immigration of premature cells to the spleen, or lymphocyte proliferation and differentiation. Compensatory mechanisms may exist to overcome immune deficiencies, if the relationship between NA nerve terminals and lymphocytes is impaired. Finally, the differential effects of sympathectomy depending on sex, and the loss of the effects of sympathectomy after puberty suggest that sex hormones may also be contributing factors in NE regulation of lymphoid development.

We postulate that NE may perform multiple duties in the developing spleen, by acting through multiple cell types. A reciprocal relationship may also exist, whereby lymphocyte and monocyte products act to sustain or support NA innervation and to control neurotransmitter release. To more clearly define the role of NE, we need to know more about the release and availability of NE, although determining the NE concentration cells are exposed to in specific compartmental microenvironments *in vivo* may be very difficult. It will also be important to determine the spleen cell subsets influenced by NE throughout development. Measurements of ß-and a-adrenoceptor density and determination of the efficiency of effector coupling on purified lymphocyte populations will contribute to our understanding of the developmental process. *In vitro* studies with adrenergic agonists will be helpful in identifying those lymphocyte and monocyte functions regulated directly by NE and other co-localized peptides released by NA nerve terminals. Elucidation of the mechanisms by which NE modulates cells of the immune system during development of the spleen and other lymphoid organs will contribute to our understanding of these interactions and their changing dynamics throughout the lifespan of the adult. This information will help determine methods of manipulating the sympathetic nervous system to beneficially modulate immune function in disease states precipitated by an overactive or suppressed immune system.

REFERENCES

Abrass CK, O'Connor SW, Scarpace PJ, Abrass IB (1985). Characterization of the ß-adrenergic receptor of the rat peritoneal macrophage. J Immunol 135:1338-1341.

Ackerman D, Bellinger DL, Felten SY, Felten DL (1990). Ontogeny and senescence of noradrenergic innervation of the rodent thymus and spleen. In R. Ader, DL Felten, N Cohen (Eds.): "Psychoneuroimmunology II", New York: Academic Press, (in press).

Ackerman KD, Felten SY, Bellinger DL, Livnat S, Felten DL (1987). Noradrenergic sympathetic innervation of spleen and lymph nodes in relation to specific cellular compartments. Prog Immunol 6:588-600.

Ackerman KD, Felten SY, Dijkstra CD, Livnat S, Felten DL (1989). Parallel development of noradrenergic innervation and cellular compartmentation in the rat spleen. Exp Neurol 103:239-255.

Ackerman KD, Madden KS, Felten SY, Felten DL (1990). Neonatal sympathetic denervation alters the ontogeny of *in vitro* spleen cell proliferation, differentiation, and NK cell activity in F344 rats. (submitted).

Ader R, Felten DL, Cohen N (eds) (1990). Psychoneuroimmunology II. New York: Academic Press (in press).

Besedovsky HO, del Rey A, Sorkin E, Da Prada M, Keller HH (1979). Immunoregulation mediated by the sympathetic nervous system. Cell Immunol 48:346-355.

Brodde OE, Engel G, Hoyer D, Block KD, Weber F (1981). The beta-adrenergic receptor in human lymphocytes - Subclassification by the use of a new radio-ligand (±)[125 Iodo]cyanopindolol. Life Sci 29:2189-2198.

Dempsey WL, Ross LL, Taylor CE (1987). Sympathetic nervous system modulation of antibody responses to streptococcus pneumoniae. Fed Proc 46:623.

Ernström U, Sandberg G (1973). Effects of adrenergic alpha- and beta-receptor stimulation on the release of lymphocytes and granulocytes from the spleen. Scand J Haematol 11:275-286.

Ernström U, Sandberg G (1974). Stimulation of lymphocyte release from the spleen by theophylline and isoproterenol. Acta Physiol Scand 90:202-209.

Felten DL, Felten SY, Carlson SL, Olschowka JA, Livnat S (1985). Noradrenergic and peptidergic innervation of lymphoid tissue. J Immunol 135:755s-765s.

Felten DL, Ackerman KD, Wiegand SJ, Felten SY (1987). Noradrenergic sympathetic innervation of the spleen: I. Nerve fibers associate with lymphocytes and macrophages in specific compartments of the splenic white pulp. J Neurosci Res 18:28-36.

Felten DL, Felten SY, Bellinger DL, Carlson SL, Ackerman KD, Madden KS, Olschowka JA, Livnat S (1987). Noradrenergic sympathetic neural interactions with the immune system: Structure and Function. Immunol Rev 100:225-260.

Felten SY, Felten DL, Bellinger DL, Carlson SL, Ackerman KD, Madden KS, Olschowka JA, Livnat S (1988). Noradrenergic sympathetic innervation of lymphoid organs. Prog Allergy 43:14-36.

Felten SY, Olschowka JA (1987). Noradrenergic sympathetic innervation of the spleen: II. Tyrosine hydroxylase (TH)-positive nerve terminals form synaptic-like contacts on lymphocytes in the splenic white pulp. J Neurosci Res 18:37-48.

Hadden JW, Hadden EM, Middleton E Jr (1970). Lymphocyte blast transformation. I. Demonstration of adrenergic receptors in human peripheral lymphocytes. Cell Immunol 1:583-595.

Hall NR, McClure JE, Hu S-K, Tare NS, Seals CM, Goldstein AL (1982). Effects of 6-hydroxydopamine upon primary and secondary thymus dependent immune responses. Immunopharmacol 5:39-48.

Hatfield SM, Petersen BH, DiMicco JA (1986). Beta adrenoceptor modulation of the generation of murine cytotoxic T lymphocytes in vitro. J Pharmacol Exp Ther 239:460-466.

Johnson DL, Ashmore RC, Gordon MA (1981). Effects of beta-adrenergic agents on the murine lymphocyte response to mitogen stimulation. J Immunopharmacol 3 :205-219.

Kasahara K, Tanaka S, Ito R, Hamashima Y (1977). Suppression of the primary immune response by chemical sympathectomy. Res Commun Chem Pthl Pharmacol 16:687-694.

Kostrzewa RM, Jacobwitz DM (1974). Pharmacological actions of 6-hydroxydopamine. Pharmacol Rev 26:199-288.

Livnat S, Felten SY, Carlson SL, Bellinger DL, Felten DL (1985). Involvement of peripheral and central catecholamine systems in neural-immune interactions. J Neuroimmunol 10:5-30.

Madden KS, Felten SY, Felten DL, Livnat S (1989). Sympathetic neural modulation of the immune system. I. Depression of T cell immunity in vivo and in vitro following chemical sympathectomy. Brain Behav Immun 3:72-89.

Melmon KL, Bourne HR, Weinstein Y, Shearer GM, Kram J, Bauminger S (1974). Hemolytic plaque formation by leukocytes in vitro. Control by vasoactive hormones. J Clin Invest 53:13-21.

Middleton PA Bullock WW (1984). Ontogeny of T-cell mitogen response in Lewis rats: III. Juvenile adherent suppressor cells block adult mitogen responses. Cell Immunol 88:421-435.

Miles K (1984). The sympathetic nerous system and the immune response in mice. Ph.D. Dissertation. Chicago: Unversity of Chicago.

Motulsky HJ, Insel PA (1982). Adrenergic receptors in man. Direction identification, physiologic regulation, and clinical alterations. N Engl J Med 307:18-29.

Reilly FD (1985). Innervation and vascular pharmacodynamics of the mammalian spleen. Experientia 41:187-192.

Sanders VM, Munson AE (1984a). Kinetics of the enhancing effect produced by norepinephrine and terbutaline on the murine primary antibody response *in vitro*. J Pharmacol Exp Ther 231:527-531.

Sanders VM, Munson AE (1984b). Beta adrenoceptor mediation of the enhancing effect of norepinephrine on the murine primary antibody response *in vitro*. J Pharmacol Exp Ther 230:183-192.

Sanders VM, Munson AE (1985). Norepinephrine and the antibody response. Pharmacol Rev 37:229-248.

Strom TB, Carpenter CB, Garovoy MR, Austen KF, Merrill JP, Kaliner M (1973). The modulating influence of cyclic nucleotides upon lymphocyte-mediated cytotoxicity. J Exp Med 138:381-393.

Sundaresan PR, Fortin TL, Kelvie SL (1987). α- and ß-adrenergic receptors in proximal tubules of rat kidney. Am J Physiol 253:F848-F856.

Sundaresan PR, Sharma PR, Gingold SI, Banerjee SP (1984). Decreased ß-adrenergic receptors in rat heart in streptozotocin-induced diabetes: Role of thyroid hormones. Endocrinology 114:1358-1363.

Williams JM, Peterson RG, Shea PA, Schmedtje JF, Bauer DC, Felten DL (1981). Sympathetic innervation of murine thymus and spleen: Evidence for a functional link between the nervous and immune systems. Brain Res Bull 6:83-94.

(Chapter by invitation)

SYNOPSIS

It is evident that during early maturation of the nervous system, the genetic directives can only be completely executed if the nutritional status of the mother is satisfactory. However, that requires some nutritional wisdom on the part of the mother and, furthermore, it is influenced by her emotional health. Up to the time of birth, the foetus has a one to one relationship to the mother. Its physical comfort and, possibly, some sense of emotional security are provided by, largely, automatic physiological processes over which neither mother nor child has much conscious control. In addition, the continuously changing chemical composition of the umbilical circulation and its proportional regulation, is so complex that this dietary and hormonal source is almost impossible to reconstitute artificially. The category of infants most at risk during the period will be the premature, and those which are carried to term but whose mothers are suffering from severe chemical imbalance. The correlation between premature birth and poor health of the mother is not coincidental. Perhaps more than in any other period of development, there is need for an enlighted community to invest in the welfare of the mother to assure a successful outcome of pregnancy.

Following birth, the infant enters the most dangerous period. Not yet able to regulate its own dietary intake, dependent entirely for food and shelter on one or more members of the community, its growing nervous system increasingly demands sensory (environmental) input for proper development. With a minimum of health care and emotional welfare provided to the mother, a breast fed infant receives, still almost automatically, most of the environmental and nutritional cues needed for continuing maturation of the brain. Under similar circumstances but without breast feeding, the present-day formulas when properly reconstituted seemingly can effectively meet nutritional requirements, although other factors such as immunological resistance, hormonal requirements and, no doubt, as yet unspecified essential nutritional components may be lacking in the infant's diet.

Contrast this then to communities where chronic malnutrition and undernutrition are the norm. During pregnancy, automatic physiological regulatory mechanisms will provide the foetus with the minimum nutrient requirements at the expense of maternal health and nutritional status. Such an infant when born carries no nutritional reserves and needs, if anything, a more enriched diet than other babies. However, as many of the reports presented here and elsewhere indicate, the mothers in poor communities suffer from several other disadvantages which pose a risk to the neonate. Not only the quantity but also, as is now known, the quality of milk provided by such mothers is deficient.

Partly because of poor hygienic conditions but also because of insufficient milk of poor quality, the increased susceptibility to infections, intestinal absorption problems, a lack of essential amino acids, vitamins, essential fatty acids and ketone bodies conspire to slow down CNS development. Such slowing down may take the form of underdevelopment of certain growth processes restricted to narrow time windows, developmental miscueing because the quantitative threshold to trigger a growth sequence is not reached, and it may affect different brain regions or functions more severely than others. Finally, aside from these direct physiological insults, nutritional insufficiencies are accompanied by physical and intellectual lethargy, in the child as well as in the mother or surrogate caretaker. This narrows the range of environmental experiences, which decreases and slows learning-dependent synaptogenesis. Perhaps the greatest wonder is that so many infants still survive and develop successfully under these adverse emotional and physiological conditions.

As postnatal maturation progresses and genetic directives for neuronal growth diminish as they exceed their time window, rehabilitation becomes more difficult. With biological development slowing down, the environmental cues which are needed to fine-tune the intellectual capacity of the brain assume a dominant importance. The evidence suggests that such cues in the form of emotional and experientially enriched environments can to a large extent compensate for nutritional underdevelopment. This implies that sensory cues are able to stimulate the anatomical, physiological and neurochemical substrates for intelligence and that they are essential for brain development. There may however be a qualitative difference between these cues, and nutrients, in terms of their ability to promote brain function.

With maturation, brain function becomes increasingly resistant to the potential benefits of a diet or, conversely, nutritional adversity; by 3-4 years of age the dietary effects on further biological development of the brain may be minimal. In contrast, emerging evidence indicates that environmental cues, i.e. the process of learning itself, may continue to alter or, at least, maintain the biological parameters of the brain throughout the entire life span of an individual. Unfortunate experiences with sensory isolation conditions have clearly demonstrated as much. To what extent, however, the biological plasticity is retained during life, which cues are most beneficial, the nature of the alteration, and the natural duration of the changes, are all questions which at this time remain unanswered.

In the face of still so many uncertainties, perhaps the safest policies to set for the community is to provide adequate nutrition, health and psychological wellfare to the pregnant and nursing mother, and to exert a large effort to allow the growing child every opportunity to interact socially and intellectually with its environment. This does not represent charity; on the contrary, the wellfare, stability, and progress of the entire community depends on maximizing the intellectual and social development of the next generation. Hence, if the bells do not seem to toll for ourselves, then assuredly they toll for our neighbors; and without them life can become very precarious and unpleasant. Such policies also give us time to refine our knowledge regarding the social and nutritional requirements which will promote optimal brain development, without at the same time penalizing the child for our own, as yet, large degree of scientific ignorance.

Nico M. van Gelder

Index

329